Perspectives on the Intersection of Multiculturalism and Positive Psychology

Cross-Cultural Advancements in Positive Psychology

Volume 7

The aim of the *Cross Cultural Advancements in Positive Psychology* book series is to spread a universal and culture-fair perspective on good life promotion. The series will advance a deeper understanding of the cross-cultural differences in well-being conceptualization. A deeper understanding can affect psychological theories, interventions and social policies in various domains, from health to education, from work to leisure. Books in the series will investigate such issues as enhanced mobility of people across nations, ethnic conflicts and the challenges faced by traditional communities due to the pervasive spreading of modernization trends. New instruments and models will be proposed to identify the crucial components of well-being in the process of acculturation. This series will also explore dimensions and components of happiness that are currently overlooked because happiness research is grounded in the Western tradition, and these dimensions do not belong to the Western cultural frame of mind and values.

For further volumes:
http://www.springer.com/series/8420

Jennifer Teramoto Pedrotti • Lisa M. Edwards
Editors

Perspectives on the Intersection of Multiculturalism and Positive Psychology

Springer

Editors
Jennifer Teramoto Pedrotti
Department of Psychology & Child Development
California Polytechnic State University
San Luis Obispo, CA, USA

Lisa M. Edwards
Department of Counselor Education and Counseling Psychology
Marquette University
Milwaukee, WI, USA

ISSN 2210-5417 ISSN 2210-5425 (electronic)
ISBN 978-94-017-7852-7 ISBN 978-94-017-8654-6 (eBook)
DOI 10.1007/978-94-017-8654-6
Springer Dordrecht Heidelberg New York London

Softcover reprint of the hardcover 1st edition 2014

Printed on acid-free paper

Springer is part of Springer Science+Business Media (www.springer.com)

For my family, of whom I am always sure.
For my children, Ben, Cate, and Chloe.
And for Brian, as always.

–JTP

To my familia *in the United States and Colombia, who has taught me about strengths, culture and love.*

–LME

Foreword

My grandfather was a *traiteur*, a Cajun faith healer. When I was a little kid, I would sit at the dining room table and watch him put his hands on the crowns of children, field workers, and old people who were crippled with headaches that wouldn't go away. They would cry and he would pray. They would cry and he would pray. He would pray until they stopped crying…and then some.

Growing up, I thought everyone went to traiteurs. I saw every grandfather as having special powers. I made assumptions about people and the world that were based on my limited experiences. They were far from true.

As a practicing psychologist and social scientist, I still make assumptions about people and their behavior, but now I call them hypotheses. I have tried to make sense out of how suffering, healing, and culture mix. The more I learn, the less I know for sure, and the more I want to think about how and why our differences and similarities affect how we live.

A treasure trove of data has helped me examine some hypotheses that I have made about people in America and across the world. Specifically, the Gallup Student Poll and the Gallup World Poll have given me the chance to ask and answer questions about what contributes to the well-being of all people. Two findings and a review of *Perspectives on the Intersection of Multiculturalism and Positive Psychology* edited by Jennifer Teramoto Pedrotti and Lisa M. Edwards have convinced me that we are too confident about what we think we know about optimal human functioning.

Let me start by sharing the two findings that many psychologists, particularly those who study what is right with people, consider to be givens. One involves money and happiness. Studies worldwide suggest that income has a small but positive correlation with happiness. The second finding links positive emotions and health. Joy and physical health seem to go together no matter who you are.

Regarding money buying happiness, I examined the subjective well-being of a representative sample of United States high school students and their parents' income. A quick literature review suggested that this had not been done before. But, given the evidence of the link taken from research on adults, I had hypothesized that there would be a small, significant correlation. To my surprise, there was a zero correlation, no link between child well-being and parent income.

Reflecting on the finding for months, I realized that I had assumed that the "life-world" of child was the same as an adult's. A read of Nakamura et al.'s chapter on "Positive Psychology Across the Lifespan" suggests that significant age differences do exist in the "positive" and that determinants of health and well-being may differ for children, adults, and older adults. So, whatever you think you know about the positive psychology of one group of people, don't think it necessarily applies to another group.

The finding about the link between joy and health was based on a representative sample of the world's citizens. That's right, the Gallup World Poll covers more than 95 % of the world's population via sophisticated sampling techniques. Not surprisingly, we did find a link between positive emotions and subjective health. But, we did not anticipate that the link would be strongest in countries where the people were the poorest. That means that the connection between joy and health is stronger in Malawi than America. Why that is I am not exactly sure, but reading Sheu, Robitschek et al., Campos and Shenhav will help me develop possible explanations.

This book subtly reminds us all that we are at times overconfident in our understanding of culture and this gives us the inspiration we need to become more skilled at making sense of psychology in a complex, diverse world. Chapters by Downey and Chang, Rasmussen and Lavish, Ho, and Capielo et al., as well as other contributors to this book give us the tools we need to properly examine hypotheses in a cultural context. Englar-Carlson and Smart, Farb and Pargament, Liu and Allmon, Wehmeyer and Shogren, and Horne et al. teach us about how particular groups of people pursue the good life. Finally, Holtz and Martinez, Youssef-Morgan and Hardy, and Magyar-Moe show us how to apply what we learn to promote the good life of others and, finally, Christopher and Howe caution us against slipping back into an oblivious confidence.

The Teramoto Pedrotti and Edwards volume is a carefully constructed, thoughtfully executed collection of chapters that challenges what we think we know and teaches us how to seek new knowledge about the intersection of multiculturalism and positive psychology.

Lawrence, KS, USA Shane J. Lopez

Acknowledgments

Numerous people have been involved in the development of this book, and we are grateful to all of them for their time and efforts. First, we thank Springer Science, Esther Otten and Hendrikje Tuerlings for their belief in the importance of this topic, and for their publishing support. We also extend our heartfelt thanks to all the authors who contributed chapters to the volume; their expertise and strong writing made this project possible.

We extend gratitude to our institutions, California Polytechnic State University, San Luis Obispo and Marquette University, which have provided the space and support for our academic efforts over the past years.

We also wish to thank our colleagues, students, clients and friends who have shaped our thinking about multiculturalism and positive psychology over the years, and who have helped to promote our own well-being. Our mentor, Shane Lopez, has provided continued guidance and encouragement which we never take for granted.

Finally, and most importantly, we give thanks to our families for their patience, encouragement and pride in our work. Special thanks go to our children who provide us with inspiration every day.

California Polytechnic State University
San Luis Obispo, CA, USA
Jennifer Teramoto Pedrotti

Marquette University
Milwaukee, WI, USA
Lisa M. Edwards

Contents

About the Editors

Jennifer Teramoto Pedrotti, Ph.D. received her doctorate and masters degrees in counseling psychology at the University of Kansas. She is currently Professor in the Department of Psychology and Child Development at California Polytechnic State University, San Luis Obispo where she teaches courses in positive psychology, multicultural psychology, clinical and counseling psychology, intergroup dialogues, and research methods. Dr. Teramoto Pedrotti's current research includes projects measuring the effectiveness of multicultural psychology courses in increasing ethnocultural empathy in students. Dr. Teramoto Pedrotti spoke on the intersection of positive psychology and culture as a keynote speaker at the 2014 Asian Pacific Conference on Applied Positive Psychology in Hong Kong. Her work on this subject and others has appeared in many journals including the *Journal of Counseling Psychology*, the *Journal of Positive Psychology*, and *Professional Psychology: Research & Practice*. She is co-author of the textbook *Positive Psychology: The Scientific and Practical Explorations of Human Strengths* (with Lopez and Snyder), the 3rd edition of which will be in print in the summer of 2014.

Lisa M. Edwards, Ph.D. is an Associate Professor in the Department of Counselor Education and Counseling Psychology at Marquette University. She received her masters and doctoral degrees in Counseling Psychology from the University of Kansas, and was a postdoctoral research associate at the University of Notre Dame. In her current position, Dr. Edwards is the Director of Counselor Education and teaches courses in multicultural counseling, group counseling, and supervision. She directs the Culture and Well-Being Research Lab and is a licensed psychologist in the state of Wisconsin. Dr. Edwards' research focuses on how cultural variables such as familism, religiosity, and ethnic identity influence well-being among Latino/as and multiracial populations. Dr. Edwards' work has appeared in several journals, including the *Journal of Counseling Psychology*, the *Hispanic Journal of Behavioral Sciences*, and *Professional Psychology: Research and Practice*. She is also co-author of *Preventing Adolescent Depression and Suicide among Latinas* (2013, SpringerBriefs in Psychology).

Perspectives on the Intersection of Multiculturalism and Positive Psychology: An Introduction

As our society becomes increasingly diverse, the importance of understanding the influence of culture is essential. Culture is a determinant in our identities, our views of self and others, and formative in the development of our unique worldview. It is also, in part, responsible for what we view as healthy, valuable, and worthwhile. As a field, psychology has historically ignored cultural facets in theory development and assessment, often leading to members of non-majority cultures being pathologized (Sue and Sue 2013). Psychology has also largely focused on the deficits of all individuals, excluding discussions of positive development and strengths (Seligman and Csikszentmihalyi 2000). In effect, this means that individuals from non-majority cultures deal with a sort of double-jeopardy; they are "branded as pathological in comparison to the majority group, and within a system that only acknowledges weakness and leaves no room for a balanced description of behavior" (Pedrotti and Edwards 2010, p. 166).

While large strides have been made in addressing the dearth of research about strengths among individuals through the positive psychology movement, the lion's share of this research has paralleled a lack of balance with regard to culture, instead primarily focusing on White, Western viewpoints as "normal" and "beneficial" as opposed to integrating ideas from a more multicultural population (Sue and Constantine 2003). A more multiculturally competent approach to positive psychology seems to necessitate identifying strengths in diverse groups as opposed to setting up deficit models across various theories.

The field of positive psychology has begun to recognize that to be viable, it must become more inclusive to the topic of culture with regard to discussion of strengths and weakness (Pedrotti et al. 2009). As such, more research within the area of positive psychology is currently being conducted on populations from non-majority and other underrepresented backgrounds. New information is emerging, providing evidence that culture is a major determinant in how one ranks various strengths, defines certain constructs, and manifests and judges healthy and positive behavior (Lu and Gilmour 2004; Pedrotti 2013; Uchida et al. 2004). Much of this research, however, has been conducted with samples comparing one country to another. While this information is invaluable, there is an even greater dearth of research aimed toward looking at differences within one cultural context (Chang and Banks 2007), and with regard to a broad range of facets as opposed to simply nation of origin. This volume is an effort to compile this research and theory across cultural facets including race, ethnicity, gender, disability, age, religion, sexual orientation, and social class within the cultural context of the United States.

Before going further, some general definitions may be necessary. Triandis (1996) discussed *culture* as passing from generation to generation, allowing for adaptations as other aspects shift over time and as a determinant for the development of worldviews. These worldviews may include "unexamined assumptions" (Triandis 1996, p. 408) that a cultural group takes for granted as part of their existence and may derive from a variety of sources. In addition, a distinction must be drawn between differences between various countries or home cultures, and those differences that occur within one context. Mio et al. (2012) define *cross-cultural psychology* as "comparisons across cultures or countries, as opposed to comparisons of groups within one society" (p. 13), while using the term *multicultural psychology* to refer to interactions among different cultural groups within one context. While cross-cultural differences and distinctions may inform and impact various multicultural issues, we cannot assume that differences that exist at a country level are also present at a racial or ethnic level. For example, research studying views or behaviors of individuals in Japan or Mexico may not necessarily translate to experiences of Japanese or Mexican Americans within the United States.

In addition, both broad and narrow definitions of culture exist throughout the literature. While some focus solely on the important facets of race, ethnicity, and nation of origin, others broaden to include such equally important facets as gender, disability, sexual orientation, social class, age, and religion (Hays 2008). This broad treatment of culture allows us to look at intersectionality of these facets as well and to determine both personal and environmental lacks and assets in a variety of individuals. Finally, the investigation of the effects of these pieces of our identity within a strength-based context might allow us to see benefit in practices and viewpoints that are different from our own, thus leading to a broader pool of strengths from which to draw.

The United States is somewhat unique in the sense that so many different groups of individuals from different backgrounds reside in one context. As a country, our history of navigating relationships amongst these different populations has unfortunately been fraught with misunderstandings, ignoring or negating the worldviews of those unlike us, and pathologizing those who lacked power. A multiculturally competent positive psychology, one that effectively embraces, values, and works to understand these differences and values, has the potential to provide a salve for the wounds we have suffered at the hands of each other across our nation.

Overview of This Volume

The chapters in this volume represent different perspectives about the intersection of Multiculturalism and Positive Psychology. Some authors address conceptual and methodological issues in studying these topics, while others review literature about certain constructs and populations. Together they provide an overview of the latest research and theory, and pose questions for readers about ways in which this unique intersection of different pieces in the field can inform future research and application.

The volume is organized around four main topics: Part I Theoretical underpinnings and research issues, Part II Specific constructs, Part III Specific populations, and Part IV Applications of positive psychology in multicultural contexts. Part I includes a history of cultural context in the study of positive psychology by Christina Downey and Edward Chang, and definitional considerations by Heather Rasmussen and Lea Lavish. Cristalis Capielo and colleagues address measurement issues within this portion of the field, and Samuel Ho and colleagues address methodological approaches to studying positive psychology and culture. Part II focuses on three main sets of constructs: Hung-Bin Sheu addresses affective constructs, Christine Robitschek and colleagues investigate cognitive aspects, and Belinda Campos and Sharon Shenhav discuss constructs that are interpersonal in nature. In each of these chapters, the authors discuss some of the prominent positive psychological constructs within a cultural context, particularly involving racial and ethnic diversity.

Part III includes an exploration of aspects of diversity in addition to race and ethnicity, including age by Jeanne Nakamura and colleagues, gender by Matt Englar-Carlson and Rebekah Smart, religion and spirituality by Melissa Falb and Kenneth Pargament, social class by William Liu and Allison Allmon, disability by Michael Wehmeyer and Karrie Shogren, and finally sexual orientation by Sharon Horne and colleagues. These chapters provide a review of the research that has been conducted in this area, noting the intersectionality of different identity facets. Lastly, Part IV addresses how the research and theory about multiculturalism and positive psychology can be applied in a variety of settings, including schools by Casey Holtz and Michael Martinez, work by Carolyn Youssef-Morgan and James Hardy, and psychotherapy by Jeana Magyar-Moe. The volume concludes with an insightful look from John Chambers Christopher and Katie Lynn Howe at where we are today, noting potential areas of growth and ways to recognize and address biases and blind spots regarding culture and positive psychology.

California Polytechnic State University
San Luis Obispo, CA, USA
Jennifer Teramoto Pedrotti

Marquette University
Milwaukee, WI, USA
Lisa M. Edwards

References

Chang, E. C., & Banks, K. H. (2007). The color and texture of hope: Some preliminary findings and implications for hope theory and counseling among diverse racial/ethnic groups. *Cultural Diversity & Ethnic Minority Psychology*, *13*, 94–103.

Hays, P.A. (2008). *Addressing cultural complexities in practice: A framework for clinicians and counselors*. Washington, DC: American Psychological Association.

Lu, L., & Gilmour, R. (2004). Culture and conceptions of happiness: Individual oriented and social oriented SWB. *Journal of Happiness Studies, 5*, 269–291.

Mio, J. S., Barker, L. A., & Tumambing, J. S. (2012). *Multicultural psychology: Understanding our diverse communities*. New York: Oxford University Press.

Pedrotti, J. T. (2013). Positive psychology, social class, and counseling. In W. M. Liu (Ed.), *Oxford handbook of social class in counseling* (pp. 131–143). New York: Oxford University Press.

Pedrotti, J. T., & Edwards, L. M. (2010). The intersection of positive psychology and multiculturalism in counseling. In J. G. Ponterotto, J. M. Casas, Suzuki, L. A., & Alexander, C. M. (Eds.), *Handbook of multicultural counseling* (pp. 165–174). Thousand Oaks: Sage.

Pedrotti, J. T., Edwards, L. M., & Lopez, S. J. (2009). Positive psychology within a cultural context. In S. J. Lopez & C. R. Snyder (Eds.), *Oxford handbook of positive psychology* (pp. 49–57). New York: Oxford University Press.

Seligman, M. E. P., & Csikszentmihalyi, M. (2000). Positive psychology: An introduction. *American Psychologist, 55*, 5–14.

Sue, D. W., & Constantine, M. G. (2003). Optimal human functioning in people of color in the United States. In W. B. Walsh (Ed.), *Counseling psychology and optimal human functioning* (pp. 151–169). Mahwah: Lawrence Erlbaum.

Sue, D. W., & Sue, D. (2013). *Counseling the culturally diverse: Theory and practice.* Hoboken: Wiley.

Triandis, H. C. (1996). The psychological measurement of cultural syndromes. *American Psychologist, 51*, 407–415.

Uchida, Y, Norasakkunkit, V., & Kitayama, S. (2004). Cultural constructions of happiness: Theory and empirical evidence. *Journal of Happiness Studies, 5*, 223–239.

Part I
Theoretical Underpinnings and Research Issues

Chapter 1
History of Cultural Context in Positive Psychology: We Finally Come to the Start of the Journey

Christina A. Downey and Edward C. Chang

1.1 History of Cultural Context in Positive Psychology

> "Wherever a process of life communicates an eagerness to him who lives it, there the life becomes genuinely significant…there is the zest, the tingle, the excitement of reality; and there is 'importance' in the only real and positive sense in which importance ever anywhere can be." – William James (1899, p. 139; excerpted from James 2007)

It is fitting to open a history of culture in positive psychology with these words of William James, not only because he was discussing what is best in life, but also because he actually was speaking directly about cultural factors in well-being. James in this piece was describing how on a visit to rural North Carolina, he viewed an area of felled forest upon which a rough homestead and meager farm had been erected. He saw the way of life exemplified there as miserable by his contemporary standards. However, James was informed by his driver that such toil was considered the only path to true happiness for the local people, representing freedom, self-sufficiency, and productivity in that place. Immediately James realized that the nature of personal fulfillment varied with cultural factors, and that his reflexive negative judgment of people different from himself had been deeply flawed.

When the field of positive psychology was officially introduced in lectures and writings (e.g., Seligman and Csikszentmihalyi 2000), its stated aim was to counterbalance the prevailing scientific emphasis on psychopathology through rigorous empirical study of wellness, positive experiences and traits, and prosocial engagement with others and society. However, positive psychology has since been

C.A. Downey, Ph.D. (✉)
Department of Psychology, Indiana University Kokomo,
2300 S. Washington St., P.O. Box 9003, Kokomo, IN 46904-9003, USA
e-mail: downeyca@iuk.edu

E.C. Chang
Department of Psychology, University of Michigan at Ann Arbor,
Ann Arbor, MI, USA

J. Teramoto Pedrotti and L.M. Edwards (eds.), *Perspectives on the Intersection of Multiculturalism and Positive Psychology*, Cross-Cultural Advancements in Positive Psychology 7, DOI 10.1007/978-94-017-8654-6_1,

criticized as not only denigrating the contributions of established fields such as humanistic psychology (Taylor 2001), but also of promoting certain culturally-biased approaches, strengths, and morals – in particular those of Western majority (e.g., White male) culture (Becker and Marecek 2008; Christopher and Hickinbottom 2008; Christopher et al. 2008; McDonald and O'Callaghan 2008; Sandage et al. 2003). In essence, regarding culture, positive psychologists were accused of committing James' (1899) prejudicial error again. It is our aim in this chapter to explore such criticisms, by reviewing how positive functioning has been approached over psychology's history; how other areas of psychology laid the foundation for the rise of positive psychology; and how culture has been approached both within psychology generally, and within positive psychology specifically.

1.2 Historical and Philosophical Roots of Positive Psychology

Critics of positive psychology are correct to assert that global interest in individual well-being long precedes the twenty-first century. For example, ancient philosophical and religious texts from places as diverse as China, India, Greece, and the Middle East contain guidelines about behavior thought to optimize functioning and experience, such as the practice of courage, justice, humanity, temperance, wisdom, and transcendence (Dahlsgaard et al. 2005). The connections between such cultural traditions and psychology have been rarely acknowledged (Segall et al. 1998), and this situation also holds for positive psychology (Roysircar 2012; Segall et al. 1998), despite the fact that philosophy and psychology were essentially synonymous until the late nineteenth and early twentieth centuries (White 1992).

1.2.1 The First Century of Western Psychology and Well-Being

When increased emphasis on the scientific method contributed to Western psychology spinning off from philosophy (White 1992), the focus of psychology was on increasingly sophisticated empirical understanding of mental processes (e.g., consciousness and mental structure), divorced from making moralistic recommendations about desirable behavior. Therefore, little scholarly exploration of the meaning of "the good life" in early psychology was undertaken. However, constructs now considered related to positive psychology were occasionally addressed or implied. For example, in addition to William James' (1899) writings on the positive outcomes of education, Sigmund Freud and his successors discussed how *Eros*, or life energy, provided vitality and positive dynamism to experience when unblocked through psychoanalysis (Ryan and Frederick 1997); Wilhelm Wundt expounded on pleasant emotions and their connections to cognition, memory, and volition (Blumenthal 1975); G. Stanley Hall investigated the functions of playful childhood behaviors in development (e.g., fun, tickling, wit, and humor;

White 1992); and John Dewey discussed how personal goal pursuit and empowerment foster intellectual and moral growth (Dewey 1900).

With the rise of behaviorism after John Watson's (1913) classic paper, psychology shifted away from studying the nature of consciousness to understanding and controlling the external drivers of observable behavior (to the dismay of Titchener 1914, and others). Thus, subjective experiences of well-being (or anything else, for that matter) were deemed by many unable to be studied (Tolman 1922). However, the behaviorists' wish to produce findings that were immediately applicable in real-world settings spoke to an intention to improve the human condition (e.g., Skinner's *Walden Two*, originally published in 1948; Skinner 2005). Their idea of positive functioning was optimal adaptation to one's circumstances, and because behavior could be (at least in great part) controlled externally, improving the lot of humankind was simply a matter of arranging the appropriate stimuli to create the appropriate responses (Rich 2001). Of course, it was soon recognized that any substantial attempt to apply principles of operant conditioning to the betterment of real individuals or societies would carry a host of problems (Stillman 1975), and thus were never instituted to the behaviorists' satisfaction.

Though behaviorism held prominence from about 1920 to 1950, the study of some aspects of cognition were always of interest to psychologists – namely, intelligence and intellectual ability (Flanigan and Harrison 2005). The assumption underlying this research was that high intelligence, particularly strong perceptual and problem-solving abilities, would be advantageous to people throughout schooling and into adulthood (and therefore comprise an individual strength). Critiques of intelligence assessment have focused on the validity of the various tests developed, rather than on the worthiness of being able to measure individual intelligence at all (Boake 2002; Flanigan and Harrison 2005). The so-called "cognitive revolution," which then began in the 1950s, brought an increasing number of other mental processes back into the purview of psychological study (Miller 2003). However, it was not until the 1980s that a steady stream of papers began to define and explore positive cognitive variables such as subjective well-being, self-efficacy, and happiness. These cognitive variables, and others, are those now most identified with positive psychology, largely due to Seligman and Csikszentmihalyi's (2000) emphasis on such constructs.

Developmental psychology is unique within Western psychology, in that it has both had a long empirical history and consistently been interested in understanding well-being. A few decades after Hall's investigations into various childhood behaviors (White 1992), John Bowlby began developing his landmark theory of how *attachment* to caregivers was essential to good psychological health in young children (Breatherton 1992; van der Horst and van der Veer 2010) and fellow psychoanalysts such as Spitz concurred (Vicedo 2009). The mid-1950s saw a great increase in study of attachment theory, both through Bowlby's work, and through the international prominence acquired by scholars such as Harry Harlow and Mary Ainsworth (Breatherton 1992). Harlow examined seemingly innate and adaptive needs for attachment in infant rhesus monkeys, positing similar needs in human children (Vicedo 2009), and Mary Ainsworth (a student and collaborator of

Bowlby's) developed the well-known "Strange Situation" test of attachment quality, concluding that young children who showed secure attachment to their caregivers were more likely to show healthy emotional development than were children showing insecure attachments (Ainsworth and Bowlby 1991). The influence of such findings led Seligman and Csikszentmihalyi (2000) to lay claim to attachment for their new positive psychology, though developmental psychology and positive psychology remain distinct.

1.2.2 *Other Important Predecessors to Positive Psychology*

Various other movements within and outside of Western psychology have connections to positive psychology. For example, Becker and Marecek (2008) discussed how the spiritual-philosophical movement of New Thought (which began in the early nineteenth century) emphasized positive thinking as a means of promoting wellness, enjoyment of life, and improving people's relations with one another. Similarly, the mental hygiene movement, associated most closely with the early practice of psychiatry, focused on the prevention of mental illness, hoping to repeat the earlier success of public campaigns against communicable diseases like tuberculosis. Its Freudian and early behaviorist assumptions led proponents to claim that inappropriate parenting drove disturbances in personality, which in turn caused maladjustment (Cohen 1983). Like positive psychology, then, it aimed to improve individual adjustment to circumstances, albeit through often-misguided approaches (Becker and Marecek 2008). For example, mental hygienists targeted certain members of society (e.g., criminals, prostitutes, and "vagrants") for the identification of "mental deficiency," ignoring the ways in which societal inequalities could influence those behaviors (Toms 2010).

The early area of humanistic psychology known as *personology* (founded by Henry Murray) also emphasized personality characteristics in adjustment, noting as early as 1938 that positive and desirable personal characteristics were not yet receiving their due attention in psychology (Taylor 2001). Indeed, it is the scholars and practitioners of humanistic psychology that have argued most strongly for having been the main progenitors of positive psychology. Humanistic psychology, which arose in the 1960s, emphasizes "a view of the human being as irreducible to parts, needing connection, meaning, and creativity…[and] offering tools for personal and spiritual transformation" (Resnick et al. 2001, p. 75). Carl Rogers and Abraham Maslow (among others) are credited with trying to push study of human flourishing to the forefront of psychology (Resnick et al. 2001; Taylor 2001), and when Division 32 (humanistic psychology) of the American Psychological Association was founded, its first brochure stated its adherence to the tenets of science in its effort to understand human experience (Aanstoos et al. 2000). It came as an unwelcome surprise to many humanistic psychologists, then, when Seligman and Csikszentmihalyi (2000) asserted that positive psychology was needed to correct the inability of humanistic psychology to contribute reliable and valid knowledge of human wellness to scientific discourse. Humanistic psychologists took particular offense to the suggestion that the main legacy of humanistic psychology is not scientifically-useful findings, but rather popular self-absorption and "kooky" self-help practices (Friedman 2008; Held 2004; McDonald and O'Callaghan 2008; Resnick et al. 2001; Taylor 2001). By contrast, humanistic psychologists consider their discipline vibrant and productive, with qualitative and quantitative findings being continuously disseminated and applied to advance human wellness (McDonald and O'Callaghan 2008; Taylor 2001). While effort has been made to heal the wounds that Seligman and Csikszentmihalyi's (2000) comments inflicted upon humanistic psychology (e.g., Linley et al. 2006; Seligman 2005), there remains a painful rift between the fields (Robbins 2008).

The discipline of counseling psychology (and a closely-related field, social work) has also objected strongly to what it sees as reluctance from positive psychologists to acknowledge their shared roots (Linley 2006; Lopez and Magyar-Moe 2006). As described by Frazier et al. (2006), "focusing on strengths and positive adaptation is a central aspect of counseling psychology's identity" (p. 293), a claim which has been empirically verified. In a content analysis of publications in counseling psychology journals, Lopez et al. (2006) concluded that counseling psychologists since 1954 have studied many constructs associated with positive psychology, including adaptability, hope, love, motivation, optimism, positive emotions, and values/ethics. Counseling psychologists have also highlighted their early emphasis on multiculturalism as an important factor in both research and practice in well-being (Constantine and Sue 2006; Frazier et al. 2006; Gerstein 2006; Lopez et al. 2006), a strength which they feel distinguishes counseling psychology from other fields.

It is clear that the twenty-first century positive psychology movement has captured the imagination of many within psychology and in popular culture. However, we conclude that the roots of the movement are so deep and broad that it cannot be considered unprecedented. We appreciate why a number of scholars may have felt snubbed when positive psychology was founded; however, we also see that empirical interest in well-being has been reinvigorated by its sudden prominence. We believe that the interdisciplinary origins of positive psychology give us reason to look forward to its interdisciplinary future, and that scientific discourse among diverse fields will further the shared goal of understanding and promoting wellness.

1.3 Issues of Race and Culture in Psychology's First Century

Unfortunately, when culture arose in Western psychology prior to the 1980s (when counseling psychologists first articulated the benefits of recognizing cultural differences), it was not in the context of discussing strengths or positive experiences. Instead, we bear the scars of a shameful past, where supposedly scientific investigations into differences between Anglo-Saxon Whites and peoples of color progressed on a deeply misguided path for nearly 100 years, advancing oppression ranging from denigration, to eugenics, to slavery (Leong et al. 2012; Tucker 1994). Early studies investigating racial differences in variables such as IQ or personality characteristics nearly always concluded that non-Whites differ in unfavorable ways from Whites, even when data were unclear or contradictory (e.g., Goodenough 1926; Tucker 1994). For the first few decades of Western psychology, there was an assumption that non-White, non-Western peoples possessed inherent biological deficiencies (e.g., Watson's [1913] reference to members of Aboriginal tribes as "savages" whose behavioral repertoires were far simpler than that of "educated Europeans," p. 168). The tools of early psychology were too often put to nefarious use when dealing with issues of cultural difference during this period (Leong et al. 2012; Richards 1997; Tucker 1994; Winston 2004), and by the mid-1920s, objections to the *deficit model* of racial minority psychology were growing louder (Kantor 1925; Leong et al. 2012; Sanchez 1932). In its place, though, arose the assumption that observed racial differences in personality variables, achievement, or IQ scores were due to socialization into inferior cultural values, and lack of access to the institutions of majority culture (e.g., "differences…being probably due to nurture," Garth 1930, p. 331; Tucker 1994). This *deprivations model*, though perhaps developed as a well-intentioned response to the deficit model, served to perpetuate negatively biased assumptions about minority groups (Dreger and Miller 1960; Tucker 1994).

Most recently, a minority of researchers have maintained a focus on supposed genetic differences between racial groups (e.g., differences in mean IQ scores; Rushton and Jensen 2005). However, most recent work has converged on a view of race, ethnicity, and culture in psychology that assumes that a combination of historical oppression, institutional disadvantage, implicit and/or explicit discrimination, and cultural differences in worldview offers the best explanation for group differences in behavior (Tucker 1994). There is also a clear effort to balance acknowledgement of group differences, with emphasis on within-group variability, as well as with aspects of behavior and experience that might be universal (Frazier et al. 2006). Still, knowledge of the psychological benefits associated with cultural background remains limited, as much more work has gone into understanding the negative impact of oppression (almost as an atonement for past harms perpetrated in the name of science). Therefore, recent interest in *multicultural positive psychology* is seen as long overdue (Roysircar 2012; Sandage et al. 2003).

1.4 Highlighting Culture in Twenty-First Century Positive Psychology

Our last goal is to explore culture within positive psychology in its first decade (roughly 2000–2010). Most positive psychology research has addressed positive emotion, and/or related cognitive constructs (such as creativity, emotional intelligence, and flow). A thorough review of all relevant constructs is impossible here; therefore, we focus the remainder of this review on hope, mindfulness, and optimism, and aspects of multiculturalism related to these constructs.

1.4.1 Hope

Hope research is closely aligned with positive psychology (Cheavens et al. 2006). In its most widely-known form, hope is conceived as a set of self-directed cognitions regarding one's ability to create goals, produce pathways (or plans to achieve those goals), and agency (or the motivation that sustains pursuit of those goals; Snyder 1989; Snyder et al. 2006). High levels of hope are associated with greater engaged coping behaviors (Chang and DeSimone 2001; Danoff-Burg et al. 2004), and more adaptive problem solving (Chang 1998b), as well as with a greater sense of life purpose and coherence (Feldman and Snyder 2005) and lower depressive symptomology (Chang 2003). Higher hope in college students is predictive of academic success (Rand 2009; Snyder et al. 2002), and attainment of personal goals (Feldman et al. 2009); similarly, higher hope among mental health patients is associated with greater belief in psychotherapy efficacy, and predictive of more positive treatment outcomes (Irving et al. 2004). As such, hope would seem to be a powerful cognitive construct to promote in times of intellectual, psychological, or physical struggle.

Hope theory has been applied not only in White Western cultures, but also in American racial minority groups, and in various non-Western societies such as South Africa (Luthans et al. 2004) and in the Philippines (Bernardo 2010). Danoff-Burg et al. (2004) examined hope in a sample of African American college students, and found that students high in hope reported more use of active coping with race-related stressors than students low in hope did (though active coping was actually most helpful to the low-hope students). Chang and Hudson Banks (2007) examined possible racial group differences in hope, and concluded that though levels and correlates of hope do not differ across U.S. racial groups (specifically European American, African American, Asian American, and Latino American college students), the strongest predictors of agency and pathways thinking in these groups varied. For example, the strongest predictor of agentic thinking in European Americans was life satisfaction; in African Americans, it was negative problem orientation (i.e., poor self-efficacy and a tendency to view problems in one's social world as a threat to well-being); in Asian Americans, it was positive affect; and in Latino Americans, it was rational problem solving. Therefore, members of diverse groups may experience similar levels of hope, but the origins of hope may differ among members of different racial groups.

1.4.2 Mindfulness

Mindfulness is "intentional and nonjudgmental awareness of moment-to-moment experience" (Shapiro et al. 2008, p. 841). Self-report studies of mindfulness using measures like the Mindful Attention Awareness Scale (MAAS; Brown and Ryan 2003) with predominantly White samples have indicated that greater tendencies towards mindfulness are associated with greater self-esteem (Thompson and

Waltz 2008), greater openness to experience, and greater optimism, as well as less neuroticism, lower anxiety, and less depressive symptomology (Brown and Ryan 2003), even controlling for other maladaptive variables such as perfectionism or poor social problem solving (Argus and Thompson 2008). Much of the knowledge on the benefits of mindfulness has come from empirical studies of interventions meant to foster mindfulness (e.g., Baer 2003; Carmody and Baer 2007; Kabat-Zinn 2003; Shapiro et al. 2008). For example, engagement in mindfulness-based stress reduction (MBSR) may improve psychological well-being (Carmody and Baer 2007), increase one's capacity to forgive others (Shapiro et al. 2008), and decrease psychological symptoms of distress, possibly via increases in cognitive, emotional, and behavioral flexibility (Carmody et al. 2009) or decreases in maladaptive cognitive distortions (Sears and Kraus 2009).

Mindfulness, with its roots in Buddhist spirituality, is a good example of how non-Western thought can be applied meaningfully in Western settings (Kabat-Zinn 2003). However, studies of mindfulness in various non-White racial groups have been few; where race has been examined as a potential covariate in linear analyses, significant differences across groups have not emerged (Creswell et al. 2007; Roemer et al. 2009). Some evidence has been found for cross-cultural understanding of mindfulness (Christopher et al. 2009a, b; Ghorbani et al. 2008; Jermann et al. 2009), though there appear to be some differences in how Western vs. non-Western individuals conceptualize and assess their own mindfulness.

1.4.3 Optimism

According to Scheier and Carver's (1985) widely-used definition, the optimist holds a *generalized positive outcome expectancy* about his or her future, typically believing that situational outcomes will be favorable to himself or herself. Optimism carries benefits such as greater life satisfaction, more positive affect and fewer depressive symptoms (Chang 1998a; Chang and Sanna 2001; Marshall et al. 1992), and may interact with factors like life stress to affect outcome. For example, Chang and Sanna (2003) found that when faced with life hassles, optimistic adolescents developed significantly less depressive symptoms and hopelessness than those who were pessimistic. Optimists also tend to use more active or problem-focused methods to cope with stressors (Nes and Segerstrom 2006) and exhibit more persistence in mastering difficult tasks (Nes et al. 2005; Segerstrom 2001) than pessimists. Still, there is evidence that not all correlates and consequences of optimism are positive, an important point to consider within and outside of the positive psychology movement (Chang et al. 2008).

The multicultural applicability of optimism has been shown in a number of studies; for example, among African Americans, optimism has been associated with greater resilience and reduced psychological distress (Baldwin et al. 2011), while experiencing racism has been associated with decreased optimism in this group (Mattis et al. 2003). Other studies, though, find that African Americans and European

Americans may not differ significantly in optimism (Brown et al. 2006) despite their different experiences of racism and life stress. Studies have also examined differences between Asian/Asian Americans and (most often) European Americans on optimism, with studies often showing few group differences on optimism levels (e.g., Chang 1996; Hardin and Leong 2005). Interestingly, Chang (1996) showed that while Asians/Asian Americans did not differ from European Americans in optimism, Asians/Asian Americans showed greater levels of pessimism; however, this pessimism was not accompanied by increased negative mood or negative problem orientation (as it was in European Americans). This indicates that the optimism-pessimism dichotomy may hold significantly different meaning among different racial and ethnic groups. Optimistic bias (the tendency to believe positive events are likely to happen to the self, and negative events are likely to happen to others) has also been examined in these groups. For example, Japanese college students have been found to be less optimistic than European Americans about their own chances of experiencing negative life events (Chang and Asakawa 2003; Chang et al. 2001).

1.5 Conclusion: A Look Back, and the Path Ahead

Frankly, we find it stunning to realize how long the road is behind us, which has now led to the very beginning of multicultural positive psychology. While it may now seem simple to ask, "What do members of various cultures possess or experience that assists their wellness?" the rocky and halting history behind that question indicates it is not simple at all. Multicultural positive psychology has gradually woven threads from many sectors of psychology together with a spirit of social justice, to start a tapestry of great potential beauty. However, it is incumbent upon present and future generations of researchers in this area to acknowledge the depth and breadth of their roots, as well as to advocate for positive and collaborative applications of findings to individuals, groups, and communities (Downey and Chang 2012). There have certainly been past errors, and the cynics may take that as reason to criticize present work in this area as "too little, too late." However, it is our belief that the only meaningful way to correct past errors is to accelerate the search for knowledge that will outshine the past darkness. We are glad to say that we see many reasons to hope for just such an outcome.

References

Aanstoos, C., Serlin, I. A., & Greening, T. (2000). History of Division 32 (humanistic psychology) of the American Psychological Association. In D. Dewsbury (Ed.), *Unification through division: Histories of the divisions of the American Psychological Association: Vol. V*. Washington, DC: American Psychological Association.

Ainsworth, M. D. S., & Bowlby, J. (1991). An ethological approach to personality development. *American Psychologist, 46*, 333–341. doi:10.1037/0003-066X.46.4.333.

Argus, G., & Thompson, M. (2008). Perceived social problem solving, perfectionism, and mindful awareness in clinical depression: An exploratory study. *Cognitive Therapy and Research, 32*, 745–757. doi:10.1007/s10608-006-9102-1.

Baer, R. A. (2003). Mindfulness training as a clinical intervention: A conceptual and empirical review. *Clinical Psychology: Science & Practice, 10*, 125–143. doi:10.1002/jclp.

Baldwin, D. R., Jackson, D., Okoh, I., & Cannon, R. L. (2011). Resiliency and optimism: An African American senior citizen's perspective. *Journal of Black Psychology, 37*, 24–41. doi:10.1177/0095798410364394.

Becker, D., & Marecek, J. (2008). Positive psychology: History in the remaking? *Theory and Psychology, 18*, 591–604. doi:10.1177/0959354308093397.

Bernardo, A. B. I. (2010). Extending hope theory: Internal and external locus of trait hope. *Personality and Individual Differences, 49*, 944–949. doi:10.1016/j.paid.2010.07.036.

Blumenthal, A. L. (1975). A reappraisal of Wilhelm Wundt. *American Psychologist, 30*, 1081–1088. doi:10.1037/0003-066X.30.11.1081.

Boake, C. (2002). From the Binet-Simon to the Wechsler-Bellevue: Tracing the history of intelligence testing. *Journal of Clinical and Experimental Neuropsychology, 24*, 383–405.

Breatherton, I. (1992). The origins of attachment theory: John Bowlby and Mary Ainsworth. *Developmental Psychology, 28*, 759–775. doi:10.1037/0012-1649.28.5.759.

Brown, K. W., & Ryan, R. M. (2003). The benefits of being present: Mindfulness and its role in psychological well-being. *Journal of Personality and Social Psychology, 84*, 822–848. doi:10.1037/0022-3514.84.4.822.

Brown, C., Matthews, K. A., & Bromberger, J. (2006). How do African American and Caucasian women view themselves at midlife? *Journal of Applied Social Psychology, 35*, 2057–2075. doi:10.1111/j.1559-1816.2005.tb02209.x.

Carmody, J., & Baer, R. (2007). Relationships between mindfulness practice and levels of mindfulness, medical and psychological symptoms and well-being in a mindfulness-based stress reduction program. *Journal of Behavioral Medicine, 31*, 23–33. doi:10.1007/s10865-007-9130-7.

Carmody, J., Baer, R. A., Lykins, E. L. B., & Olendzki, N. (2009). An empirical study of the mechanisms of mindfulness in a Mindfulness-Based Stress Reduction program. *Journal of Clinical Psychology, 65*, 613–626. doi:10.1002/jclp.20579.

Chang, E. C. (1996). Evidence for the cultural specificity of pessimism in Asians vs. Caucasians: A test of the general negativity hypothesis. *Personality and Individual Differences, 21*, 819–822.

Chang, E. C. (1998a). Does dispositional optimism moderate the relation between perceived stress and psychological well-being?: A preliminary investigation. *Personality and Individual Differences, 25*, 233–240.

Chang, E. C. (1998b). Hope, problem-solving ability, and coping in a college student population: Some implications for theory and practice. *Journal of Clinical Psychology, 54*, 953–962.

Chang, E. C. (2003). A critical appraisal and extension of hope theory in middle-aged men and women: Is it important to distinguish agency and pathways components? *Journal of Social and Clinical Psychology, 22*, 121–143.

Chang, E. C., & Asakawa, K. (2003). Cultural variations on optimistic and pessimistic bias for self versus a sibling: Is there evidence for self-enhancement in the West and for self-criticism in the East when the referent group is specified? *Journal of Personality and Social Psychology, 84*, 569–581. doi:10.1037/0022-3514.84.3.569.

Chang, E. C., & DeSimone, S. L. (2001). The influence of hope on appraisals, coping, and dysphoria: A test of hope theory. *Journal of Social and Clinical Psychology, 20*, 116–128.

Chang, E. C., & Hudson Banks, K. (2007). The color and texture of hope: Some preliminary findings and implications for hope theory and counseling among diverse racial/ethnic groups. *Cultural Diversity and Ethnic Minority Psychology, 13*, 94–103. doi:10.1037/1099-9809.13.2.94.

Chang, E. C., & Sanna, L. J. (2001). Optimism, pessimism, and positive and negative affectivity in middle-aged adults: A test of a cognitive-affective model of psychological adjustment. *Psychology and Aging, 16*, 524–531.

Chang, E. C., & Sanna, L. J. (2003). Experience of life hassles and psychological adjustment among adolescents: Does it make a difference if one is optimistic or pessimistic? *Personality and Individual Differences, 34*, 867–879.

Chang, E. C., Asakawa, K., & Sanna, L. J. (2001). Cultural variations in optimistic and pessimistic bias: Do Easterners really expect the worst and Westerners really expect the best when predicting future life events? *Journal of Personality and Social Psychology, 81*, 476–491. doi:10.1037//0022-3514.81.3.476.

Chang, R., Chang, E. C., Sanna, L. J., & Hatcher, R. L. (2008). Optimism and pessimism as personality variables linked to adjustment. In G. J. Boyle, G. Matthews, & D. H. Saklofske (Eds.), *SAGE handbooks of personality theory and assessment: Personality measurement and testing* (Vol. 1, pp. 470–485). London: Sage.

Cheavens, J. S., Feldman, D. B., Woodward, J. T., & Snyder, C. R. (2006). Hope in cognitive psychotherapies: On working with client strengths. *Journal of Cognitive Psychotherapy: An International Quarterly, 20*, 135–145.

Christopher, J. C., & Hickinbottom, S. (2008). Positive psychology, ethnocentrism, and the disguised ideology of individualism. *Theory and Psychology, 18*, 563–589. doi:10.1177/0959354308093395.

Christopher, J. C., Richardson, F. C., & Slife, B. D. (2008). Thinking through positive psychology. *Theory and Psychology, 18*, 555–561. doi:10.1177/0959354308093395.

Christopher, M. S., Charoensuk, S., Gilbert, B. D., Neary, T. J., & Pearce, K. L. (2009a). Mindfulness in Thailand and the United States: A case of apples versus oranges? *Journal of Clinical Psychology, 65*, 590–612. doi:10.1002/jclp.20580.

Christopher, M. S., Christopher, V., & Charoensuk, S. (2009b). Assessing "Western" mindfulness among Thai Theravada Buddhist monks. *Mental Health, Religion, & Culture, 12*, 303–314. doi:10.1080/13674670802651487.

Cohen, S. (1983). The mental hygiene movement, the development of personality and the medicalization of American education. *History of Education Quarterly, 23*, 123–149. Stable URL: http://www.jstor.org/stable/368156

Constantine, M. G., & Sue, D. W. (2006). Factors contributing to optimal human functioning in people of color in the United States. *The Counseling Psychologist, 34*, 228–244.

Creswell, J. D., Way, B. M., Eisenberger, N. I., & Lieberman, M. D. (2007). Neural correlates of dispositional mindfulness during affect labeling. *Psychosomatic Medicine, 69*, 560–565. doi:10.1097/PSY.0b013e3180f6171f.

Dahlsgaard, K., Peterson, C., & Seligman, M. E. P. (2005). Shared virtue: The convergence of valued human strengths across culture and history. *Review of General Psychology, 9*, 203–213. doi:10.1037/1089-2680.9.3.203.

Danoff-Burg, S., Prelow, H. M., & Swenson, R. R. (2004). Hope and life satisfaction in Black college students coping with race-related stress. *Journal of Black Psychology, 30*, 208–228. doi:10.1177/0095798403260725.

Dewey, J. (1900). Psychology and social practice. *Psychological Review, 7*, 105–124. doi:10.1037/h0066152.

Downey, C. A., & Chang, E. C. (2012). Multidimensional clinical competence: Considering racial group, development, and the positive psychology movement in clinical practice. In E. C. Chang & C. A. Downey (Eds.), *Handbook of race and development in mental health* (pp. 355–382). New York: Springer.

Dreger, R. M., & Miller, K. S. (1960). Comparative psychological studies of Negroes and whites in the United States. *Psychological Bulletin, 57*, 361–402. doi:10.1037/h0047639.

Feldman, D. B., & Snyder, C. R. (2005). Hope and the meaningful life: Theoretical and empirical associations between goal-directed thinking and life meaning. *Journal of Social and Clinical Psychology, 24*, 401–421.

Feldman, D. B., Rand, K. L., & Kahle-Wrobleski, K. (2009). Hope and goal attainment: Testing a basic predication of hope theory. *Journal of Clinical Psychology, 28*, 479–497.

Flanigan, D. P., & Harrison, P. L. (Eds.). (2005). *Contemporary intellectual assessment: Theories, tests, and issues*. New York: Guilford Press.

Frazier, P. A., Lee, R. M., & Steger, M. F. (2006). What can counseling psychology contribute to the study of optimal human functioning? *The Counseling Psychologist, 34*, 292–303. doi:10.1177/0011000005283521.

Friedman, H. (2008). Humanistic and positive psychology: The methodological and epistemological divide. *The Humanistic Psychologist, 36*, 113–126. doi:10.1080/08873260802111036.

Garth, T. R. (1930). A review of race in psychology. *Psychological Bulletin, 27*, 329–356. doi:10.1037/h0075064.
Gerstein, L. H. (2006). Counseling psychology's commitment to strengths: Rhetoric or reality? *The Counseling Psychologist, 34*, 276–292. doi:10.1177/0011000005283518.
Ghorbani, N., Watson, P. J., & Hargis, M. B. (2008). Integrative Self-Knowledge Scale: Correlations and incremental validity of a cross-cultural measure developed in Iran and the United States. *Journal of Psychology, 142*, 395–412.
Goodenough, F. L. (1926). Racial differences in the intelligence of school children. *Journal of Experimental Psychology, 9*, 388–397. doi:10.1037/h0073325.
Hardin, E. E., & Leong, F. T. L. (2005). Optimism and pessimism as mediators of the relations between self-discrepancies and distress among Asian and European Americans. *Journal of Counseling Psychology, 52*, 25–35. doi:10.1037/0022-0167.52.1.25.
Held, B. S. (2004). The negative side of positive psychology. *Journal of Humanistic Psychology, 2004*, 9–46. doi:10.1177/0022167803259645.
Irving, L. M., Snyder, C. R., Cheavens, J., Gravel, L., Hanke, J., Hilberg, P., & Nelson, N. (2004). The relationships between hope and outcomes at the pretreatment, beginning, and later phases of psychotherapy. *Journal of Psychotherapy Integration, 14*, 419–443. doi:10.1037/1053-0479.14.4.419.
James, W. (2007). *Talks to teachers on psychology: And to students on some of life's ideals*. Charleson: Bibliobazaar.
Jermann, F., Billieux, J., Laroi, F., d'Argembeau, A., Bondolfi, G., & Zermatten, A. (2009). Mindful Attention Awareness Scale (MAAS): Psychometric properties of the French translation and exploration of its relations with emotion regulation strategies. *Psychological Assessment, 21*, 506–514. doi:10.1037/a0017032.
Kabat-Zinn, J. (2003). Mindfulness-based interventions in context: Past, present, and future. *Clinical Psychology: Science and Practice, 10*, 144–156. doi:10.1093/clipsy/bpg016.
Kantor, J. R. (1925). Anthropology, race, psychology, and culture. *American Anthropologist, 27*, 267–283. Stable URL: http://www.jstor.org/stable/661207
Leong, F. T. L., Pickren, W., & Tang, L. C. (2012). A history of cross-cultural clinical psychology, and its importance to mental health today. In E. C. Chang & C. A. Downey (Eds.), *Handbook of race and development in mental health* (pp. 11–26). New York: Springer.
Linley, P. A. (2006). Counseling psychology's positive psychological agenda: A model for integration and inspiration. *The Counseling Psychologist, 34*, 313–322. doi:10.1177/0011000005284393.
Linley, P. A., Joseph, S., Harrington, S., & Wood, A. M. (2006). Positive psychology: Past, present, and (possible) future. *The Journal of Positive Psychology, 1*, 3–16. doi:10.1080/17439760500372796.
Lopez, S. J., & Magyar-Moe, J. L. (2006). A positive psychology that matters. *The Counseling Psychologist, 34*, 323–330. doi:10.1177/0011000005284392.
Lopez, S. J., Magyar-Moe, J. L., Petersen, S. E., Ryder, J. A., Krieshok, T. S., Koetting O'Byrne, K., Lichtenberg, J. W., & Fry, N. A. (2006). Counseling psychology's focus on positive aspects of human functioning. *The Counseling Psychologist, 34*, 205–227. doi:10.1177/0011000005283393.
Luthans, F., Van Wyk, R., & Walumbwa, F. O. (2004). Recognition and development of hope for South African organizational leaders. *The Leadership and Organization Development Journal, 25*, 512–527. doi:10.1108/01437730410556752.
Marshall, G. N., Wortman, C. B., Kusulas, J. W., Hervig, L. K., & Vickers, R. R. (1992). Distinguishing optimism from pessimism: Relations to fundamental dimensions of mood and personality. *Journal of Personality and Social Psychology, 62*, 1067–1074.
Mattis, J. S., Fontenot, D. L., & Hatcher-Kay, C. A. (2003). Religiosity, racism, and dispositional optimism among African Americans. *Personality and Individual Differences, 34*, 1025–1038.
McDonald, M., & O'Callaghan, J. (2008). Positive psychology: A Foucauldian critique. *The Humanistic Psychologist, 36*, 127–142. doi:10.1080/08873260802111119.
Miller, G. A. (2003). The cognitive revolution: A historical perspective. *TRENDS in Cognitive Sciences, 7*, 141–144. doi:10.1016/S1364-6613(03)00029-9.
Nes, L. S., & Segerstrom, S. C. (2006). Dispositional optimism and coping: A meta-analytic review. *Personality and Social Psychology Review, 10*, 235–251.

Nes, L. S., Segerstrom, S. C., & Sephton, S. E. (2005). Engagement and arousal: Optimism's effects during a brief stressor. *Personality and Social Psychology Bulletin, 31*, 111–120.
Rand, K. L. (2009). Hope and optimism: Latent structures and influences on grade expectancy and academic performance. *Journal of Personality, 77*, 231–260. doi:10.1111/j.1467-6494.2008.00544.x.
Resnick, S., Warmoth, A., & Serlin, I. A. (2001). The humanistic psychology and positive psychology connection: Implications for psychotherapy. *Journal of Humanistic Psychology, 41*, 73–101.
Rich, G. J. (2001). Positive psychology: An introduction. *Journal of Humanistic Psychology, 41*, 8–12.
Richards, G. (1997). *Race, racism, and psychology: Towards a reflexive history*. New York: Routledge.
Robbins, B. D. (2008). What is the good life?: Positive psychology and the renaissance of humanistic psychology. *The Humanistic Psychologist, 36*, 96–112. doi:10.1080/08873260802110988.
Roemer, L., Lee, J. K., Salters-Pedneault, K., Erisman, S. M., Orsillo, S. M., & Mennin, D. S. (2009). Mindfulness and emotion regulation difficulties in generalized anxiety disorder: Preliminary evidence for independent and overlapping contributions. *Behavior Therapy, 40*, 142–154. doi:10.1016/j.beth.2008.04.001.
Roysircar, G. (2012). Foreword. In E. C. Chang & C. A. Downey (Eds.), *Handbook of race and development in mental health* (pp. v–x). New York: Springer.
Rushton, J. P., & Jensen, A. R. (2005). Thirty years of research on race differences in cognitive ability. *Psychology, Public Policy, and Law, 11*, 235–294. doi:10.1037/1076-8971.11.2.235.
Ryan, R. M., & Frederick, C. (1997). Subjective vitality as a dynamic reflection of well-being. *Journal of Personality, 65*, 529–565. doi:10.1111/1467-6494.ep9710314567.
Sanchez, G. I. (1932). Group differences and Spanish-speaking children: A critical review. *Journal of Applied Psychology, 16*, 549–558. doi:10.1037/h0072844.
Sandage, S. J., Hill, P. C., & Vang, H. C. (2003). Toward a multicultural positive psychology: Indigenous forgiveness and Hmong culture. *The Counseling Psychologist, 31*, 564–592. doi:10.1177/0011000003256350.
Scheier, M. F., & Carver, C. S. (1985). Optimism, coping, and health: Assessment and implications of generalized outcome expectancies. *Health Psychology, 4*, 219–247.
Sears, S., & Kraus, S. (2009). I think therefore I Om: Cognitive distortions and coping style as mediators for the effects of mindfulness meditation on anxiety, positive and negative affect, and hope. *Journal of Clinical Psychology, 65*, 561–573. doi:10.1002/jclp.20543.
Segall, M. H., Lonner, W. J., & Berry, J. W. (1998). Cross-cultural psychology as a scholarly discipline: On the flowering of culture in behavioral research. *American Psychologist, 53*, 1101–1110. doi:10.1037/0003-066X.53.10.1101.
Segerstrom, S. C. (2001). Optimism, goal conflict, and stressor-related immune change. *Journal of Behavioral Medicine, 24*, 441–467.
Seligman, M. E. P. (2005). Positive psychology, positive prevention, and positive therapy. In C. R. Snyder & S. J. Lopez (Eds.), *Handbook of positive psychology* (pp. 3–9). Oxford: Oxford University Press.
Seligman, M. E. P., & Csikszentmihalyi, M. (2000). Positive psychology: An introduction. *American Psychologist, 55*, 5–14. doi:10.1037//0003-066X.55.1.5.
Shapiro, S. L., Oman, D., Thoresen, C. E., Plante, T. G., & Flinders, T. (2008). Cultivating mindfulness: Effects on well-being. *Journal of Clinical Psychology, 64*, 840–862. doi:10.1002/jclp.20491.
Skinner, B. F. (2005). *Walden two*. Indianapolis: Hackett Publishing.
Snyder, C. R. (1989). Reality negotiation: From excuses to hope and beyond. *Journal of Social and Clinical Psychology, 8*, 130–157.
Snyder, C. R., Shorey, H. S., Cheavens, J., Pulvers, K. M., Adams, V. H., III, & Wiklund, C. (2002). Hope and academic success in college. *Journal of Educational Psychology, 94*, 820–826. doi:10.1037//0022-0663.94.4.820.
Snyder, C. R., Lehman, K. A., Kluck, B., & Monsson, Y. (2006). Hope for rehabilitation and vice versa. *Rehabilitation Psychology, 51*, 89–112. doi:10.1037/0090-5550.51.2.89.
Stillman, P. G. (1975). The limits of behaviorism: A review essay on B. F. Skinner's social and political thought. *American Political Science Review, 69*, 202–213. Stable URL: http://www.jstor.org/stable/1957901

Taylor, E. (2001). Positive psychology and humanistic psychology: A reply to Seligman. *Journal of Humanistic Psychology, 41*, 13–29.
Thompson, B. L., & Waltz, J. A. (2008). Mindfulness, self-esteem, and unconditional self-acceptance. *Journal of Rational-Emotive & Cognitive-Behavior Therapy, 26*, 119–126. doi:10.1007/s10942-007-0059-0.
Titchener, E. B. (1914). On "Psychology as the behaviorist views it." *Proceedings of the American Philosophical Society, 53*, 1–17. Stable URL: http://www.jstor.org/stable/984126
Tolman, E. C. (1922). A new formula for behaviorism. *Psychological Review, 29*, 44–53. doi:10.1037/h0070289.
Toms, J. J. (2010). Mind the gap: MIND, the mental hygiene movement and the trapdoor in measurements of intellect. *Journal of Intellectual Disability Research, 54*, 16–27. doi:10.1111/j.1365-2788.2009.01234.x.
Tucker, W. H. (1994). *The science and politics of racial research*. Urbana: University of Illinois Press.
van der Horst, F. C. P., & van der Veer, R. (2010). The ontogeny of an idea: John Bowlby and contemporaries on mother-child separation. *History of Psychology, 13*, 25–45. doi:10.1037/a0017660.
Vicedo, M. (2009). Mothers, machines, and morals: Harry Harlow's work on primate love from lab to legend. *Journal of the History of Behavioral Sciences, 45*, 193–219. doi:10.1002/jhbs.20378.
Watson, J. B. (1913). Psychology as the behaviorist views it. *Psychological Review, 20*, 158–177. doi:10.1037/h0074428.
White, S. H. (1992). G. Stanley Hall: From philosophy to developmental psychology. *Developmental Psychology, 28*, 25–34. doi:10.1037/0012-1649.28.1.25.
Winston, A. S. (2004). Introduction: Histories of psychology and race. In A. S. Winston (Ed.), *Defining difference: Race and racism in the history of psychology* (pp. 3–18). Washington, DC: American Psychological Association.

Chapter 2
Broad Definitions of Culture in the Field of Multicultural Psychology

Heather N. Rasmussen and Lea Lavish

2.1 Multicultural Positive Psychology

An increasing number of scientists and theorists are devoting attention to the intersection of optimal human functioning and culture. While older theoretical models and frameworks conceptualized human behavior and functioning from a deficit viewpoint and without cultural considerations, contemporary models not only focus on a balance between deficient and optimal functioning, but also are culturally responsive. Indeed, recent work in positive psychology considers both the investigation of cultural representations of optimal human functioning, as well as the importance of the relationship between individuals and their environments (Delle Fave and Bassi 2009; Lopez et al. 2002; Pedrotti et al. 2009; Uchida et al. 2004). Other chapters in this volume will provide reviews of specific positive psychology constructs and their application to multiculturalism. In this chapter, we first provide an overview of definitions of culture and then discuss the importance of considering different ways of integrating cross-cultural thinking into our everyday work as researchers or helping professionals. We utilize the ADDRESSING framework (Hays 2008) as a guide to integrate thinking about multiculturalism, identity, and human strengths.

H.N. Rasmussen, Ph.D. (✉)
Northcentral University, Living Healthy Solutions, Prescott Valley, AZ, USA

Living Healthy Solutions, 1045 Stonecreek Drive, Lawrence, KS 66049, USA
e-mail: Heather_rasmussen@yahoo.com

L. Lavish, Ph.D.
Dwight D. Eisenhower VA Medical Center, Leavenworth, KS, USA

J. Teramoto Pedrotti and L.M. Edwards (eds.), *Perspectives on the Intersection of Multiculturalism and Positive Psychology*, Cross-Cultural Advancements in Positive Psychology 7, DOI 10.1007/978-94-017-8654-6_2,

2.1.1 Overview of Multiculturalism

The study of culture cannot be separated from our understanding of the *self,* which is not a fixed phenomenon but rather a series of complex, dynamic interactions with our environment (Huitt 2004). This view of a dynamic self is central to the work of social scientists that recognize that multiple levels exist at which change can be initiated. In summary, how we view ourselves is the total sum of our affective, cognitive, instinctual, environmental, and behavioral experiences (Judge et al. 1997), and is influenced by the specific evidence we gather from our cultural values and norms (Harter 1999). Some researchers note that at a deeper level, culture is also an evolving process that is mutually agreed upon by a specific social group, which is transmitted through our chosen language, customs and social institutions (Wong et al. 2006). According to Wong and colleagues (2006): "In many important ways cultures are the expressions of human nature in all its complexity and duality – fears and hopes, cravings and aspirations, selfishness and generosity, cruelty and compassion." (p. 1). Culture is a fluid phenomenon in a constant state of flux, being shaped by our environment, social and political events along with the interaction of individual and group differences.

In fact, there is a long history and multiple definitions attempting to capture the nuances of what culture includes. Culture was first defined by Cicero as a cultivation of the soul (i.e., *cultura animi*) and culture was more widely used in the eighteenth century as an agricultural term to describe improvements in cultivation (Kroeber and Kluckhohn 1952). In the nineteenth century, culture was used to describe the refinement, or the education of an individual. In simple terms, culture means the customs, language and practices attributable to specific group membership (Ben-Shalom and Horenczyk 2003; Snauwert et al. 2003). More recently, there have been multiple, and even controversial definitions of culture (Triandis 1996). While the definitions vary widely, there is consensus that culture is comprised of *shared* elements (Shweder and LeVine 1984), such as standards for believing and communicating "among those who share a language, a historic period, and a geographic location" (Triandis 1996, p. 408). These elements are passed through generations with modifications, including "unexamined assumptions and standard operating procedures reflecting what have worked at one point in the history of a cultural group" (Triandis 1996, p. 408). Culture can be thought of as a specific way to view the world based on a socially constructed set of beliefs, values, and norms.

It is clear there are multiple definitions of culture and a wide range of disciplines have attempted to capture the richness of this phenomenon. While there does not seem to be a unified definition, there are certain agreed upon commonalities. The most vital is its acceptance as a felt phenomenon that is best described and discussed rather than forced into a single inflexible definition (Axelson 1985). For our purposes we will combine multiple definitions to create a broad base to begin our discussion. *Culture describes the whole of an individual's learned behaviors, thoughts and perceptions that have been transmitted throughout generations from institutions, organizations, or group membership.*

2.1.2 *Moving from Culture-Free to Culturally Embedded Thinking*

Two approaches to the integration of culture and positive psychology have been proposed. Some scholars advocate for a culture-free approach to research. To support this view, they cite positive psychology researchers who propose to have identified strengths that are common across cultures. As an example, Peterson and Seligman (2004) developed the *Character Strengths and Virtues: A Handbook and Classification* (*CSV*). They used the *Diagnostic and Statistical Manual of Mental Disorders* (*DSM*; American Psychiatric Association 1994) as a model, but rather than describing psychological disorders, the *CSV* is intended to describe and classify human strengths. In developing the CSV, the authors state that they relied on overarching strengths that "almost every culture across the world endorses" (Seligman et al. 2005, p. 411). They note that there is a similarity in the endorsement of the 24 strengths across 40 countries, with correlations from nation to nation ranging in the 1980s, which defies cultural, ethnic, and religious differences (Seligman et al. 2005). Embedded within this culture-free approach is the assumption that a researcher also is culture-free. In other words, the researcher is assumed to be objective, with the values of their own culture not entering into their professional work (Pedrotti et al. 2009).

Another approach is the culturally-embedded perspective, which is the approach taken by the editors of this volume and the authors of the chapters herein. A culturally-embedded perspective suggests that strengths should be viewed within a cultural context and that our cultures and worldviews do indeed affect our work (Pedrotti et al. 2009). In addition, the question must be asked, does mere presence of a behavior/attitude in a variety of cultures tell us enough about how that strength behaves, if it has the same definition as the one we are providing, or if it is valued as a strength at all (see Pedrotti 2013 for an expanded discussion of the different manifestations of positive characteristics)? We too, believe that a key to understanding strengths and cultural influences is to start by examining one's personal views on specific cultural dimensions. It is also important to understand where those with whom we work and interact fall on these dimensions. For example we might want to ask ourselves and others about: our beliefs about the concept of "self;" how do we feel most comfortable communicating and relating to others; what value do we place on appearance and things like meal time; what does time mean to us; which do we value more, the individual or the group; how do we feel about handling disagreements; what are our beliefs about the meaning of existence; and finally how do we view such things as work and play. It is important for both clinicians and scholars to not only see the similarities between ourselves and those with whom we work, but to take the time to notice the differences that may be due to cultural influences coming from multiple sources.

As Pedrotti and colleagues (2009) noted, the field of psychology has often used deficit models in the past that explain pathology as a function of non-White racial and ethnic differences. Deficit models were formed to support the White or dominant cultures source of privilege (McIntosh 1998). These entitlements and privileges are unearned, unacknowledged, or some would argue unconscious standards and norms, which have been created from what is considered acceptable by the group with the majority of the power (McIntosh 1998). When other cultures are measured by these dominant cultural standards and norms, they are often found to be deficient at best and abnormal by those with an extreme view. While there has been a great deal of research conducted on positive psychological constructs, it is imperative that the shift from fixing what is unhealthy to fostering strengths also focuses on the contextual influences of the individual. Instead of viewing a person through the lens of diagnosis or to viewing behaviors or rituals of an entire group as aberrant or deficient because they are viewed as such within our own personal cultural context, we must first consider the information provided by the individual's cultural context from which the behavior/action originated and then note whether the behavior/action contributes to healthy functioning. Our goal, within this shift is to move toward explanatory models that acknowledge cultural factors and then recognize that they also can contribute to healthy functioning.

2.1.3 *Making Meaning out of Cultural Context*

Indeed, it seems clear that people are influenced by multiple contextual factors and it is important to consider how context affects our daily decision-making, as well as those with whom we work. In addition, it is important to remember that individuals not only have multiple personal identities and strengths, but environments also provide strengths and resources upon which individuals can draw from. Professionals are compelled to integrate their thinking to consider how a person's values, worldview, culture, and environment contribute to optimal functioning. When we begin to integrate our thinking in such a way, we gain a richer, broader, and more complex understanding of ourselves and the individuals with whom we interact, as well as a deeper field of study with regard to research possibilities.

Bronfenbrenner's ecological theory (1977, 1992) has been a widely applied framework to understand the complex interactions between an individual and sociocultural systems. Briefly, ecological systems theory explains that individuals are influenced by five environmental systems: (1) the microsystem, which includes the individual's family, peers, school, and neighborhood; (2) the mesosystem, which is the quality of the relationships among the different contexts, such as between the family and the school; (3) the exosystem, which is the environmental systems and contexts for which the individual is not directly a part of, but which affect the individual; (4) the macrosystem, which is the culture in which the individual lives. The latter system includes societal values, socioeconomic status, poverty, and ethnicity; and (5) the chronosystem, which includes the transitions over the life course, such as divorce. It is important to note that the influences between these systems are bidirectional (Bronfenbrenner 1977, 1992). Each experience and developmental process affects an individual's functioning across various contexts

(Yakushko et al. 2009). Thus, individuals are influenced and shaped by multiple interacting contexts (Yakushko et al. 2009). Keeping the influence of these contexts in mind, multicultural researchers suggest that when attempting to understand an individual we must examine the context in which psychological traits and behaviors occur (Constantine and Sue 2006; Pedrotti and Edwards 2009). Therefore, it is imperative that we consider every individual's experience as a series of fluctuating contexts and connections to multiple cultural identities. Theorists have assumed that an individual can have varying levels of identification and involvement with multiple cultures (Kvernmo and Heyerdahl 2003). It could be said that our cultural identity is inherently *multicultural* (Gamst et al. 2002; Kvernmo and Heyerdahl 2003; Lopez-Class et al. 2011; Phinney et al. 1997; Ward and Kus 2012). Shifts in culture occur when individuals from one culture are exposed to a new culture, resulting in changes in behavior and attitude (Ben-Shalom and Horenczyk 2003; Berry 1979; Flannery et al. 2001; Lopez-Class et al. 2011; Miranda and Umhoefer; 1998; Sattler 2001; Snauwert et al. 2003; Ward and Kus 2012). All cultures have distinct patterns of affective, cognitive, and behavioral expression. Cultural diversity occurs when the interaction of a unique set of social environments, geographical locations, historical context, political events, dominant religions, and philosophies combine (Wong et al. 2006). These distinctions may gradually diminish as cultures blend, coexist or when the domination of one culture supersedes all others.

Each individual can be seen as behaving, thinking, and feeling from multiple cultural influences. This same individual is then interacting and reacting to the multiple cultural influences of other individuals which results in an infinite number of astounding combinations (Axelson 1985). This cultural similarity or dissimilarity, which is based on each individual's background and experience, must therefore be the starting point for clinicians and scholars to examine their own cultural context in order to effectively communicate and relate. Multiculturalism implies an approval or celebration of diversity based on either the right of different groups to respect, recognize, or to acknowledge the benefits of membership to the larger cultural society (Heywood 2007). Multiculturalism is closely associated with the concept of cultural pluralism which is defined by Axelson (1985) as the benefits received by the dominant culture "...from coexistence and interaction with the culture of adjunct groups" (p. 13).

In order to better understand the multiple cultural influences that shape individuals' identities and conceptualize personal and environmental strengths, several strategies or heuristics can be utilized. We will now describe the ADDRESSING Framework (Hays 2008) and the four-front approach (Wright and Lopez 2009).

2.2 Hays ADDRESSING Framework

Hays (2008) has developed an approach to help researchers and clinicians assess and examine their own values, beliefs, and contexts in order to better understand the impact of culture on our work. Hays (2008) has identified several cultural influences and identities that affect our human experience. Clinicians must first recognize and then assume responsibility for our own cultural influences as they shape such factors as our decision-making, communication style, case conceptualization, or the client's to whom we are drawn. Researchers must also consider their own cultural influences as these affect development of theory, hypothesis formation, and even the topics we choose to explore. These influences are denoted through the use of the ADDRESSING acronym, along with sample questions a clinician or researcher could ask herself:

- **A**ge-related issues and generational influences: What are my age-related issues or generational influences or experiences that may affect my work with clients, students or research?
- **D**evelopmental disability or **d**isability that occurred later in life: What is the influence on disability on my life? How does my invisible disability affect my work? or How does my family member with a disability influences my understanding and interaction with others?
- **R**eligion and spiritual orientation: How does my religious upbringing or spiritual orientation affect my work? What are my current beliefs and how might they affect my work with individuals from different backgrounds?
- **E**thnic or racial identity: How does my racial or ethnic identity influence my work?
- **S**ocioeconomic status: What is my socioeconomic status and beliefs associated with my current status? How does this influence my work with others of a different status?
- **S**exual orientation: How does my sexual orientation affect my work with others? What are my views regarding people who have a sexual orientation that is different from my own?
- **I**ndigenous heritage: Do I have an indigenous heritage that is part of my identity? In what ways does my heritage influence my work?
- **N**ational identity or origin and primary language: What is my national identity and primary language and how does this influence work with others?
- **G**ender-related information: What gender-related information is significant and how is this intertwined with my cultural identity and heritage? How do my roles and expectations, such as parenting status, marital status, and other family relationships, influence my worldview?

It should be apparent after reviewing the aforementioned questions that a person's identity will evolve over time. As we age, our identity and worldview change. We may become more aware and educated about certain types of acquired disabilities, for example, as our friends and families face these challenges. If we become parents or grandparents or have relationships with partners and end these relationships, each of these life transitions has an effect on our identity, work, and worldview. Cultural identities and influences are complex and fluid. Bronfenbrenner (1992) would suggest that this fluid movement from one system to another is the natural and complex course of our human experiences. Cultural change requires an open examination of the interactions between the individual and their multiple social systems. It is only through this awareness that our own cultural identity, as well as the cultural identity of others, can be fully understood and appreciated.

2.2.1 *Self-Assessment*

Hays (2008) notes that it is important for us to first engage in a self-assessment, which requires critical thinking skills, as well as a lens of humility and compassion. Her approach to this self-assessment begins with an examination of how privilege affects relationships between those who have privilege and those who do not. McIntosh (1998) defines privilege as the advantages that one has because they belong to a dominant group. She notes that privilege is like having an invisible knapsack that individuals with privilege often are not aware that they possess. McIntosh goes on to state that the invisible knapsack includes unearned positive advantages and power that a person is given in society due to membership in the dominant group. As an example of privilege, she states that, as a White woman, she is confident that she could move to most neighborhoods without worrying about whether she would be allowed to rent or purchase property. Furthermore, she could be fairly confident that her neighbors will accept her or at least be neutral to her presence in the neighborhood. McIntosh states that awareness of the magnitude of these advantages possessed as a result of privileged status is elusive, as people who have these advantages are taught to remain oblivious to privilege in their daily lives. McIntosh argues that because of this, those who are privileged must be vigilant about bringing their awareness to the forefront, lest they fall back into being unaware of the unearned advantages that are inherent via membership in a dominant group. Similarly, the self-examination in the ADDRESSING model (Hays 2008) is an ongoing process which partly takes place during sessions with clients or in the tasks related to research; however, the majority of the learning takes place through introspection, readings, research, and learning about diverse people outside the working environment. This can involve activities such as attending community events and developing relationships with people of diverse identities. The emphasis here is to explore and understand the effect of cultural influences on our own worldviews, as well as how our group membership(s) can affect others.

2.2.2 *Interpersonal Engagement*

The second category in the ADDRESSING framework (Hays 2008) is engaging in interpersonal work. This is where we begin to recognize that it is not only ourselves that are complex beings experiencing multiple influences on our lives and worldview, but that others also are complex and constantly adjusting, changing. No one is a static unidimensional being. Once we realize and appreciate the complexity of ourselves and others, the better we are able to understand those who are different from us. Such recognition can clarify how our decision-making in our professional work is affected by our various cultural values, influences, and worldviews. Similar to the process of identifying the multiple memberships and influences on our worldview, we can utilize the ADDRESSING framework to uncover the cultural complexity of our clients and within our scientific inquiry. By doing this, we can avoid making generalizations based on physical appearance or primary language (Hays 2008). For example, the curriculum we choose to teach and the research questions we formulate are affected by our complex experiences, cultural environment, and values that are salient in our life (Constantine and Sue 2006; Pedrotti et al. 2009; Snyder et al. 2011). As stated previously, we often identify strongly with more than one cultural group. For example, our society is becoming increasingly multiracial and it is common to find people who identify simultaneously with minority and majority identities (Edwards and Pedrotti 2008). Self, culture, identity, all of these constructs cannot be understood as a static process, though, as over time and depending on the context, an individual may identify more strongly with different groups than at other times during their lives.

2.3 The Four-Front Approach

Other frameworks exist that can be used to understand the complex and diverse strengths that can be found in individuals, as well as environments. Scholars have noted that a common error of professional psychology is the primary focus on the deficiencies of the person when making diagnostic, treatment, and policy decisions without regard to the strengths *and* deficits of both the individual *and* the environment (Wright and Lopez 2009). This is a fundamental negative bias that can lead us astray in practice and research by ignoring the strengths and resources that could be developed to increase optimal human functioning. Wright (1991) developed the four-front approach when attempting to understand strengths and deficiencies in others and the environments within which they exist. This approach encourages gathering of comprehensive information about a client's strengths and weaknesses, as well as the influence of environmental stressors and resources. We see this approach as one that can be applied to gathering culturally-relevant strengths and undermining characteristics as well. Wright and Lopez (2009) suggest the following four areas be covered, and in parentheses, we have identified examples of how the approach could be used to identify culturally-relevant variables: (1) resources and opportunities in the environment (such as supportive extended family, a strong church community or other organizations that provide support to the individual, or a workplace that is supportive of the individual's identity, such as being a parent, or being a gay individual); (2) lacks and destructive factors in the environment (such as a workplace that discriminates against the individual, violence in the home or community, or a community that lacks supports for an individual with a disability); (3) strengths and assets of the person (strong ethnic identity, pride in one's culture, or being multilingual); and (4) deficiencies and undermining characteristics of the person (such as confusion about identity or problems in daily living due to age-related factors). Researchers and clinicians are encouraged to consider the multiple cultural identities via the ADDRESSING model, and to integrate this with the four-front approach similar to our previous examples. This process can be challenging, but is important to understand how an individual's multiple identities, strengths, and limitations influence each other, but also to understand that the individual's behavior and environment are also mutually dependent. Some may argue that this approach will encourage the focus to swing from negative and deficiencies to focusing solely on positive cultural characteristics. To remedy this, Wright (1991) proposed that researchers and clinicians give equal time and space as a reminder to attend to both the negatives and strengths in clinical work and research. Since our current practice in psychology tends to already focus on the negatives and lacks, we, along with others (i.e., Wright and Lopez 2009), encourage clinicians and researchers to spend as much time and effort on uncovering the positives as is spent on the negatives. Adding to this, "culture counts" (Pedrotti et al. 2009) and we urge professionals to integrate the identification and investigation of cultural influences and strengths into their professional practice.

2.3.1 *Identifying Individual, Interpersonal, and Contextual Culturally-Relevant Strengths*

As mentioned, professionals can integrate the ADDRESSING model and the four-front approach in order to provide a more balanced conceptualization of individuals and their functioning. Once one is aware of the potential cultural influences that may exist, researchers and clinicians can also identify and recognize individual, interpersonal, and cultural strengths as an important part of the complex human experience via the lens of these frameworks.

From a research standpoint, knowledge of the facets of the ADDRESSING framework and the four-front approach might assist in developing interesting areas of study. As an example, researchers have investigated how personal identification with certain cultural facets may have an impact on the effects of stressors. Indeed, a strong ethnic identity may be a protective factor by helping individuals appreciate and understand the positive qualities of their ethnic group, thus minimizing negative influences such as discrimination. Support for this hypothesis can be found in the literature. Stronger ethnic identification has been found to be related to higher self-esteem in some cultural groups (Phinney and Chavira 1992; Phinney et al. 1997; Pieterse and Carter 2010; Smith and Silva 2011) and self-efficacy (Phinney et al. 1997; Whitsell et al. 2006), and to buffer against stressors (Lee 2005). Similar to the studies on self-esteem and self-efficacy, researchers can use their knowledge of the ADDRESSING model and the four-front approach to identify variables that emerge from a certain cultural background and environmental context to investigate whether these facets are protective against stress and/or promote optimal human functioning. For example, individual strengths that could be investigated include bilingualism, pride in one's sexual orientation, or personal growth stemming from facing a disability. Interpersonal strengths include a strong religious community, extended family supports, or culture-specific celebrations. Finally, environmental resources include a religious or spiritual space (Pedrotti et al. 2009) and supports in the school and stable work environments. Scholars turning their attention to individual, interpersonal, and environment strengths rather than solely focusing on the lacks or negatives help balance the research focus as suggested by Wright and Lopez (2009).

As a second example, bicultural identification (i.e., individuals who have intimate knowledge of the norms and customs of more than one cultural group) has been associated with higher global-self-esteem (Oetting and Beauvis 1991; Walters 1999). Bicultural individuals who found themselves immersed in multicultural systems were also more likely to feel a sense of positive psychological well-being and greater self-esteem (Phinney et al. 1997). Brendtro et al. (1990) suggested that individuals who do not feel like an authentic member of the majority group, must find a sense of mastery, belonging, and autonomy in both worlds while maintaining identification with their own group. As a specific example, when asked about American Indian culture, Red Horse, a tribal leader, insisted that his people must remain rooted in American Indian culture while developing ways to find harmony with the majority culture, thus holding a "foot in both worlds" (Hill 1991, p. 85). The ability to live in two worlds has been cited by multiple social scientists as necessary to foster positive growth (Bryant and LaFromboise 2005; Chang et al. 1996; Herring 1994; Hill 1991; Kunitz and Levy 1994; Moncher et al. 1990; Stewart 1984); thus, it appears that understanding the norms of two different cultures could be a strength.

Finally, other researchers have studied how sociocultural environments and cultural diversity may facilitate strengths. Hays (2008) has provided three sources of cultural strengths; personal (i.e., strengths attributed to self), interpersonal (i.e., strengths attributed to our relationships) and environmental (i.e., strengths attributed to our external world) that might be attended to in therapy. Pedrotti and Edwards (2009) provided multiple examples of each strength-based category. These examples should be viewed as a starting point and are not exhaustive. A personal cultural strength may be bilingual ability, culturally grounded craft or skill, spiritual or religious belief system, a sense of pride in one's heritage, life experience (Pedrotti and Edwards 2009). Interpersonal supports might include a broad view and definition of family; culturally centered festivals, gatherings and celebrations; meaningful rituals and identification as a member if a specific cultural group (Pedrotti and Edwards 2009). Finally, environmental strengths are culturally based choices of food, clothing, housing and decoration; spaces dedicated to prayer, honoring deceased ancestors, or honoring relationship to other living things such as animals (Pedrotti and Edwards 2009).

In using Hays's (2008) delineations in combination with the four-front, researchers are also able to more easily view individuals as complex beings whose environments also play a role in their development. Simonton (1997, 2000) notes that creative activity increases after societies and individuals open up to various cultural influences such as immigration or travel abroad. Thus, in considering the role of environment (both lacks and resources) one may gain a better understanding of the origin of a particular strength. It is clear that cultural strengths can come from personal, interpersonal, and environmental contexts. Researchers should continue to work to provide additional descriptions of how individual and environmental resources are related to well-being and other positive health markers. Similar to Wright and Lopez (2009), our hope is that clinicians, educators, and researchers will take a more balanced view by assessing for strengths and environmental resources, rather than just focusing on deficiencies (see also the following for expanded discussions of focusing on strengths in the environment: Lopez et al. 2003; Rasmussen et al. 2003).

2.4 Conclusion

The need to integrate multicultural competence more fully into the field of positive psychology is beyond argument. We are complex beings with multiple identities and influences living in a world that is continually more globally connected and interdependent (Gerstein et al. 2009). Other authors have called for taking a more balanced view of others, considering not only deficiencies, but also strengths and environmental resources (Wright and Lopez 2009; Pedrotti et al. 2009; Rasmussen et al. 2003). It is our hope that providing a broad definition of culture and integrating the ADDRESSING framework (Hays 2008) with the four-front approach (Wright and Lopez 2009) as one model to become more aware of the complexity of human experience and strengths and resources, will help us identify ways in which we can increase the adaptive functioning of those with whom we work. Working from such a lens will help us strive toward becoming culturally competent psychologists.

References

American Psychiatric Association. (1994). *Diagnostic and statistical manual of mental disorders* (4th ed.). Washington, DC: Author.

Axelson, J. A. (1985). *Counseling and development in a multicultural society*. Monterey: Brooks/Cole Publishing Company.

Ben-Shalom, U., & Horenczyk, G. (2003). Acculturation orientations: A facet theory perspective on the bi-dimensional model. *Journal of Cross-Cultural Psychology, 34*, 176–188.

Berry, J. W. (1979). Research in multicultural societies: Implications of cross-cultural methods. *Journal of Cross-Cultural Psychology, 10*, 415–434.

Brendtro, L. K., Brokenleg, M., & Van Brokern, S. (1990). *Reclaiming youth at risk: Our hope for the future*. Bloomington: National Education Services.

Bronfenbrenner, U. (1977). Toward an experimental ecological of human development. *American Psychologist, 32*, 513–531.

Bronfenbrenner, U. (1992). Ecological systems theory. In R. Vasta (Ed.), *Six theories of child development* (pp. 187–250). London: Jessica Kingsley Publishers Ltd.

Bryant, A., Jr., & LaFromboise, T. D. (2005). The racial identity and cultural orientation of Lumbee American Indian high school students. *Cultural Diversity and Ethnic Minority Psychology, 11*, 82–89.

Chang, I., Lapham, S. C., & Barton, K. J. (1996). Drinking environment and sociodemographic factors among DWI offenders. *Journal of Studies on Alcohol, 57*, 659–668.

Constantine, M., & Sue, D. W. (2006). Factors contributing to optimal human functioning of people of color in the United States. *The Counseling Psychologist, 34*, 228–244.

Delle Fave, A., & Bassi, M. (2009). Sharing optimal experiences and promoting good community life in a multicultural society. *The Journal of Positive Psychology, 4*, 280–289.

Edwards, L. A., & Pedrotti, J. T. (2008). A content and methodological review of articles concerning multiracial issues in six major counseling journals. *Journal of Counseling Psychology, 55*, 411–418.

Flannery, W. P., Reise, S. P., & Yu, J. (2001). An empirical comparison of acculturation models. *Personality and Social Psychology Bulletin, 27*, 1035–1045.

Gamst, G., Dana, R. H., Der-Karabetian, A., Aragon, M., Arellano, L. M., & Kramer, T. (2002). Effects of Latino acculturation and ethnic identity on mental health outcomes. *Hispanic Journal of Behavioral Sciences, 24*, 479–504.

Gerstein, L. H., Heppner, P. P., Egisdottir, S., Leung, S. M. A., & Norsworthy, K. L. (Eds.). (2009). *International handbook of cross-cultural counseling: Cultural assumptions and practices worldwide*. Thousand Oaks: Sage.

Harter, S. (1999). Symbolic interactionism revisited: Potential liabilities for the self-constructed in the crucible of interpersonal relationships. *Merrill-Palmer Quarterly, 45*, 677–703.

Hays, P. A. (2008). *Addressing cultural complexities in practice: Assessment, diagnosis, and therapy* (2nd ed.). Washington, DC: American Psychological Association.

Herring, R. D. (1994). The clown or contrary figure as a counseling intervention strategy with Native American Indian clients. *Journal of Multicultural Counseling and Development, 22*(3), 153–164.

Heywood, A. (2007). *Political ideologies* (4th ed.). Basingstoke: Palgrave Macmillan. 313.

Hill, N. (1991). A college intervention program that works. *Change, 23*, 24.

Huitt, W. (2004). Self-concept and self-esteem. *Educational Psychology Interactive*. Valdosta: Valdosta State University. Retrieved January 4, 2006, from http://chiron.valdosta.edu/whuitt/col/regsys/self.html

Judge, T. A., Locke, E. A., Durham, C. C., & Kluger, A. N. (1997). Dispositional effects on job and life satisfaction: The role of core evaluations. *Journal o f Applied Psychology, 83*, 17–34.

Kroeber, A. L., & Kluckhohn, C. (1952). Culture: A critical review of concepts and definitions. *Paper of the Peabody Museum of American Archaeology and Ethnology, 41*. Cambridge, MA: Harvard University.

Kunitz, S. J., & Levy, J. E. (1994). Drinking careers: A twenty-five year study of three Navajo populations. *American Indian Culture and Research Journal, 21*, 204–225.

Kvernmo, S., & Heyerdahl, S. (2003). Acculturation strategies and ethnic identity as predictors of behavior problems in Arctic minority adolescents. *Journal of the American Academy of Child and Adolescent Psychiatry, 42*, 57–65.

Lee, D. G. (2005). Calls for multiple indices incorporating multiculturalism in content analysis. *The Counseling Psychologist, 33*(3), 349–357.

Lopez, S. J., Prosser, E. C., Edwards, L. M., Magyar-Moe, J. L., Neufeld, J. E., & Rasmussen, H. N. (2002). Putting positive psychology in a multicultural context. In C. R. Snyder & S. J. Lopez (Eds.), *Handbook of positive psychology* (pp. 700–714). Washington, DC: American Psychological Association.

Lopez, S. J., Snyder, C. R., & Rasmussen, H. N. (2003). Striking a vital balance: Developing a complementary focus on human weakness and strength through positive psychological assessment. In S. J. Lopez & C. R. Snyder (Eds.), *Positive psychological assessment: A handbook of models and measures* (pp. 3–20). Washington, DC: American Psychological Association.

Lopez-Class, M., Felipe González, C., & Ramirez, A. G. (2011). Conceptions of acculturation: A review and statement of critical issues. *Social Science & Medicine, 72*, 1555–1562. doi:10.1016/j.socscimed.2011.03.011.

McIntosh, P. (1998). White privilege: Unpacking the invisible knapsack. In P. S. Rothenberg (Ed.), *Race, class, and gender in the United States: An integrated study* (pp. 188–191). New York: Worth Publishers.

Miranda, A. O., & Umhoefer, D. L. (1998). Acculturation, language use, and demographic variables as predictor of career self-efficacy of Latino career counseling clients. *Journal of Multicultural Counseling and Development, 26*, 39–51.

Moncher, M. S., Holden, G. W., & Trimble, J. E. (1990). Substance abuse among Native American youth. *Journal of Consulting and Clinical Psychology, 58*, 408–415.

Oetting, E. R., & Beauvis, F. (1991). Adolescent drug use: Findings of national and local surveys. *Journal of Consulting and Clinical Psychology, 58*, 385–394.

Pedrotti, J. T. (2013). Taking culture into account with positive psychological interventions. In A. C. Parks (Ed.), *The handbook of positive psychological interventions*. Hoboken: Wiley-Blackwell.

Pedrotti, J. T., & Edwards, L. M. (2009). The intersection of positive psychology and multiculturalism in counseling. In J. Ponterotto, M. Casas, L. Suzuki, & C. Alexander (Eds.), *Handbook of multicultural counseling* (3rd ed.). Thousand Oaks: Sage.

Pedrotti, J. T., Edwards, L. M., & Lopez, S. J. (2009). Putting positive psychology within a cultural context. In S. J. Lopez & C. R. Snyder (Eds.), *The Oxford handbook of positive psychology* (pp. 49–57). New York: Oxford.

Peterson, C., & Seligman, M. E. P. (2004). *Character strengths and virtues: A handbook and classification*. Washington, DC: American Psychological Association.

Phinney, J. S., & Chavira, V. (1992). Ethnic identity and self-esteem: An exploratory longitudinal study. *Journal of Adolescence, 18*, 271–281.

Phinney, J. S., Cantu, C. L., & Kurtz, D. A. (1997). Ethnic and American identity as predictors of self-esteem among African American, Latino, and White adolescents. *Journal of Youth and Adolescence, 26*, 165–185.

Pieterse, A. L., & Carter, R. T. (2010). The role of racial identity in perceived racism and psychological stress among Black American adults: Exploring traditional and alternative approaches. *Journal of Applied Social Psychology, 40*, 1028–1053.

Rasmussen, H. N., Nuefeld, J. E., Bouwkamp, J. C., Edwards, L. M., Ito, A., Magyar-Moe, J. L., Ryder, J. A., & Lopez, S. J. (2003). Environmental assessment: Examining influences on optimal human functioning. In S. J. Lopez & C. R. Snyder (Eds.), *Positive psychological assessment: A handbook of models and measures* (pp. 443–458). Washington, DC: American Psychological Association.

Sattler, J. M. (2001). Assessment of culturally and linguistically diverse children: Background considerations and dynamics. In J. M. Sattler (Ed.), *Assessment of children cognitive applications* (4th ed., pp. 635–656). San Diego: Jerome M. Sattler Inc.

Seligman, M. E. P., Steen, T. A., Park, N., & Peterson, C. (2005). Positive psychology progress: Empirical validation of interventions. *American Psychologist, 60*(5), 410–421.

Shweder, R., & LeVine, R. A. (1984). *Culture theory: Essays on mind, self, and emotion*. Cambridge, England: Cambridge University Press.

Simonton, D. K. (1997). Foreign influence and national achievement: The impact of open milieus on Japanese civilization. *Journal of Personality and Social Psychology, 72*, 86–94.

Simonton, D. K. (2000). Creativity: Cognitive, personal, developmental, and social aspects. *American Psychologist, 55*, 151–158.

Smith, T. B., & Silva, L. (2011). Ethnic identity and personal well-being of people of color: A meta-analysis. *Journal of Counseling Psychology, 58*, 42–60.

Snauwert, B., Soenens, B., Vanbeselaere, N., & Boen, F. (2003). When integration does not necessarily imply integration: Different conceptualizations of acculturation orientations lead to different classifications. *Journal of Cross-Cultural Psychology, 34*, 231–239.

Snyder, C. R., Lopez, S. J., & Pedrotti, J. T. (2011). *Positive psychology: The scientific and practical explorations of human strengths* (2nd ed.). Thousand Oaks: Sage.

Stewart, O. C. (1984). Taos factionalism. *American Indian Culture and Research, 18*, 37–57.

Triandis, H. C. (1996). The psychological measurement of cultural syndromes. *American Psychologist, 51*, 407–415.

Uchida, Y., Norasakkunkit, V., & Kitayama, S. (2004). Cultural constructions of happiness: Theory and empirical evidence. *Journal of Happiness Studies, 5*, 223–239.

Walters, K. L. (1999). Urban American Indian identity attitudes and acculturation styles. *Journal of Human Behavior in the Social Environment, 2*, 163–179.

Ward, C., & Kus, L. (2012). Back to and beyond Berry's basics: The conceptualization, operationalization and classification of acculturation. *International Journal of Intercultural Relations, 36*, 471–485.

Whitsell, N., Mitchell, C., Kaufman, C., & Spicer, P. (2006). Developmental trajectories of personal collective self-concept among American Indian adolescents. *Child Development, 77*, 1487–1503.

Wong, P. T. P., Wong, L. C. J., & Scott, C. (2006). The positive psychology of transformation: Beyond stress and coping. In P. T. P. Wong & L. C. J. Wong (Eds.), *Handbook of multicultural perspectives on stress and coping*. New York: Springer.

Wright, B. A. (1991). Labeling: The need for greater person-environment individuation. In C. R. Snyder & D. R. Forsyth (Eds.), *The handbook of social and clinical psychology* (pp. 469–487). New York: Pergamon.

Wright, B. A., & Lopez, S. J. (2009). Widening the diagnostic focus: A case for including human strengths and environmental resources. In S. J. Lopez & C. R. Snyder (Eds.), *Oxford handbook of positive psychology* (pp. 71–87). New York: Oxford University Press.

Yakushko, O., Davidson, M. M., & Williams, E. N. (2009). Clinical work with limited English proficiency clients: A phenomenological exploration. *Psychotherapy Theory, Research, Practice, Training, 46*, 180–192.

Chapter 3
Multicultural Considerations in Measurement and Classification of Positive Psychology

Cristalis Capielo, Lauren Mann, Bailey Nevels, and Edward Delgado-Romero

Ligaya is a 33 year-old Filipina attorney practicing in a large northeast metropolitan area. Despite Ligaya's professional successes, she often feels lonely and guilty. Ligaya immigrated to the U.S. in her mid-twenties to attend law school, but her immediate family is still in the Philippines. She is currently single and living with a female roommate who is her best friend from Law School. Ligaya has many friends and a good support network at her job. Her friends tell her she has bright future ahead of her and should enjoy being single. In contrast, whenever Ligaya calls home, her mother is critical that she is single and insists that she should meet a man and get married or return home to the Philippines. According to Ligaya's family, she should have married long ago, and the longer she waits, the harder it will be for Ligaya to find a husband. Ligaya has become increasingly frustrated and her roommate suggests that Ligaya should speak to a therapist.

As part of the intake assessment, Ligaya's counselor, a positive psychologist, gives Ligaya the Values In Action Inventory of Strengths (VIA-IS). She completes the measure and scores low in certain leadership and teamwork constructs, but high on constructs of gratitude and humor. When discussing the results of the assessment Ligaya tells her counselor that she feels that she is a great leader, as she is the first in her family to move away from the Philippines, and the first to obtain a graduate degree. In addition, she reports that collaboration is an important piece of her identity as she often takes into account the opinions and views of her family members when making decisions. Ligaya reports that she doesn't understand her test results and that maybe the test is wrong. The counselor struggles to understand Ligaya's difficulty with the assessment, as he has successfully used the assessment with culturally diverse clients previously.

C. Capielo, M.S. • L. Mann • B. Nevels • E. Delgado-Romero (✉)
Department of Counseling and Human Development Services, The University of Georgia, 402 Aderhold Hall, Athens, GA 30602, USA
e-mail: edelgado@uga.edu

J. Teramoto Pedrotti and L.M. Edwards (eds.), *Perspectives on the Intersection of Multiculturalism and Positive Psychology*, Cross-Cultural Advancements in Positive Psychology 7, DOI 10.1007/978-94-017-8654-6_3,

3.1 Introduction

Positive psychology encourages psychologists to focus research efforts on the prevention of disease, the development of strengths, and virtues that lead to optimal human functioning (Pedrotti and Edwards 2010; Sandage et al. 2003). The joining of strengths, virtues and multiculturalism "is both logical and necessary" (p. 166) as multiculturalism becomes a strength in and of itself (Pedrotti and Edwards 2010). Although the combination of strengths, virtues and multiculturalism is logical, it is also important to consider variance in cross-cultural applications and definitions of positive psychology constructs and subsequent measurements of these constructs. For example, in the case above, Ligaya's unique perspective and cross-cultural experiences may lead her to view strengths differently than someone from the dominant culture in the United States. Although successfully navigating the dominant culture, Ligaya is struggling to integrate the strengths and virtues of her culture of origin with those of the mainstream. Her ability to mediate these often competing values, although frustrating, can be viewed as a strength in and of itself. Ligaya's case will be revisited at the end chapter to illustrate how to incorporate multicultural considerations in measurement of positive psychology into the therapeutic process.

Carter (1991) stated, "mismatches in cultural values may affect the delivery of mental health and educational services, the communication process, and interactional dynamics" (p. 165). Carter's point is also applicable to the way that positive psychological constructs are operationalized across diverse groups. That is, strengths and virtues derived from the experiences of a subset of the U.S. population (e.g., Euro-Americans) are not necessarily generalizable to either U.S. minority populations or the 95 % of human beings who live outside the U.S. Additionally, given Carter's (1991) statement that differing cultural values impact mental healthcare services, and given that assessment and measurement are important aspects of mental healthcare service, it is important to consider how differing cultural values may affect the assessment and measurement of positive psychological constructs.

This chapter will give a broad overview of measurement in positive psychology and multicultural applications of these measurements. In addition, we will discuss strengths and limitations of assessment in positive psychology especially in terms of how they address equivalence of measures including linguistic and construct equivalence. Examples of specific measures will be given to illustrate applicability to cross-cultural populations. Finally, we will suggest future research areas for these measures including creating cultures-specific measures and utilizing qualitative and innovative research methods.

3.2 Critical Issues with Multicultural Populations in Research and Practice

Multicultural perspectives raise important concerns about the connection between cultural specificity, definitions and expressions of strengths and virtues (Sandage et al. 2003). Before discussing the cultural implications of positive psychology, it is critical to first consider the issues that continue to permeate multicultural research: conceptualization of race and ethnicity; within-groups differences; exclusion of diverse population from research and exclusion of data related to race and ethnicity of samples; and the use of White control groups.

Understanding the relationship between race, ethnicity, and culture to human functioning can positively impact interventions that promote growth and change (Delgado-Romero et al. 2005). However, defining race and ethnicity when examining psychological phenomena, has also been problematic. Race is a widely used social identity construct use to assign people to distinct groups based on phenomenological resulting in "caste-like" (Robinson, p. 128) categories (Helms and Talleyrand 1997; Robinson 2005). In the United States, Whites have often benefited from this style of categorization; as the dominant group, Whites enjoy numerical, political, economic, and social power (Delgado-Romero et al. 2005). Although Phinney (1996) argued that race and ethnicity be used interchangeably, Helms and Talleyrand (1997) contended that although "crudely assessed" (p. 1246) race has a clear meaning. Though ethnicity has been conceptualized as shared culture, traditions and values (Phinney 1996), it is an imposed construct that continues to perpetuate minority status and inferiority (Trimble et al. 2002). Given that race and ethnicity are concepts that are grounded in political and not scientific rationales, social scientists that blindly use these categorical variables as constructs often produce research that is of questionable scientific merit and in fact may cause harm by reinforcing political or social prejudice. Thus, it is no surprise that many researchers often avoid the issue of race and ethnicity altogether, and this avoidance is problematic in and of itself (see Delgado-Romero et al. 2005).

A common practice by researchers is to use broad and generic labels ignoring important within-group differences. An example of this questionable action is the usage of the term Latino. Latino subgroups in the United States share commonalities such as the use of the Spanish language, Catholic religious roots, and a history of Spanish colonialism (Baker 2002). Despite similarities, important economical and sociopolitical distinctions exist among Latinos. For example, in the U.S. the three largest Latino subgroups, Mexicans, Puerto Ricans, and Cubans, represent a broad range of diversity both across and within these subcategories. These differences are often blurred when the Latino or Hispanic label is used. Portés and Truelove (1987) called this label "a term of convenience for administrative agencies and scholarly researchers" (p. 359). This continued practice further perpetuates the myth of homogeneity (Rinderle and Montoya 2008) among Latinos/as in the United States. Trimble and Dickson (2001) called this practice ethnic gloss and posited that the "use of an ethnic glosses provides little or no information on the richness and cultural variation within ethnocultural groups" (Trimble and Dickson 2001). Data disaggregation by relevant contextual factors (e.g., time in the U.S., historical factors, circumstances of immigration) will help explain examine within group differences (Delgado-Romero et al. 2005).

In social science research, the burden to obtain high internal validity regularly supplants the also important need for external validity (Sue 1999). Recruitment difficulties and funding constraints are often cited as reasons to exclude diverse groups from experimental and non-experimental designs (Delgado-Romero et al. 2005;

Sue 1999). In addition, the omission of the racial and ethnic characteristics of the sample investigated is another frequent solution. This failure was highlighted by Delgado-Romero and colleagues (2005), which found that 43 % (N=796) of the studies published in three main counseling journals did not provide racial or ethnic information on their participants at all. These methodologies result in the inadequate generalization of psychological findings across different racial, ethnic and cultural groups and fail to understand the role of culture on psychological functioning (Delgado-Romero et al. 2005; Sue 1999).

Racial and ethnic diverse groups continue to be compared to the White standard or White sample groups without consideration of equivalence before comparisons are made (more on this in a later section). Studies interested in racial and ethnic minority groups are often rejected for publication if a White control group is not included in the sample (Sue 1999). This idea continues to portray individuals of non-majority backgrounds in a model of deficiency (Sue and Sue 2008) and they continued to be discussed "in relation to their weaknesses much more often than their strengths and branded as pathological in comparison to the majority group" (Pedrotti and Edwards 2010, p. 166).

3.3 Defining Strengths and Virtues: Value Orientation Differences

Constructs associated with optimal human functioning like self-efficacy, individuality, optimisms, hope and happiness are highly valued by Euro-American individuals including researchers and clinicians (Wong et al. 2006). However, these definitions might not tap into how other cultures define or express optimal functioning (Constantine and Sue 2006). For positive psychology to be relevant to racial and ethnic minority groups, it is pivotal that researchers and clinicians examine the role of culture in the diverse expression of strengths and virtues (Sandage et al. 2003). To understand definitions of strengths and virtues we must attend to the value orientations of different cultures, including relational, time, spirituality, and activity orientations.

Relational orientation concerns how we relate to others (Wong et al. 2006). Individuals with an individualistic relational orientation may value self-efficacy, autonomy, and personal achievement over group goals (Wong et al. 2006; Sandage et al. 2003; Constantine and Sue 2006). Those with a collectivistic relational orientation on the other hand, are more likely to give priority to family and group goals over individual goals (Sandage et al. 2003). For example, among Latinos/as, relational orientation may be expressed through *personalismo* (a preference for close personal relationships), *respeto* (respect for elders and authority), *familismo* (an emphasis on the family, including the extended family and friends), *simpatia* (need for behaviors that promote pleasant and non-conflicting social relationships), and *allocentrism* (high levels of conformity, mutual empathy, willingness to sacrifice for the welfare of the group, and high levels of personal interdependence;

Delgado-Romero et al. 2013; Marín and Marín 1991). In the case of Latinas specifically, self-sacrificing and submissiveness may be expected (Arredondo 2002). These attitudes should not be dismissed as weaknesses, however, as there are also strengths inherent in female gender roles, such as having a family orientation and being a keeper of tradition (Delgado-Romero et al. 2013). Dismissing these cultural values as weaknesses because they do not match Euro-American individualistic traits is clearly problematic.

A second value orientation is termed by Wong et al. (2006) as *time orientation,* and is described as the transient focus of human life; it can be divided into past, present, and future. American Indians and African Americans tend to view time in a present orientation. For instance, present orientation among some American Indian cultures is evinced by the absence of future tense in some American Indian languages (Hamme 1995) On the other hand, Asian Americans and Latinas/os have a present-past focus (Sue and Sue 2008). Individuals with a traditional Chinese background, for example, might hold a past orientation, valuing traditions, the role of ancestors and elders (Sue and Sue 2008; Wong et al. 2006). White Americans, in contrast, might relate better to future orientation thus emphasizing the importance of present sacrifices and hard work to achieve happiness in the future (Wong et al. 2006).

Spirituality orientation is concerned with the existence of a supreme being. Spirituality and religion are salient factors across different cultures but groups and individuals may differ in the way they define and express their spiritual beliefs (Schlosser et al. 2010; Sue and Sue 2008; Wong et al. 2006). For example, spirituality is central to the Hmong culture and values ancestral worship (Sandage et al. 2003). Sandage and colleagues state that in this culture ailments and suffering can result from offending ancestors or the deceased for whom they must seek forgiveness. Thus, as part of their healing process and forgiveness, Hmong individuals resort to spiritual healers who assert that suffering signifies the beginning of healing and forgiveness (Sandage et al. 2003). However, because the construct of forgiveness defined by clinicians and researchers is rooted in the Euro-American idea of forgiving others as a way to ameliorate suffering (e.g., VIA-IS measures whether or not a person can forgive other who have done wrong; Sandage et al. 2003) an individual from the Hmong culture who is asked to complete the VIA-IS might find this forgiveness item very confusing.

Finally, *activity orientation* focuses on the activities or experiences people value and thus practice in order to achieve optimal functioning (Delle Fave and Bassi 2009; Wong et al. 2006). Delle Fave and Bassi examined which activities 159 first-generation African, Indian, South American, and Eastern Europe immigrants in Italy chose as activities that symbolized optimal living. Participants could select from four activities: productivity (work, study, volunteer work), social relations (family, relating with friends), leisure (hobbies, use of media), and personal care (resting, body care, and self-care). Results showed that Indians and Africans highly endorsed productivity and leisure activities while South Americans and East Europeans preferred productivity and social activities (Delle Fave and Bassi 2009). U.S. clinicians and researchers must also be aware of potential multicultural implications of activity orientation that can be derived from such cross-cultural studies. Activities that are compatible with the person's activity orientation are salient and important. Ignoring these differences might lead a clinician from a productivity activity orientation judge a client from a personal care activity orientation as apathetic and unambitious. We present these value orientations as important considerations to address when attempting to measure positive psychological constructs in diverse populations. It is within the context of these differing value orientations that we will provide an overview of existing measures of positive psychological constructs and their strengths and weaknesses.

3.4 Overview of Assessments in Positive Psychology

Duckworth et al. (2005) noted that the assumptions of positive psychology are only as valid as their measures. Therefore, developing assessments that measure human strengths has been an important step in the positive psychology movement. Historically, negative symptoms of psychological disorders have been perceived as clinically informative, whereas a person's strengths are considered to be the "by-products of symptom relief or clinical peripheries that do not need assessment" (Rashid and Ostermann 2009, p. 489). However, in the past three decades we have seen an increase in the development and use of assessments related to human strengths. In fact, as a result of an increased focus on positive qualities, an Axis VI for the DSM has been proposed to evaluate human strengths to gain a more comprehensive picture of a client's life in the diagnostic phase of treatment (Lopez et al. 2006).

There are clear benefits to assessing human strengths. Within the clinical realm, for example, researchers have suggested that assessing strengths provides psychologists with a holistic picture of the client and decreases negative bias in treatment. These benefits, in turn, enable psychologists and clients to enhance client strengths to increase well-being (Rashid and Ostermann 2009). The idea is to build upon the client's established strengths in order to combat psychopathology. Furthermore, assessing a client's strengths enables alternate conceptualizations to drive psychological treatment. For example, diagnoses such as anxiety or depression may not exclusively represent a presence of symptoms but a deficit in strengths and coping strategies (Rashid and Ostermann 2009). There exists great potential for positive psychological assessments to enhance psychological treatment.

Positive psychological constructs were originally conceptualized to fall into the three overarching domains: (a) subjective, (b) individual, and (c) social context (Seligman and Csikszentmihalyi 2000). As research, practice, and assessment related to positive psychology have evolved, these overarching domains have been reconceptualized into categories of positive psychological assessments. Specifically, Duckworth et al. (2005) divided strengths-based assessments into those whose purposes are measuring subjective well-being, measurement of character strengths, measurement of engagement and flow, and measurement of meaning. In addition to these broad categories, multiculturally diverse groups can also benefit from research activities investigating how specific psychological factors, such as resilience, growth and ethnic identity, relate to optimal living. Given this great potential, it is imperative that positive psychological assessments adequately assess the strengths of multicultural populations.

Psychologists can utilize both formal and informal strengths-based assessments. At present there are a variety of formal measurements that have been created to assess human strengths and subjective well-being. For example, the most popular and most researched measure of human strength assessment is the Values in Action-Inventory of Strengths (VIA-IS; Peterson and Seligman 2004). The VIA-IS is a self-report measure based on a 5-point Likert scale measuring the degree to which test-takers agree with strength based statements (ranging from 1 = very much unlike me, 5 = very much like me). Likewise, there exist other formal measurements such as the Curiosity and Exploration Inventory (CEI; Kashdan et al. 2004) which measures openness and engagement with novel experiences. However, it is important for assessors to know the psychometric properties of these instruments with multicultural populations, keeping in mind that most of these assessing tools have not had representative norming samples. For instance, many of these measures are normed on a convenience sample comprised of primarily White, undergraduate psychology majors. Some of the measures do not even report demographic characteristics of the sample; therefore, it is unclear as to the norming practices of that measure.

Multiple questionnaires developed by researchers at the University of Pennsylvania (e.g., VIA-S) are available to consumers and clients online. The consumer must have access to a computer and email address to complete some of them. Furthermore, full reports for each measure can cost up to $50 each, a price that may likely serve to exclude lower SES groups, which may have higher percentages of non-White individuals or individuals from rural communities in the U.S. This financial situation demonstrates that even if a measure can be normed for specific cultural groups the access to the measures following stringent testing may still be limited.

3.5 Cultural Equivalence of Measurement

With respect to measurement in positive psychology, scholars often have dichotomous viewpoints. Some argue that the empirical investigation of strengths can transcend cultures and approach universality (e.g., Seligman and Csikszentmihalyi 2000) while others argue that strengths, similar to other psychological constructs, must be examined within a cultural context and framework (e.g., Sue and Constantine 2006). Although the universality hypothesis and the specificity hypothesis may have relevance with regard to specific constructs, there is little current research or data to fully support either of these viewpoints. Current measurements of strengths and positive psychological constructs tend to include U.S. population normative data, that are primarily centered on White Americans, and therefore do not provide concrete evidence to bolster either viewpoint exclusively.

Historically, group differences of psychological constructs are measured using mean scores, assuming measurement equivalence across groups (Miller and Sheu 2008). This assumption is often predicated on psychometric properties such as reliability (Miller and Sheu 2008); whereas invariance is frequently overlooked (Miller and Sheu 2008). Although reliability provides information about a test's consistency across items, times and/or examiners, it does not offer evidence about the consistency of the construct (e.g. happiness, satisfaction) the test purposes to measure. In other words, if a test is found to lack invariance, the meaning of the construct will vary across groups thus confounding the interpretation of results (Cheung and Rensvold 2002). Thus ensuring that measurements operate equally across groups is imperative. Measurement invariance (also known as measurement equivalence or factorial invariance) can be defined as the equality of measurement or assessment of a construct across two or more cultural groups thus ensuring the same constructs are being assessed across groups (Chen 2008). Measurement equivalence includes construct equivalence, scalar equivalence, and linguistic equivalence. It is important to note that different facets of equivalence are discussed by different researchers in the field, and different terminology is sometimes used by different authors (please see Chap. 4, this volume, for additional discussion of equivalence issues). Miller and Sheu (2008) report that measurement invariance analyses (e.g. exploratory and confirmatory factor analyses) are powerful ways to enhance understanding of diverse cultural groups and specific multicultural constructs above and beyond the use of mean scores.

The most often cited type of measurement equivalence is construct equivalence (in scale construction this is known as factor-form equivalence), which tests the ability of similar, but not equivalent measures, to assess similar constructs. More specifically, construct equivalence is transition from theory to measurement (Hui and Triandis 1985) or the operationalization of an identified strength (e.g., self-esteem). Following the example of self-esteem, we found that much of the current research related to self-esteem measurement focuses on inner aspects of self-esteem (e.g., "I am a good person"). However, the social aspect of self-esteem (i.e. feeling accepted and valued by others) might be more important given the collectivistic orientation of certain cultural groups (e.g., "I am a good neighbor"). Chen (2008) has suggested that future research with self-esteem should address the construct in a culturally appropriate manner by including both inner- and social aspects of self-esteem.

If researchers are able to construct a scale that has similar, but equal constructs, a next step for comparisons across groups would be to establish scalar equivalence. Scalar equivalence refers to numerical equivalence from one scale to another such that the ratio scale is the same in each cultural group (Caprara et al. 2000). Specifically, a numerical value on one scale refers to the same degree, intensity, or magnitude regardless of the population to which the respondent belongs (Hui and Triandis 1985). Scalar equivalence is the most difficult to achieve as this type of equivalence requires hierarchical analyses and large sample sizes for testing, although it is ideal for cross-cultural comparisons among populations.

Another important aspect in measurement equivalence is linguistic equivalence, which refers to the process by which a scale or measure is translated to a language

Table 3.1 Sample characteristics of commonly used positive psychology measures

Measurement name	Constructs	Sample characteristics
Attributional Style Questionnaires (ASQ) (Hjelle et al. 1996)	Explanatory style for good and bad events	N=436 (ages 17–35) U.S. only 22 % male, 78 % female Race/ethnicity not reported
Meaning in Life Questionnaire (MLQ) (Steger et al. 2007)	Presence of meaning & search for meaning	N=154 (μ=21.8, s.d.=3.9) 30 % male, 70 % female 79 % White, 9 % Asian, 4 % Native American, 3 % African American, 2 % Asian American, 1 % Hispanic
Quality of Life Inventory (QOLI) (Frisch et al. 2005)	Life satisfaction and well-being	N=3,638 (μ=23, s.d.=5.42) U.S. only 43 % male, 57 % female 86 % white, 5.5 % International students, 4.7 % African American, 2.2 % Hispanic, 1.3 % Asian American, .3 % Native American
Subjective Happiness Scale (SHS) (Lyubomirsky and Lepper 1999)	Global characterization of subjective happiness	N=2,732 (ages 14–94) U.S. and Russia sample 36 % male, 64 % female, >1 % unknown Race/ethnicity not reported
Values in Action Inventory of Strengths (VIA-IS) (Park et al. 2006)	Character strengths and core virtues	N=117,676 (ages 18–65+) U.S. and 54 Countries (English speakers only) 28 % male, 72 % female (U.S.) 38 % male, 62 % female (non-U.S.) Race/ethnicity not reported

other than the language to which a measure was originally normed and tested (for example translating from English to Spanish). Language affects the meaning of scales, thus possibly preventing comparisons between linguistically diverse groups (Sanchez et al. 2006). When using self-report measures is it crucial for psychologists to determine whether the endorsement of different values and or virtues (e.g. happiness, forgiveness) are equivalent, meaning that psychologists need to question whether these claims convey the same meaning across languages and cultures different from the ones from which they were originally conceptualized (Caprara et al. 2000). For instance, when translating an English Likert-scale response with the word 'slightly' to Spanish, might be a difficult task, as there is not direct translation for this word. Hui and Triandis (1985) were among the first to examine cross-cultural differences in measurement and to propose future directions for assessment and research to better facilitate development of measurement equivalence. Given that most of the scales related to positive psychological constructs (e.g. VIA-IS; Peterson and Seligman 2004) were created in the U.S. and normed with U.S. samples, basic English language skills are required to complete the assessments (see Table 3.1).

3.6 Future Directions and Conclusions

Returning to our original example of Ligaya, there are many potential implications of this case with respect to understanding and interpreting strengths within a cultural context. For the clinician working with Ligaya it is important to allow Ligaya to subjectively define her perception of strengths by asking open-ended questions during an intake or assessment phases in addition to the use of the VIA-IS. Doing so provides additional, more in-depth, measurement of Ligaya's strengths that will prove helpful in conceptualizing her concerns. Questions might include, "*What qualities do you see as strengths in yourself*?, *What would your friends and family members consider to be your strengths*?, and *Who or what can support you throughout the process of therapy*?" The clinician should consider addressing how his/her cultural values differ from Ligaya's, and what impact those differences may have on the therapeutic process.

When interpreting the VIA-IS the therapist should consider inviting Ligaya to be a collaborator in discussing the results so that she can report which results she considers to be relevant and useful. Psycho-education about what the results mean, strengths and weaknesses of the assessment, and how Ligaya's values may manifest themselves in the results may also be important to address. The counselor should also ask Ligaya if including friends or family members in the assessment or treatment process would be helpful. Finally, it is imperative that the counselor continuously conducts self-assessments of his/her own potential biases. While the notion of error in psychological testing is often related to instrumentation, accurate assessment interpretation is also predicated upon clinical errors, including bias and ethnocentricity (Suzuki et al. 2005). For example, if the counselor working with Ligaya comes from a European-American background, his or her interpretation of Ligaya's assessment results will likely reflect this background. Therefore to minimize these clinician errors in interpretation of results, it is imperative that the clinician include self-evaluation of biases when interpreting measures (Pieterse and Miller 2010).

Our understanding of diverse definitions and manifestations of optimal functioning can further be strengthened by focusing on how untoward circumstances can lead to growth. Constantine and Sue (2006) postulate that these unique stressors have led to a unique strength-based resilience, which they have termed "strengths gained through adversity" (p. 231). Diverse cultural groups within the United States (e.g., African Americans during the Civil Rights Movement) have been faced with unique challenges that have resulted in distinct strengths and virtues not currently recognized by positive psychology assessment. For example, an area of research that has received little attention is the history of immigration in the United States and its effects on mental health and wellness (Weiss and Berger 2006). Immigration has been associated with acculturative stress and negative mental health outcomes (Henkin et al. 2011). However, challenging situations associated with immigration can also create opportunities for development of strengths and resiliency (Weiss and Berger 2006). For instance, the Latino health paradox states that Latino/as with stronger Latino/a cultural orientation experience better mental and physical health outcomes compared to those who have a more American orientation (Torres 2010).

This example illustrates how ethnic and cultural pride may facilitate a sense of belonging and community within those groups (Constantine and Sue 2006).

Research and measurement development with positive psychological instruments and constructs can be divided into three important areas of future study: adaptation of measurements, creation of culturally specific instruments, and use of qualitative and innovate methods. Specifically, research in positive psychological assessment should involve testing existing measures on diverse populations in order to demonstrate external validity of these assessments. Sue (1999) noted that the United States produces the majority of research and represents the majority of participants in that research. This trend is problematic in that we cannot assume data from United States samples generalize to the population at large. If external validity of positive psychological measures cannot be established, then adapting measures to incorporate differing cultural values would be the next step for research. For example, if a study were to reveal that different results emerge when strengths-based instruments such as the Satisfaction with Life Scale (Diener et al. 1985) are administered to people from differing cultures, economic levels, and educational levels, then scale construction research could be conducted to adapt the measure so that it could be generalized to different cultures. Given the impact that cultural differences may have on assessment performance, it could be beneficial for future research to address the benefit of adapting existing instruments so that one's cultural identity does not negatively impact assessment results.

Additionally, as we have demonstrated, culture informs our definition and expressions of strengths and virtues. Thus, positive psychology researchers and clinicians must avoid imposing their own culture's values and theoretical constructs as the standard to study in other cultural groups (Wong et al. 2006) and instead they should identify and understand unique factors that contribute to optimal living in people of color (Constantine and Sue 2006; Sandage et al. 2003). To meet this goal, Constantine and Sue posited that positive psychology conceptualizations should include: collectivism; racial and ethnic pride; spirituality and religion; interconnectedness of mind, body, and spirit, and; family and community. The addition of these constructs is not meant to supplant already established constructs. Instead, researchers and clinicians can help by making these constructs more reflective of the life experiences of individuals belonging to different groups (Pedrotti and Edwards 2010).

In addition to cultural adaptation and creation of culture specific measurement, Sue (1999) suggested that ethnic minority research should include a variety of research methodologies such as qualitative and ethnographic studies. Over time, there has been a shift away from logical positivism and blind acceptance of the objectivity of quantitative assessment (Duran et al. 2008). The movement toward applied research and more socially and culturally derived research has led to an increase in qualitative and mixed-methods research promoting a more culture sensitive, subjective, and emancipatory approach to studying strength-based behaviors and social relationships (Tashakkori and Teddlie 2003). In relation to measurement with positive psychology and culturally diverse groups, exploratory qualitative research could offer scholars and clinicians a better understanding of culturally defined strengths.

Overall, there will likely be continued discrepancy between the cultural specificity and cultural universality hypotheses related to assessment of positive psychological constructs, as the constructs are generally broad, continuous variables. In essence, most strength-based constructs can have individual, subjective meanings, and can be treated as such using innovative or qualitative measurement methods. However, this is not to say that specific constructs cannot be measured or evaluated for specific populations or universally. We merely attempt to show the scope of the task at hand for researchers and clinicians within the positive psychology movement.

References

Arredondo, P. (2002). Mujeres Latinas-santas y marquesas. *Cultural Diversity and Ethnic Minority Psychology, 8*(4), 308–319. doi:10.1037/1099-9809.8.4.308.

Baker, S. S. (2002). *Understanding mainland Puerto Rican Poverty*. Philadelphia: Temple University Press.

Caprara, G. V., Barbaranelli, C. B., Bermudez, J., Maslach, C., & Ruch, W. (2000). Multivariate methods for the comparison of factor structures in cross cultural research: An illustration with the big five questionnaire. *Journal of Cross-Cultural Research, 31*(4), 437–464.

Carter, R. T. (1991). Cultural values: A review of the empirical research and implications for counseling. *Journal of Counseling and Development, 69*(1), 46–50.

Chen, F. F. (2008). What happens if we compare chopsticks with forks? The impact of making inappropriate comparisons in cross-cultural research. *Journal of Personality and Social Psychology, 95*(5), 1005–1018. doi:10.1037/a0013193.

Cheung, G. W., & Rensvold, R. B. (2002). Evaluating goodness of fit indexes for testing measurement invariance. *Structural Equation Modeling, 9*(2), 233–255.

Constantine, M. G., & Sue, D. W. (2006). Factors contributing to optimal human functioning in people of color in the United States. *The Counseling Psychologist, 34*(2), 228–244. doi:10.1177/0011000005281318.

Delgado-Romero, E. A., Galván, N., Maschino, P., & Rowland, M. (2005). Race and ethnicity in empirical counseling and counseling psychology research: A 10-year review. *The Counseling Psychologist, 33*(4), 419–448. doi:10.1177/0011000004268637.

Delgado-Romero, E. A., Nevels, B. N., Capielo, C., Galván, N., Hunter, M. R., & Torres, V. (2013). Latino/a Americans. In G. McAuliffe (Ed.), *Culturally alert counseling: A comprehensive introduction*. Thousand Oaks: Sage.

Delle Fave, A., & Bassi, M. (2009). Sharing optimal experiences and promoting good community life in a multicultural society. *The Journal of Positive Psychology, 4*(4), 280–289. doi:10.1080/17439760902933716.

Diener, E., Emmons, R. A., Larson, R. J., & Griffin, S. (1985). The satisfaction with life scale. *Journal of Personality Assessment, 49*, 71–75.

Duckworth, A. L., Steen, T. A., & Seligman, M. E. P. (2005). Positive psychology in clinical practice. *Annual Review of Clinical Psychology, 1*, 629–651. doi:10.1146/annurev.clinpsy.1.102803.144154.

Duran, E., Firehammer, J., & Gonzalez, J. (2008). Liberation psychology as the path toward healing cultural soul wounds. *Journal of Counseling & Development, 86*, 288–295.

Frisch, M. B., Clark, M. P., Rouse, S. V., Rudd, M. D., Paweleck, J., & Greenstone, A. (2005). Predictive and treatment validity of life satisfaction and the Quality of Life Inventory. *Assessment, 12*(1), 66–78. doi:10.1177/1073191104268006.

Hamme, L. V. (1995). American Indian culture and the classroom. *Journal of American Indian Education, 35*(2), 21–36.

Helms, J. E., & Talleyrand, R. M. (1997). Race is not ethnicity. *American Psychologist, 52*(11), 1246–1247. doi:10.1037/0003-066X.52.11.1246.

Henkin, S., Tucker, K. L., Gao, X., Falcon, L. M., Qawi, I., & Brugge, D. (2011). Association of depression, psycho-social stress and acculturation with respiratory disease among Puerto Rican adults in Massachusetts. *Journal of Immigrant and Minority Health, 13*(2), 214–223. doi:10.1007/s10903-009-9307-y.

Hjelle, L., Belongia, C., & Nesser, J. (1996). Psychometric properties of the life orientation test and attributional style questionnaire. *Psychological Reports, 78*, 507–515. doi:10.2466/pr0.1996.78.2.507.

Hui, C. H., & Triandis, H. C. (1985). Measurement in cross-cultural psychology. *Journal of Cross-Cultural Psychology, 16*(1), 131–152. doi:10.1177/0022002185016002001.

Kashdan, T. B., Rose, P., & Fincham, F. D. (2004). Curiosity and exploration: Facilitating positive subjective experiences and personal growth opportunities. *Journal of Personality Assessment, 82*(3), 291–305. doi:10.1207/s15327752jpa8203_05.

Lopez, S. J., Magyar-Moe, J. L., Petersen, S. E., Ryder, J. A., Krieshok, T. S., O'Byrne, K. K., Lichtenberg, J. W., & Fry, N. A. (2006). Counseling psychology's focus on positive aspects of human functioning. *The Counseling Psychologist, 34*(2), 205–227. doi:10.1177/0011000005283393.

Lyubomirsky, S., & Lepper, H. S. (1999). A measure of subjective happiness: Preliminary reliability and construct validation. *Social Indicators Research, 46*, 137–155. doi:10.1023/A:1006824100041.

Marín, G., & Marín, B. V. (1991). *Research with Hispanic populations*. Newbury Park: Sage.

Miller, M. J., & Sheu, H. (2008). Conceptual and measurement issues in multicultural psychology research. In S. D. Brown & R. W. Lent (Eds.), *Handbook of counseling psychology*. Hoboken: Wiley.

Park, N., Peterson, C., & Seligman, M. E. P. (2006). Character strengths in fifty-four nations and the fifty US states. *The Journal of Positive Psychology, 1*(3), 118–129. doi:10.1080/17439760600619567.

Pedrotti, J. T., & Edwards, L. M. (2010). The intersection of positive psychology and multiculturalism in counseling. In J. G. Ponterotto, J. M. Casas, L. A. Suzuki, & C. M. Alexander (Eds.), *The handbook of multicultural counseling* (3rd ed.). Thousand Oaks: Sage.

Peterson, C., & Seligman, M. E. P. (2004). *Character strengths and virtues: A handbook and classification*. New York: Oxford University Press.

Phinney, J. S. (1996). When we talk about American ethnic groups, what do we mean? *American Psychologist, 51*, 918–927. doi:10.1037/0003-066X.51.9.918.

Pieterse, A. L., & Miller, M. J. (2010). Current considerations in the assessment of adults: A review and extension of culturally inclusive models. In J. G. Ponterotto, J. M. Casas, L. A. Suzuki, & C. M. Alexander (Eds.), *The handbook of multicultural counseling* (3rd ed.). Thousand Oaks: Sage.

Portes, A., & Truelove, C. (1987). Making sense of diversity: Recent research on Hispanic minorities in the United States. *Annual Review of Sociology, 13*, 359–385. doi:10.0360-0572/87/0815-0359.

Rashid, T., & Ostermann, R. F. (2009). Strengths-based assessment in clinical practice. *Journal of Clinical Psychology, 65*(5), 488–498. doi:10.1002/jclp.20595.

Rinderle, A. D., & Montoya, S. R. (2008). Hispanic/Latino identity labels: An examination of cultural values and personal experiences. *The Howard Journal of Communications, 19*, 145–164. doi:10.1080/10646170801990953.

Robinson, T. L. (2005). *The convergence of race, ethnicity, and gender: Multiple identities in counseling* (2nd ed.). Upper Saddle River: Pearson.

Sanchez, J. I., Spector, P. E., & Cooper, C. L. (2006). Frequently ignored methodological issues in cross-cultural stress research. In P. T. P. Wong & L. C. J. Wong (Eds.), *Handbook of multicultural perspectives on stress and coping*. New York: Springer.

Sandage, S. J., Hill, P. C., & Vang, H. C. (2003). Toward a multicultural positive psychology: Indigenous forgiveness and Hmong culture. *The Counseling Psychologist, 31*(5), 564–591. doi:10.1177/0011000003256350.

Schlosser, L. Z., Foley, P. F., Stein, E. P., & Holmwood, J. R. (2010). Why does counseling psychology exclude religion?: A content analysis and methodological critique. In J. G. Ponterotto,

J. M. Casas, L. A. Suzuki, & C. M. Alexander (Eds.), *The handbook of multicultural counseling* (3rd ed.). Thousand Oaks: Sage.

Seligman, M. E. P., & Csikszentmihalyi, M. (2000). Positive psychology: An introduction. *American Psychologist, 55*(1), 410–421. doi:10.1037/0003-066X.60.5.410.

Steger, M. F., Kawabata, Y., Shimai, S., & Otake, K. (2007). The meaningful life in Japan and the United States: Levels and correlates of meaning in life. *Journal of Research in Personality, 42*(1), 660–678. doi:10.1016/j.jrp.2007.09.003.

Sue, S. (1999). Science, ethnicity, and bias. *American Psychologist, 54*(12), 1070–1077. doi:10.1037//0003-066X.54.12.1070.

Sue, D. W., & Sue, D. (2008). *Counseling the culturally diverse: Theory and practice* (5th ed.). Hoboken: Wiley.

Suzuki, L. A., Kugler, J. F., & Aguiar, L. J. (2005). Assessment practices in racial-cultural psychology. In R. T. Carter (Ed.), *Handbook of racial-cultural psychology and counseling* (Vol. 2). Thousand Oaks: Sage.

Tashakkori, A., & Teddlie, C. (2003). *Handbook of mixed methods in social and behavioral research*. Thousand Oaks: Sage.

Torres, L. (2010). Predicting levels of Latino depression: Acculturation, acculturative stress, and coping. *Cultural Diversity and Ethnic Minority Psychology, 16*(2), 256–263. doi:10.1037/a0017357.

Trimble, J., & Dickson, R. (2001). *Ethnic gloss*. Retrieved from http://pandora.cii.wwu.edu/trimble/research_themes/ethnic_gloss.htm

Trimble, J., Helms, J., & Root, M. (2002). Social and psychological perspectives on ethnic and racial identity. In G. Bernal, J. Trimble, K. Burlew, & F. Leong (Eds.), *Handbook of racial and ethnic minority psychology*. Thousand Oaks: Sage.

Weiss, T., & Berger, R. (2006). Reliability and validity of a Spanish version of the posttraumatic growth disorder. *Research and Social Work Practice, 16*(2), 191–199. doi:10.1177/1049731505281374.

Wong, P. T. P., Wong, L. C. J., & Scott, C. (2006). Stress and coping: The positive psychology of transformation. In P. T. P. Wong & L. C. J. Wong (Eds.), *Handbook of multicultural perspective in stress*. New York: Springer.

Chapter 4
Methodological Issues in Positive Psychology Research with Diverse Populations: Exploring Strengths Among Chinese Adults

Samuel M.Y. Ho, Tina L. Rochelle, Lawrence S.C. Law, Wenjie Duan, Yu Bai, and Shih-Ming Shih

4.1 Introduction

Positive psychology is the study of the conditions and processes that contribute to the optimal functioning of people, groups, and institutions (Gable and Haidt 2005). Positive psychology is a relatively new area in psychology, with its roots in the West. As positive psychology gains momentum, both within the greater field of psychology and in the broader context of society and culture, one major challenge in non-Western cultures is how to measure positive psychological constructs properly, in ways that are culturally-relevant. Of the numerous and varied problems with cross-cultural and multicultural research, one fundamental, recurring problem concerns the measurement of equality in measures (Berry 1980; Leong et al. 2010). The most straightforward and possibly easiest method is to simply translate instruments designed to be used on Western populations and use them directly on non-Western

S.M.Y. Ho, Ph.D. (✉) • T.L. Rochelle
Department of Applied Social Studies, City University of Hong Kong,
Office: Y7315, Tat Chee Avenue, Kowloon Tong, Hong Kong
e-mail: munyinho@cityu.edu.hk

L.S.C. Law
Centre for Quantitative Medicine, Duke-NUS Graduate Medical School,
Singapore, Singapore

W. Duan
Department of Applied Social Studies, City University of Hong Kong, Hong Kong, China

Y. Bai
Tsinghua-Rocfly Academy of Education, Institute of Education,
Tsinghua University, Beijing, China

S.-M. Shih
Department of Palliative Medicine, Koo Foundation Sun
Yat-Sen Cancer Center, Taipei, Taiwan

J. Teramoto Pedrotti and L.M. Edwards (eds.), *Perspectives on the Intersection of Multiculturalism and Positive Psychology*, Cross-Cultural Advancements in Positive Psychology 7, DOI 10.1007/978-94-017-8654-6_4,

groups. However, a number of issues have been raised by researchers concerning the comparability of the instruments across cultures (Kankaraš and Moors 2010). Key issues regarding the comparability of instruments across cultures include linguistic equivalence, conceptual equivalence, metric equivalence, and functional equivalence (Hui and Triandis 1985; Lonner and Berry 1986).

4.1.1 Evaluating and Establishing Equivalence in Cross-Cultural and Multicultural Measurements

With the increase in multicultural societies comes the inevitable rise in individuals wanting to conduct positive psychology research across cultures as well as among multicultural populations (e.g., African Americans, Hispanic and Latino Americans, Asian Americans and White Americans within the U.S.). This is probably a reflection of rapid societal changes across the globe. The rise in globalization and migration, to name just two, are moving cultural boundaries and transforming local and regional issues into global factors. However, despite the rise in interest in multicultural studies, standard procedures for conducting such research are much less well-established than the procedures for mono-cultural research (Church 2010). Since the same instruments are used for all involved groups, it is all-too-often assumed that results are comparable among groups. However, as each cultural context reflects a mixture of numerous factors, processes and attributes, instrument items may have different meanings for different people, particularly across cultures (Greenfield 1997). This is particularly worrying given the stark increase in multicultural research over recent years.

The steady rise in psychological research across nations parallels the significant development in research on the cultural and ethnic groups within nations (Leong et al. 2010). Studies of populations in their original cultures will inform the ethnic populations in other contexts. For example, psychological studies of British Chinese and Hong Kong Chinese show similar patterns in terms of health behaviours (Rochelle and Marks 2011; Rochelle et al. 2009). The continuity of cultural roots of British Chinese is often maintained through parental or familial socialisation, even after several generations of acculturation (Cheung 2002; Rochelle and Marks 2010). Similarly, studies of populations in original cultures (e.g., Chinese) can inform work on individuals who live within the United States (e.g., Chinese Americans), which is the focus of the current volume.

4.1.2 Cultural Measurement Equivalence

Cultural measurement equivalence refers to the possibility that interpretations of psychological measurements, assessments and observations are similar if not equal across different cultural groups. It is important to note that different facets of equivalence are discussed by different researchers in the field, and different terminology is sometimes used by different authors. Please see Chap. 3, this volume, for additional discussion of equivalence issues. While more than 50 types of measurement equivalence have been identified, there are four types of measurement equivalence commonly used by researchers conducting cross-cultural studies: linguistic, conceptual, metric, and functional (Johnson 1998). *Linguistic equivalence* refers to whether words included in psychological instruments and measurements have the same meaning across cultures, the linguistic accuracy of instrument items. It is primarily concerned with the translation of psychological measures from one language into another for use in another country and culture. Direct simple translation is perceived to be an inadequate procedure to provide support for this type of equivalence. Back-translation has become the standard procedure and technique of choice among cross-cultural researchers. However, it has been described to be subjective and it only attempts to achieve linguistic equivalence (Mallinckrodt and Wang 2004). Of course, the aim of the translation process and adaptation of instruments is to achieve different linguistic versions of the original instrument that are conceptually equivalent in the target country or culture. Factors affecting translation of instruments the most are cultural and linguistic in nature.

Besides linguistic equivalence, three other measurement equivalences should be considered in multicultural research: *conceptual equivalence*, *metric equivalence*, and *functional equivalence* (Johnson 1998). Conceptual equivalence is when the meaning of factors, concepts etc., are comparable or the same for culturally different groups/cohorts established by a common set of behaviours that define a construct. Metric equivalence, perceived as more technical and complex to evaluate/assess is demonstrated if the psychometric properties of two sets of data are the same for different cultural groups. Functional equivalence is established by demonstrating that two or more behaviours in different cultures are functionally related to the same problem.

4.2 Cross-Cultural Approaches to Instrument Development

Since many instruments are developed in the West, one of the common issues facing cross-cultural researchers is how to measure similar constructs in non-Western cultures. Possibly the most renowned work in this area was conducted by Hofstede (1980), who famously classified Western countries as being more individualistic while many Eastern countries were classified as collectivistic. There are three main approaches to developing psychological instruments in non-Western cultures: (1) Etic approach; (2) Emic approach; and (3) Combined etic-emic approach.

The underlying theory of the etic approach is that theories developed in the West are universal and generalizable. Thus, researchers simply translate an instrument developed in the West and apply the measure directly on a non-Western target population without considering any cultural implications of directly applying the measure to a non-Western audience. Although the etic approach has dominated, there have been attempts to develop emic or indigenous instruments. The emic approach suggests that behaviours are culturally-specific. The combined etic-emic approach enables researchers to develop theories and instruments that are sensitive and relevant to the local context in order to increase ecological validity (Ho and Cheung 2007).

4.3 Lessons from Positive Psychology Research with Chinese Populations

In the following sections, we will use three positive psychology studies conducted among Chinese populations to illustrate the approaches to establish linguistic equivalence, conceptual equivalence, metric equivalence, and functional equivalence.

4.3.1 Linguistic Equivalence: Applications from "Positive Psychology" to Chinese Populations

First, we will briefly discuss the issue of linguistic equivalence. Over the years, we have used the forward-translation and back-translation method as a gold standard for developing successful non-English versions of positive psychology inventories. We have also followed published guidelines (Wild et al. 2005; World Health Organization 2011) to achieve equivalent meanings between different cultures' questionnaire versions. The steps we typically follow include the forward-translation of the English questionnaire into the second language by a bilingual translator; the back-translation of the questionnaire into English by another bilingual translator with no knowledge of the original English version; a triangulation meeting between the two translators and other experts with a proven understanding of positive psychology to resolve any inadequate expressions/concepts produced by the translation process; and qualitative interviewing and pre-testing to determine the final version. One requirement is that the translators and expert panel members should aim for the conceptual rather than literal equivalent of a word or phrase (World Health Organization 2011). Accordingly, the researchers must possess a working knowledge of the concepts involved to achieve this requirement. This situation, however, could become complicated when applied to positive psychology, because some of the terms in positive psychology are new and may not exist in other languages. More importantly, positive psychology's migration to non-Western countries is very recent, and thus it may be the case that fewer researchers in other countries have developed a comprehensive understanding of the fundamental concepts of positive psychology.

Some examples arise from work with Chinese populations in the area of positive psychology. It seems that literal translations are not uncommon in the Chinese positive psychology literature. For instance, the word "positive" is most

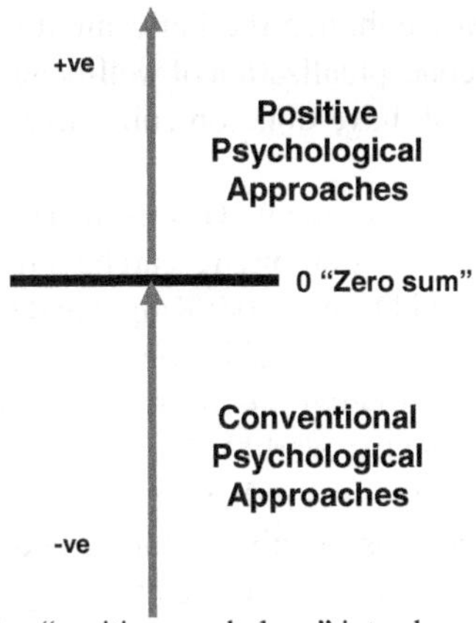

Fig. 4.1 Rationale of translating "positive psychology" into zheng xiang xīn lǐ xué (正向心理学) to capture the theme of "pointing north" in positive psychology. Positive psychological approaches, which aim at working beyond the "zero sum" towards the positive side, can be clearly distinguishable from conventional psychological approaches, which merely emphasize restoring the "zero sum" from the negative side

commonly translated as "jī jí" (積極). Nevertheless, the term "jī jí" carries particular connotations in Chinese, specifically "proactive" and "vigorous" which, in our opinion, are not consistent with the core theme of positive psychology. After prolonged discussion, those of us working in Hong Kong have decided to translate the term "positive psychology" into "zheng xiang xīn lǐ xué" (正向心理學), with "zheng xiang" capturing the connotation of "pointing north" (i.e., beyond zero sum) to distinguish this new stream of psychology from conventional approaches that focus more on rectifying psychological problems (Fig. 4.1). Although this translation has not been universally accepted in all Chinese speaking communities, we anticipate its eventual adoption in light of similar issues that have occurred with other linguistic representations of positive psychology concepts, including flow, gratitude, hope, etc.

4.3.2 *Conceptual Equivalence: What We Have Learned from Well-Being*

Well-being, with its focus on optimal functioning, is one of the cornerstones of positive psychology (Seligman and Csikszentmihalyi 2000). There are two broad perspectives on well-being: the hedonic and eudaimonic perspectives (Ryan and Deci 2001). In essence, the hedonic view defines well-being in terms of pleasure or happiness, whereas the eudaimonic view suggests that well-being is not self-happiness per se but involves the actualization of human potential (Waterman 1993). According to the eudaimonic perspective, one can engage in activities that are not pleasure producing and still experience a high level of well-being if the activities are judged "worth doing" because they enhance the betterment of the self and/or society. In positive psychology, the conceptualization of well-being can largely be represented by the work that Diener et al. have done on subjective well-being (SWB; Diener 2000; Diener and Suh 2000).

SWB is a hedonic model of well-being (Kahneman et al. 1999) that has become one of the most influential models among researchers in Chinese communities for studying well-being (Chen and Davey 2008; Knight and Gunatilaka 2009; Lu 2001; Shu and Zhu 2009). However, it is debatable whether a hedonic view is most appropriate for conceptualizing well-being among the Chinese. In an early study, Suh et al. (1998) analyzed data from the World Value Survey II and reported that positive emotion is an important factor in predicting SWB in individualistic societies (e.g. the United States), whereas positive emotion and social norms are equally important in predicting SWB in collective societies (e.g. China). Accordingly, parents who work hard and suffer to provide education for their children would have low positive emotion, but consider themselves in line with social norms. These parents may thus report a high level of well-being in a collective society, despite the presence of self-suffering. If people in different cultures (collective versus individualistic) use different sets of behaviors and values (positive emotion versus social norms) to define and construct well-being, it becomes an issue of conceptual equivalence (Leong et al. 2010), which makes cultural comparison difficult.

The Satisfaction with Life Scale (SWLS; Diener et al. 1985) and the Subjective Happiness Scale (SHS; Lyubomirsky and Lepper 1999) are the two most widely used measures of well-being in positive psychology research among the Chinese. Sample items on these scales include: "*The conditions of my life are excellent,*" (from SWLS; 1 = Strongly disagree to 7 = Strongly agree) and "*In general, I consider myself,*" (from SHS; 1 = Not a very happy person to 7 = A very happy person). Note that items in both inventories focus exclusively on self-appraisal of one's own condition, focusing on "Me" instead of "We." Ho and Cheung (2007) hypothesized that this "Me" approach may not capture the total conception of well-being among the Chinese, who are relationally "We" oriented. They argued that it would be difficult for Chinese people to judge their own level of well-being without taking the well-being of significant others into consideration. To examine the hypothesis that an interpersonal dimension of well-being exists among the Chinese, Ho and his colleagues (2007) used the combined etic-emic approach (Cheung et al. 2011) to develop a Chinese version of the Expanded Satisfaction with Life Scale (Ch-ESWLS). The original five self-oriented items from the SWLS were considered as etic items because it was assumed they were universal (Diener and Diener 1995; Diener and Suh 1999). Another five other-oriented items were added to parallel the self-oriented items from the original SWLS (e.g., "The conditions of my family members' lives are excellent"). Three independent studies were conducted to examine the existence of an interpersonal dimension of well-being among the Chinese. The first two studies conducted an exploratory factor analysis and a confirmatory factor analysis of two independent samples in Beijing (sample 1, n = 296; sample 2, n = 485) and established a 6-item Ch-ESWLS with three items measuring self-oriented well-being (e.g., "*So far I have gotten the important things I want in life*") and another three items measuring other-oriented well-being: (e.g., "*The conditions of my family members' lives are excellent*"). The researchers conducted a series of studies and the final multi-group confirmatory factor analysis showed that the two-factor well-being model measured the same construct to the same extent among participants in both Beijing and Hong Kong.

In summary, Chinese people can report a high level of well-being despite the presence of low positive emotion by fitting into social norms (Suh et al. 1998), making their significant others happy (Ho 2010) and judging that their significant others are happy (Ho and Cheung 2007). In retrospect, the two concepts of well-being mentioned above are more consistent with a eudaimonic (Ryan and Deci 2001) than a hedonic perspective. Future studies should explore to what extent the eudaimonic perspective is relevant to conceptualizing well-being among the Chinese. A combined etic-emic approach would be useful for integrating the hedonic and eudaimonic perspectives of well-being among the Chinese.

4.3.3 Metric Equivalence: What We Have Learned from Posttraumatic Growth

The term posttraumatic growth (PTG) was initially coined by Tedeschi and Calhoun (1995) to represent the positive psychological changes that may occur after a traumatic event. One of the first validated measurements of PTG (the Posttraumatic Growth Inventory [PTGI]; Tedeschi and Calhoun 1996) was found to have five factors in a sample of U.S. undergraduate students with mixed traumatic events using exploratory factor analysis (EFA). The five factors are: (I) Relating to others; (II) New possibilities; (III) Personal strength; (IV) Spiritual change; and (V) Appreciation of life. Although first developed among a non-clinical population, the five-factor structure of PTGI has been found to be applicable to other populations, such as cancer patients. For instance, a recent study conducted in Canada (n=470) reported that the above five-factor structure of the PTGI can be applied to breast cancer survivors (Brunet et al. 2010). Subsequent multi-group confirmatory factor analysis (CFA) of the same study also supported the invariance of the PTGI across age groups, treatment type, time since diagnosis, and time since last treatment. In fact, the five-factor model was found to be valid not only among cancer patients but also among samples with mixed traumatic events (Taku et al. 2008), including active duty soldiers (n=3,537) in terms of being exposed to combat in Iraq or Afghanistan (Lee et al. 2010).

In summary, the existing evidence seems to support the consistent factor structure of PTGI across different samples, including undergraduate students (Tedeschi and Calhoun 1996), community samples (Taku et al. 2008), deployed soldiers (Lee et al. 2010) and breast cancer survivors (Brunet et al. 2010). However, it should be noted that the majority of participants in the above-mentioned studies were Caucasian. For instance, in the study on breast cancer survivors (Brunet et al. 2010), 94.5 % of the patients were Caucasian. Similarly, 74.5 % of the participants in the active duty soldier study (Lee et al. 2010) were Caucasian. Further multicultural investigations are required to explore whether the findings from these studies can be generalized to other ethnic groups or other cultures.

Due to the popularity of PTG research globally in recent decades, the PTGI has been translated into numerous different languages, however, different factor structures were obtained from the studies. For instance, CFA of the PTGI-C (Chinese version) among a group of Chinese cancer patients revealed that the Chinese sample was unable to fit the five-factor model of PTGI (Ho et al. 2004). Subsequently, a four-factor model of PTGI-C was proposed after EFA and CFA. Similarly, the factor structure of PTGI-J (Japanese version) was investigated among a sample of Japanese undergraduate students with experience of various traumatic events (Taku et al. 2007). After EFA and CFA, another four-factor model of PTGI-J was suggested, though with different factors than the PTGI-C.

Thus, it seems the original factor structure of the PTGI cannot be replicated among Asian populations, nor with European populations. When the factor structure of the PTGI-G was examined on undergraduate students and patients from internal medicine clinics in Germany (Maercker and Langner 2001), only four out of the five original PTGI factors were obtained (Powell et al. 2003). Finally, in a study of the PTGI-S (Spanish version) with Latina immigrants to the U.S., a three-factor structure was obtained (Weiss and Berger 2006).

These examples highlight the issue of metric equivalence of positive psychology measures across languages and/or cultures. The above issue has another implication on positive psychology research in Chinese populations. It is well-known that even though they share the same language, Chinese in different countries can vary immensely in terms of tradition and culture. For instance, both Taiwan and Hong Kong use Traditional Chinese as their written language. The two cities, on the other hand, have very distinct histories and socio-cultural backgrounds. Thus, it is possible that the factor structure of PTGI-C established in Hong Kong may not be generalizable to people in Taiwan. This type of research demonstrates how among different groups within the same country (as would also be the case between cultural groups in the US), issues of equivalence are critical.

In order to investigate the above issue, Ho et al. (2013) examined the factorial equivalence of the PTGI-C between a sample of cancer survivors from Hong Kong ($n=223$) and Taipei ($n=248$) using multi-sample confirmatory factor analysis (MS-CFA).

First, the researchers compared the goodness-of-fit of the factor structure proposed by Tedeschi and Calhoun (1996) with that proposed by Ho et al. (2004). The samples from Hong Kong and Taiwan fitted Ho's model ($\chi^2[170]=425.40$, AGFI=0.83, CFI=0.90, RMSEA=0.06) better than Tedeschi's model ($\chi^2[358]=1{,}088.27$, AGFI=0.75, CFI=0.83, RMSEA=0.07). The above findings suggest that the emic structure developed by Ho et al. (2004) is more appropriate to both Hong Kong and Taiwan samples than the original factor structure of Tedeschi and Calhoun (1996) developed in the United States. The goodness-of-fit of the final model and the internal reliabilities of the four subscales as well as the whole 15-item PTGI-C were satisfactory.

In summary, the above findings suggest that metric equivalence cannot be assumed for different translated versions of PTGI. Nevertheless, metric equivalence is supported for the Traditional Chinese version of the PTGI among different

Chinese communities using the same language, despite having different cultural backgrounds (Ho et al. 2013). Most importantly, multi-samples confirmatory factor analysis is a useful tool to investigate metric equivalence in cross-cultural positive psychology studies.

4.3.4 Functional Equivalence: Studying Character Strengths in Chinese Samples

Character strength has aroused the interest of researchers across the globe largely because of the momentum gained by the positive psychology movement (Linley et al. 2007; Park et al. 2006; Peterson et al. 2010). Character strength is a family of positive traits manifested in an individual's thoughts, emotions and behaviors (Peterson and Seligman 2004). Twenty-four such positive traits have been identified as character strengths and it has been proposed that these 24 traits are universal across countries (Peterson and Seligman 2004; Steger et al. 2007). Moreover, these 24 character strengths are theoretically hypothesised to aggregate on the following overarching virtues: (1) Wisdom and Knowledge (creativity, curiosity, judgment, love of learning, perspective); (2) Courage (bravery, industry, honesty, zest); (3) Justice (citizenship, fairness, leadership); (4) Humanity (love, kindness, social intelligence); (5) Temperance (forgiveness, modesty, caution, self-control); and (6) Transcendence (appreciation of beauty and excellence, gratitude, hope, humour, spirituality) (Peterson and Seligman 2004; Steger et al. 2007).

Peterson and Seligman (2004) developed the *Values in Action Inventory of Strengths* (VIA-IS) to measure the character strengths of adults according to their taxonomy. The VIA-IS consists of 24 character strength subscales, with 10 items per subscale (a total of 240 items). There are two issues related to the VIA-IS when applying it to Chinese samples: the cross-cultural invariance of its factor structure and the appropriateness of each item when measuring the expected strength among Chinese populations. The first is the issue of metric equivalence discussed above. The second focuses on whether the behaviour described by the items in the VIA-IS are functionally related to similar strengths in Chinese individuals compared to their American counterparts. This is the issue of functional equivalence (Leong et al. 2010), which is discussed below.

A closer look at the VIA-IS items suggests that some of the behaviors described in the inventory may appear odd when applied to a Chinese sample, especially individuals in rural mainland China. For example, the item "*I never tell outsiders things bad about my team*" (item 108 of the VIA-IS) is a common social expectation in a collective culture such as Mainland China and may lack the sensitivity to measure the strength related to citizenship. Similarly, the item "*I practice my religion*" (item 124 of the VIA-IS) may not appropriately represent spirituality in mainland China, due to the fact that most of the people in the country are atheists. The same may apply to items not directly related to religion that carry a strong religious connotation (e.g., item 66 of the VIA-IS: "*At least once a day, I stop and count my blessings*").

Additionally, some of the items representing strength in Western culture may represent socially unacceptable behaviour in China. For example, the item "*When I hear people say something mean, I protest*" (item 199 of the VIA-IS to measure courage) may not merge well into the Chinese social context where the emphasis is on conformity rather than uniqueness (Kim and Markus 1999). Similarly, item 15 of the VIA-IS (*"I have no trouble eating healthy foods"*) may not be suitable for some Chinese, especially those in rural areas who do not have a clear concept of what eating "healthy food" entails. We believe that the above issues are not unique to the Chinese but should be relevant to other ethical groups within the U.S. as well. Two of the authors of this chapter (Duan and Ho) have conducted a series of studies using structural equation modelling (SEM) and qualitative interview strategies in Mainland China to examine both the factor structures and functional equivalence of the Chinese version of the VIA. Three theoretically meaningful virtues comparable to some virtue structures proposed in previous studies conducted in Western countries, were obtained. These three virtues are: interpersonal, vitality, and cautiousness (Duan et al. 2012). We are conducting further research to develop an emic measure of positive psychological resources among the Chinese.

4.4 Summary and Conclusion

In this chapter, we have used existing frameworks to discuss four methodological issues related to positive psychology research in Chinese populations (Johnson 1998; Leong et al. 2010). Conceptual equivalence refers to the same concept representing the same attitude and set of behaviours in targeted cultures. We argue that the hedonic view of well-being, with its focus on the self, may not be able to capture the conception of well-being among the Chinese. Using the *combined etic-emic approach*, we have provided initial support to our proposition that Chinese people may adopt a more collective view when judging their own well-being. Metric equivalence refers to the psychometric properties of the Chinese versions of positive psychology questionnaires, compared to the original English versions of the same questionnaires. Using *multi-sample CFA,* our study on Posttraumatic Growth Inventory has shown that the factor structure of the original English version of the questionnaire is not generalizable to Chinese participants. However, the factor structure of the Chinese version of the Posttraumatic Growth Inventory developed in Hong Kong can be applied to similar participants in Taiwan, although Taiwan has a distinct socio-cultural background compared to Hong Kong. Regarding functional equivalence, we have drawn on our experience and used the VIA-IS to highlight that although its 24 strengths and six virtues are considered universal across cultures, some of the behaviour that reflects strength in one culture might be sanctioned in another culture. *Qualitative research strategies*, including in-depth interviews and focus groups, may help to address such items. Finally, the standard *forward- and backward-translation* procedure remains the gold standard for developing linguistically equivalent questionnaires for different language versions.

Although we have used our research experience among Chinese to illustrate the above issues, we believe that they are highly relevant to positive psychology research among minority populations in the United States, especially among Asian Americans. It has been shown that Asian Americans have different degrees of acculturation and the extent of acculturation has important effects on their physical and psychological health (Suinn 2010). Importantly, the degree of acculturation among minority groups in the United States may also affect their responses to psychological assessments related to positive psychology, and should be considered as a critical variable.

Positive psychology was developed in the era of globalization and people all over the world have been contributing to it since its conception. We should be more aware of the roles of culture in shaping positive psychology constructs and measures in both research and applications (Kubokawa and Amber 2009). We hope more research will be conducted in future to clarify further the issues mentioned above.

References

Berry, J. W. (1980). Acculturation as varieties of adaptation. In A. M. Padilla (Ed.), *Acculturation: Theory, models and some new findings* (pp. 9–25). Boulder: Westview Press.

Brunet, J., McDonough, M. H., Hadd, V., Crocker, P. R. E., & Sabiston, C. M. (2010). The posttraumatic growth inventory: An examination of the factor structure and invariance among breast cancer survivors. *Psycho-Oncology, 19*, 830–838. doi:10.1002/pon.1640.

Chen, Z., & Davey, G. (2008). Happiness and subjective wellbeing in Mainland China. *Journal of Happiness Studies, 9*, 589–600. doi:10.1007/s10902-008-9092-7.

Cheung, F. M. (2002). Universal and indigenous dimensions of Chinese personality. In K. S. Kurasaki & S. Sue (Eds.), *Asian American Mental Health: Assessment theories and methods* (pp. 141–157). Dordrecht: Kluwer.

Cheung, F. M., van de Vijver, F. J. R., & Leong, F. T. L. (2011). Toward a new approach to the study of personality in culture. *American Psychologist, 66*, 593–603. doi:10.1037/a0022389.

Church, A. T. (2010). Measurement issues in cross-cultural research. In G. Walford, E. Tucker, & M. Viswanathan (Eds.), *The Sage handbook of measurement* (pp. 151–177). Los Angeles: Sage.

Diener, E. (2000). Subjective well-being: The science of happiness and a proposal for a national index. *American Psychologists, 55*, 34–43. doi:10.1037/0003-066X.55.1.34.

Diener, E., & Diener, M. (1995). Cross-cultural correlates of life satisfaction and self-esteem. *Journal of Personality and Social Psychology, 68*(4), 653–663. doi:10.1007/978-90-481-2352-0_4.

Diener, E., & Suh, E. M. (1999). National differences in subjective well-being. In D. Kahneman, E. Diener, & N. Schwartz (Eds.), *Well-being: The foundations of hedonic psychology* (pp. 434–450). New York: Russell Sage.

Diener, E., & Suh, E. (Eds.). (2000). *Culture and subjective well-being*. Cambridge, MA: The MIT Press.

Diener, E., Emmons, R. A., Larson, R. J., & Griffin, S. (1985). The satisfaction with life scale. *Journal of Personality Assessment, 49*, 71–75. doi:10.1207/s15327752jpa4901_13.

Duan, W., Ho, S. M. Y., Yu, B., Tang, X., Zhang, Y., Li, T., & Yuen, T. (2012). Factor structure of the Chinese Virtues Questionnaire. *Research on Social Work Practice, 22*, 680–688. doi:10.1177/1049731512450074.

Gable, S. L., & Haidt, J. (2005). What (and why) is positive psychology? *Review of General Psychology, 9*, 103–110. doi:10.1037/1089-2680.9.2.103.

Greenfield, P. M. (1997). You can't take it with you: Why ability assessments don't cross cultures. *American Psychologist, 52*(10), 1115–1124.
Ho, S. M. Y. (2010). Universal happiness. In L. Bormans (Ed.), *The world book of happiness* (pp. 253–255). Singapore: Page One Publishing.
Ho, S. M. Y., & Cheung, M. W. L. (2007). Using the combined etic-emic approach to develop a measurement of interpersonal subjective well-being in Chinese populations. In A. D. Ong & M. van Dulmen (Eds.), *Oxford handbook of methods in positive psychology* (pp. 139–152). New York: Oxford University Press.
Ho, S. M. Y., Chan, C. L. W., & Ho, R. T. H. (2004). Post-traumatic growth in Chinese cancer survivors. *Psycho-Oncology, 13*, 377–389. doi:10.1002/pon.758.
Ho, S. M. Y., Law, L. S. C., Wang, G.-L., Shih, S.-M., Hsu, S.-H., & Hou, Y.-C. (2013). Psychometric analysis of the Chinese version of the Posttraumatic Growth Inventory with cancer patients in Hong Kong and Taiwan. *Psycho-Oncology, 22*(3), 715–719. doi:10.1002/pon.3024.
Hofstede, G. (1980). *Culture's consequences: International differences in work-related values*. Beverly Hills: Sage.
Hui, C. H., & Triandis, H. (1985). Measurement in cross-cultural psychology: A review and comparison of strategies. *Journal of Cross-Cultural Psychology, 16*, 131–152. doi:10.1177/002200 2185016002001.
Johnson, T. P. (1998). Approaches to equivalence in cross-cultural and cross-national survey research. *ZUMA-Nachrichten Spezial, 3*, 1–40. Retrieved from http://www.gesis.org/fileadmin/upload/forschung/publikationen/zeitschriften/zuma_nachrichten_spezial/znspezial3.pdf
Kahneman, D., Diener, E., & Schwatz, N. (Eds.). (1999). *Well-being: The foundations of hedonic psychology*. New York: Russell Sage.
Kankaraš, M., & Moors, G. (2010). Researching measurement equivalence in cross-cultural studies. *Psihologija, 43*, 121–135. doi:10.2298/PSI1002121K.
Kim, H., & Markus, H. R. (1999). Deviance or uniqueness, harmony or conformity? A cultural analysis. *Journal of Personality and Social Psychology, 77*, 785–800. doi:10.1037/0022-3514.77.4.785.
Knight, J., & Gunatilaka, R. (2009). Great expectations? The subjective well-being of rural-urban migrants in China. *World Development, 38*, 113–124. doi:10.1016/j.worlddev.2009.03.002.
Kubokawa, A., & Amber, O. (2009). Positive psychology and cultural sensitivity: A review of the literature. *Graduate Journal of Counseling Psychology*, 1(2, Article 13). Retrieved from http://epublications.marquette.edu/gjcp/vol1/iss2/13
Lee, J. A., Luxton, D. D., Reger, G. M., & Gahm, G. A. (2010). Confirmatory factor analysis of the Posttraumatic Growth Inventory with a sample of soldiers previously deployed in support of the Iraq and Afghanistan wars. *Journal of Clinical Psychology, 66*, 813–819. doi:10.1002/jclp.20692.
Leong, F. T. L., Leung, K., & Cheung, F. M. (2010). Integrating cross-cultural psychology research methods into ethnic minority psychology. *Cultural Diversity and Ethnic Minority Psychology, 16*, 590–597. doi:10.1037/a0020127.
Linley, P. A., Maltby, J., Wood, A. M., Joseph, S., Harrington, S., Peterson, C., Park, N., & Seligman, M. E. P. (2007). Character strengths in the United Kingdom: The VIA inventory of strengths. *Personality and Individual Differences, 43*(2), 341–351. doi:10.1016/j.paid.2006.12.004.
Lonner, W. J., & Berry, J. W. (1986). *Field methods in cross-cultural research*. Beverly Hills: Sage.
Lu, L. (2001). Understanding happiness: A look into the Chinese folk psychology. *Journal of Happiness Studies, 2*, 407–432. doi:10.1023/A:1013944228205.
Lyubomirsky, S., & Lepper, H. S. (1999). A measure of subjective happiness: Preliminary reliability and construct validation. *Social Indicators Research, 46*, 137–155. doi:10.1023/A:1006824100041.
Maercker, A., & Langner, R. (2001). Posttraumatic personal growth: Validation of German versions of two questionnaires. *Diagnostics, 47*, 153–162. doi:10.1026//0012-1924.47.3.153.
Mallinckrodt, B., & Wang, C. C. (2004). Quantitative methods for verifying semantic equivalence of translated research instruments: A Chinese version of the experiences in close relationships scale. *Journal of Counseling Psychology, 51*(3), 368–379. doi:10.1037/0022-0167.51.3.368.
Park, N., Peterson, C., & Seligman, M. E. P. (2006). Character strengths in fifty-four nations and the fifty US states. *Journal of Positive Psychology, 1*, 118–129. doi:10.1080/17439760600619567.

Peterson, C., & Seligman, M. E. P. (2004). *Character strengths and virtues: A handbook and classification*. Washington, DC: American Psychological Association.

Peterson, C., Stephens, J. P., Park, N., Lee, F., & Seligman, M. E. P. (2010). Strengths of character and work. In P. A. Linley, S. Harrington, & N. Garcea (Eds.), *Oxford handbook of positive psychology and work*. New York: Oxford University Press.

Powell, S., Rosner, R., Butollo, W., Tedeschi, R. G., & Calhoun, L. G. (2003). Posttraumatic growth after war: A study with former refugees and displaced people in Sarajevo. *Journal of Clinical Psychology, 59*, 71–83. doi:10.1002/jclp.10117.

Rochelle, T. L., & Marks, D. F. (2010). Medical pluralism of the Chinese in London: An exploratory study. *British Journal of Health Psychology, 15*, 715–728. doi:10.1348/135910709X479195.

Rochelle, T. L., & Marks, D. F. (2011). Health behaviours and use of Chinese medicine among the British Chinese. *Journal of Cross-Cultural Psychology, 42*, 390–405. doi:10.1177/0022022110362745.

Rochelle, T. L., Shardlow, S. M., & Ng, S. H. (2009). Ageing in Hong Kong and the UK: A comparison of the Chinese at home and abroad. *Journal of Comparative Asian Development, 8*, 25–41. doi:10.1080/15339114.2009.9678472.

Ryan, R. M., & Deci, E. L. (2001). On happiness and human potentials: A review of research on hedonic and eudaimonic well-being. *Annual Review of Psychology, 52*, 141–166. doi:10.1146/annurev.psych.52.1.141.

Seligman, M. E. P., & Csikszentmihalyi, M. (2000). Positive psychology: An introduction. *American Psychologist, 55*, 5–14. doi:10.1037/0003-066X.55.1.5.

Shu, X., & Zhu, Y. (2009). The quality of life in China. *Social Indicators Research, 92*, 191–225. doi:10.1007/s11205-008-9350-4.

Steger, M. F., Hicks, B., Kashdan, T. B., Krueger, R. F., & Bouchard, T. J., Jr. (2007). Genetic and environmental influences on the positive traits of the values in action classification, and biometric covariance with normal personality. *Journal of Research in Personality, 41*, 524–539. doi:10.1016/j.jrp.2006.06.002.

Suh, E., Diener, E., Oishi, S., & Triandis, H. C. (1998). The shifting basis of life satisfaction judgments across cultures: Emotions versus norms. *Journal of Personality and Social Psychology, 74*, 482–493. doi:10.1037/0022-3514.74.2.482.

Suinn, R. M. (2010). Reviewing acculturation and Asian Americans: How acculturation affects health, adjustment, school achievement, and counseling. *Asian American Journal of Psychology, 1*(1), 5–17. doi:10.1037/a0018798.

Taku, K., Calhoun, L. G., Tedeschi, R. G., Gil-Rivas, V., Kilmer, R. P., & Cann, A. (2007). Examining posttraumatic growth among Japanese university students. *Anxiety, Stress and Coping: An International Journal, 20*, 353–367. doi:10.1080/10615800701295007.

Taku, K., Cann, A., Calhoun, L. G., & Tedeschi, R. G. (2008). The factor structure of the Posttraumatic Growth Inventory: A comparison of five models using confirmatory factor analysis. *Journal of Traumatic Stress, 21*, 158–164. doi:10.1002/jts.20305.

Tedeschi, R. G., & Calhoun, L. G. (1995). *Trauma and transformation: Growing in the aftermath of suffering*. Thousand Oaks: Sage.

Tedeschi, R. G., & Calhoun, L. G. (1996). The Posttraumatic Growth Inventory: Measuring the positive legacy of trauma. *Journal of Traumatic Stress, 9*, 455–471. doi:10.1002/jts.2490090305.

Waterman, A. S. (1993). Two conceptions of happiness: Contrasts of personal expressiveness (eudaimonia) and hedonic enjoyment. *Journal of Personality and Social Psychology, 64*, 678–691. doi:10.1037/0022-3514.64.4.678.

Weiss, T., & Berger, R. (2006). Reliability and validity of a Spanish version of the Posttraumatic Growth Inventory. *Research on Social Work Practice, 16*, 191–199. doi:10.1177/1049731505281374.

Wild, D., Grove, A., Martin, M., Eremenco, S., McElroy, S., Verjee-Lorenz, A., & Erikson, P. (2005). Principles of good practice for the translation and cultural adaptation process for patient-reported outcomes (PRO) measures: Report of the ISPOR task force for translation and cultural adaptation. *Value in Health, 8*, 94–104. doi:10.1111/j.1524-4733.2005.04054.x.

World Health Organization. (2011). *Process of translation and adaptation of instruments*. Retrieved November 25, 2011, from http://www.who.int/substance_abuse/research_tools/translation/en/

Part II
Specific Constructs

Chapter 5
Affective Well-Being Viewed Through a Lens of Race and Ethnicity

Hung-Bin Sheu

Since the turn of the twenty-first century, there has been a renewed interest in exploring human strengths and optimal functioning in the field of psychology. Special volumes on positive psychology and its applications in work and school settings have been published (e.g., Linley et al. 2010). Research has produced abundant findings on correlates of well-being outcomes for different cultural groups (see Diener and Suh 2000 for a review). Given the limited space, this chapter will focus primarily on racial and ethnic differences in the affective component of well-being, including subjective happiness and positive and negative emotions. Although the term "life satisfaction" is sometimes used interchangeably with happiness (e.g., Ram 2010), the variable of life satisfaction is not emphasized as much in this chapter because it is often conceptualized as a cognitive construct and is covered in greater depth in Chap. 6 of this volume. After a brief discussion on the definition of, cultural influences on, and assessment tools of well-being, research that compares happiness, positive and negative emotions of individuals with different racial and ethnic backgrounds will be reviewed. When relevant, findings of cross-cultural research will be drawn upon to shed light on racial and ethnic differences. Finally, methodological issues and recommendations for future research will be highlighted, and findings of an exemplar designed to follow some of the recommendations will be presented.

H.-B. Sheu, Ph.D. (✉)
Department of Educational and Counseling Psychology,
University at Albany, State University of New York,
Education 223, 1400 Washington Avenue, Albany, NY 12222, USA
e-mail: hsheu@albany.edu

J. Teramoto Pedrotti and L.M. Edwards (eds.), *Perspectives on the Intersection of Multiculturalism and Positive Psychology*, Cross-Cultural Advancements in Positive Psychology 7, DOI 10.1007/978-94-017-8654-6_5,

5.1 Definition of Well-Being

Research on what makes for a good life has been guided by two major philosophical perspectives: hedonics and eudaimonia. These two perspectives have led to different conceptualizations and operationalizations of well-being outcomes and predictors. Based on the *hedonic* tradition, subjective well-being (SWB) can be defined as the presence of positive affect, the absence of negative affect, and satisfaction with life (Diener 1984; Diener et al. 2002). On the other hand, following the *eudaimonic* tradition, Ryff (1989) argues that positive functioning is more than feeling good, and states that psychological well-being (PWB) consists of six overlapping but distinct dimensions: autonomy, environmental mastery, personal growth, positive relationships with others, purpose in life, and self-acceptance.

Although outcome variables derived from SWB and PWB models are often studied separately, empirical evidence shows that hedonic happiness and eudaimonic happiness are likely to represent distinct but overlapping latent dimensions (Compton et al. 1996). Researchers have continued to debate whether the distinction between hedonic and eudaimonic happiness is warranted (Kashdan et al. 2008; Keyes and Annas 2009). Given that SWB is generally conceptualized as containing two components of positive affect (and the absence of negative affect) and life satisfaction, these variables are often investigated in the same study. Therefore, although not the main focus of this chapter, life satisfaction is included in the review as well when appropriate.

5.2 Culture and Affective Well-Being

Researchers have proposed to integrate culture into our understanding of happiness and well-being. Happiness can be defined as a general positive emotional state that is not restricted to any specific circumstances or events (Kitayama et al. 1995). While this broad definition suggests that the pursuit of happiness is likely to be a universal desire, the meaning and experience of happiness are likely to be dictated by specific sociocultural norms. Conceptual and empirical attention has been given to lay conceptions of happiness and unhappiness as well as possible cultural variations in the nature and experiences of well-being. Uchida et al.'s (2004) review showed that individuals in the North American cultural context tended to define happiness in terms of personal achievement and were motivated to maximize the experience of positive affect; on the other hand, people in the East Asian cultural context tended to define happiness in terms of interpersonal connectedness and strived to maintain a balance between positive and negative affect. By analyzing essays provided by Caucasian American and Chinese participants, Lu and Gilmour (2004) compared and contrasted individually-oriented happiness (e.g., personal achievement, self-autonomy) with socially-oriented happiness (e.g., harmonious homeostasis within the individual and between the individual and his surroundings), which are similar to the distinction made by Uchida et al.

Moreover, new theoretical frameworks have been introduced to explain how personality, social, and cultural factors may predict well-being. For example, Affect Valuation Theory posits that temperament shapes actual affect (i.e., the affective states that people actually feel) more than ideal affect (i.e., the affective states that people value and would ideally like to feel) while cultural variables shape ideal affect more than actual affect (Tsai et al. 2006). Existing conceptual and empirical progress has focused on the impact of cultural group membership and outlined possible effects of characteristics associated with the individualistic and collectivistic cultural orientations. These efforts clearly indicate the important role that culture plays in illuminating how people with different backgrounds may understand and pursue the affective component of well-being.

5.3 Assessment of Affective Well-Being Constructs

Single- and multi-item assessment approaches have been developed to measure happiness. An example of the single-item approach is the Global Happiness Item with response options of "not too happy," "pretty happy," and "very happy" (Bradburn 1969). Multi-item instruments, such as the Subjective Happiness Scale (Lyubomirsky and Lepper 1999) and the Oxford Happiness Questionnaire (Hills and Argyle 2002), are also available. These measures include such items as "I am very happy," and "Life is good" (1 = strongly disagree; 6 = strongly agree).

In well-being research, assessment of emotions and affect is typically done by using the Affective Balance Scale (ABS; Bradburn 1969) or the Positive and Negative Affect Schedule (PANAS; Watson et al. 1988). Both instruments measure positive affect (e.g., "proud") and negative affect (e.g., "distressed") as separate constructs. Other researchers have also used level of agreement with a set of feeling words, such as calm and happy, to assess positive emotions (e.g., Kitayama et al. 2000). The Affect Valuation Index (Tsai et al. 2006) was recently developed for research that explores the difference between ideal affect (how one would ideally like to feel) and actual affect (how one actually feels) among people who have different cultural backgrounds.

Most of the assessment tools developed to measure the above well-being outcomes have been examined using exploratory and confirmatory factor analysis, and measurement equivalence of some of these instruments has been tested across different groups or over time. For example, factor loadings of the ABS were found to be invariant over a 3-year period, and only one factor loading differed significantly between younger adult and older adult age groups (Maitland et al. 2001). Similarly, the difference between younger (third-grade) and older (sixth-grade) children on the factor structure of the PANAS-C (a children version of the PANAS; Laurent et al. 1999) has been tested (Bushman and Crowley 2010). However, measurement equivalence of these well-being measures on happiness and affect have rarely been examined across racial and ethnic groups within the United States. In one of the few studies that tested well-being measures across racial groups, Lawrence and Liang

(1988) imposed a single subjective well-being factor on both items of the ABS and items assessing life satisfaction. They found significant differences on some factor loadings between White Americans and African Americans while such differences were absent between gender and age groups. These findings suggested that White Americans and African Americans might respond to some of the items differently due to measurement artifacts, and, therefore, meaningful interpretations of the difference in well-being between the two racial groups might not be possible.

These well-being instruments have provided useful tools for us to assess the constructs of happiness and positive/negative affect. Although they have advanced our understanding of these important well-being outcomes, their applicability to individuals with racial and ethnic backgrounds other than White/Caucasian has not been thoroughly investigated, rendering the results of cross-racial and ethnic comparisons on these variables less reliable and valid.

5.4 Racial and Ethnic Differences in Subjective Happiness and Satisfaction

Cross-cultural and cross-national research has shown that individuals in Asian cultures tend to report lower levels of life satisfaction, less pleasant emotions, and greater negative emotions compared to their counterparts in North America (Diener et al. 1995). Although some evidence shows that differences among racial and ethnic groups in the U.S. seems to echo cross-national findings with Asian Americans reporting lower SWB than European Americans, such conclusions were drawn primarily from research on negative emotions, such as depression and anxiety, rather than on positive well-being outcomes (Okazaki 1997, 2000). Compared with cross-national research, empirical attention given to exploring differences in SWB among racial and ethnic groups in the U.S. is surprisingly limited.

Differences in subjective happiness between White Americans and African Americans have received a small amount of empirical scrutiny. For example, based on the data from the General Social Survey (GSS; Hughes and Thomas 1998), African American adults were found to report lower overall happiness and life satisfaction, lower marital happiness, and worse health status than their White American counterparts after controlling for income, education, work status, marital status, and age. This study also revealed that these racial differences had persisted from 1972 to 1996. Subsequent analysis using more data (1972–2004) from the same survey continued to show that the gap between these two groups in happiness remained substantial (Yang 2008). Interestingly, research on life satisfaction with younger populations (adolescents, children) showed no difference or small effect sizes between White Americans and African Americans (Huebner 1995; Huebner et al. 2004).

Different assessment tools used in the aforementioned studies as well as developmental tasks typically encountered and coping strategies employed by African Americans and White Americans at different ages are possible explanations for differences in well-being. It is also possible that oppression and discrimination experienced by African Americans over time may be associated with lower well-being, therefore widening the gap with White Americans as they move into their adulthood. The cumulative effects of racism-related stress have been explored in public health research to account for disparities in pregnancy outcomes between these two racial groups (Collins et al. 2004). Such race-related stressors could also have cumulative impacts on well-being of racial and ethnic minorities over the life course, and longitudinal studies offer a viable way to test this hypothesis.

Furthermore, using a large high school student sample ($n = 4{,}514$), Brown et al. (2001) study showed that White American and Hispanic American students were happier and more satisfied with their lives than their African American counterparts. They also found that, regardless of racial or ethnic backgrounds, high school students who perceived racial relations between White Americans and African Americans as getting worse also reported lower levels of happiness. In spite of a large sample size, findings of Brown et al.'s study must be interpreted with caution as happiness and life satisfaction were each assessed by a single item.

In addition to being a predictor of well-being, racial and ethnic group membership has also been found to function as a moderator for the relations between well-being predictors and outcomes. Examining the relationship between happiness and role configuration (e.g., married or not, employed or not) for a sample of elderly men (55–69 years old in 1976), Burton et al. (1993) showed that being married was a significant positive predictor of changes in happiness over a 5-year period for White Americans, but not for Blacks. On the other hand, Black men who held a married/not employed role configuration reported a decline in happiness over the same 5-year period, whereas the impact of such role configuration on happiness was absent for White men. Additionally, Le et al. (2009) found that the relation of perceived school multiculturalism to subjective happiness was mediated by ethnocultural empathy for African American and Asian American youth, but not for their Hispanic counterparts. These findings suggest that individuals of different racial and ethnic groups are likely to pursue happiness through different means. More research should be devoted to identifying specific mechanisms that promote well-being for each group.

Recent development in cross-cultural well-being research may shed light on racial and ethnic differences in happiness. For example, Uchida and Kitayama (2009) used multidimensional scaling technique to analyze descriptions of happiness generated freely by American (primarily Caucasian) and Japanese college students, and found that American students associated happiness with personal achievement whereas Japanese students associated it with social harmony. Similarly, Lu and Gilmour (2004) discussed individually-oriented happiness valued by Euro-Americans versus socially-oriented happiness deemed important by Asians. Their study revealed that for Asians, routes toward happiness emphasized role obligations, harmonious relationship between self and the external world, and dialectical balance between happiness and unhappiness. On the other hand, for Euro-Americans, routes toward happiness emphasized personal accountability and explicit pursuit of happiness. These empirical efforts suffered from small sample sizes ($n < 100$) for each cultural group. Nevertheless, their findings show that culture can be a major force shaping the conception and experience of happiness. To the extent that racial and ethnic minorities conform to collectivistic or individualistic cultural norms, these cross-cultural findings may be relevant to understanding how they make sense of and pursue happiness within a U.S. context.

The above review on racial and ethnic group membership as a predictor and a moderator of well-being shows that White Americans tend to report higher levels of happiness and life satisfaction than other minority groups, and that different mechanisms may underlie the process through which different racial and ethnic groups pursue and maintain their well-being. However, this literature may not be conclusive due to the use of a single item for assessing well-being outcomes (e.g., Brown et al. 2001) and small sample sizes (e.g., Lu and Gilmour 2004). These studies also fall short of systematically investigating cultural or psychological variables that might help to explain racial and ethnic differences in well-being. These methodological and theoretical issues need to be addressed to advance our knowledge in this area.

5.5 Racial and Ethnic Differences in Positive and Negative Emotions

In addition to subjective happiness, culture norms are also likely to influence how people experience and recall their emotional states. The following review provides a summary of racial and ethnic differences in positive and negative emotions and how cultural factors may be related to emotional experiences.

With small sample sizes (ranging from 33 to 80) for each of the three racial and ethnic groups, Scollon et al. (2009) found that European American and Hispanic American young adults reported more pleasant emotions and less unpleasant emotions than Asian Americans. On the other hand, Aune and Aune (1996) collected data from college students in romantic relationships, and found that Filipino Americans rated experience, intensity, and appropriateness in positive emotions higher than Japanese Americans and Euro-Americans, but no group differences were found in reporting negative emotions. Based on Affect Valuation Theory, Tsai et al.'s (2006) study showed that European Americans and Asian Americans valued high arousal positive emotional states (e.g., excitement) more than Chinese in Hong Kong, whereas Chinese and Asian Americans valued low arousal positive states (e.g., calm) more than European Americans. This small body of literature does not offer conclusive findings on racial and ethnic differences in positive and negative emotions; however, it suggests that experience and expression of emotions may be culture-bound. More empirical inquiries are clearly needed to unravel between-group and within-group differences in the affective aspect of well-being.

Some research that compared immigrants with racial minority groups has shown that levels of acculturation might be related to how individuals experiences emotions. Leu et al. (2011) found that while positive emotions, as assessed by the PANAS-X (an extended version of the PANAS; Watson and Clark 1994), were negatively related to depression for European Americans and Asian Americans, such a relationship was absent for Asian immigrants. In their research, positive emotions also mediated the relation of perceived stress to depression symptoms only among European Americans, but not among either Asian group. Moreover, Jang et al.'s (2010) study showed that Koreans and Korean Americans were less likely than White Americans to endorse two positive affect items ("I felt hopeful," "I was happy") after controlling for depressive symptoms. Further analysis revealed that Korean Americans who were less acculturated to mainstream American culture were also less likely to endorse positive affect items than those who were more acculturated. Finally, Molix and Bettencourt's (2010) longitudinal study showed that higher levels of ethnic identity development at time 1 predicted greater psychological empowerment and positive affect at time 2 among ethnic minority students (primarily African Americans), but the prediction was the opposite for White students.

Sheldon and Hoon's (2007) study revealed that cultural membership was a significant predictor of SWB (measured by summing positive affect and life-satisfaction and subtracting negative affect) after controlling for gender, psychological need satisfaction, neuroticism, goal progress, self-esteem, and social support. Specifically, Singaporean students had lower SWB than students from a public university in the Midwestern U.S. Furthermore, when comparing 630 Japanese with 283 U.S. college students, Kitayama et al. (2000) found that positive emotions (e.g., calm, elated) were most closely related to interpersonally engaged emotions (e.g., friendly feelings) in Japan, whereas in the U.S. positive emotions were associated with interpersonally disengaged positive emotions (e.g., pride). Kitayama et al. speculated that positive emotions could be linked to independence of the self for students in the U.S. while interdependence of the self was correlated with positive emotions for Japanese students.

The above review indicates that, in addition to racial and ethnic group membership, cultural factors, such as independent/interdependent self-construal, acculturation levels, and ethnic identity could also influence how individuals experience various emotions (Jang et al. 2010, Molix and Bettencourt 2010). Due to the paucity of empirical studies in this area, how these cultural factors impact the pursuit of emotional well-being for individuals with different racial and ethnic backgrounds remain unclear.

5.6 Methodological Issues and Directions for Future Research

Literature reviews on racial and ethnic differences in well-being research evidently indicate the need to devote more empirical attention to this area. Also, several methodological issues need to be addressed to produce theoretically and scientifically sound results.

First, although well-being research has existed for decades, cross-racial validity of several key well-being measures (e.g., Subjective Happiness Scale; Lyubomirsky and Lepper 1999, ABS; Bradburn 1969) is a topic left mostly unexamined. Conceptual and measurement equivalence should be established before meaningful comparisons can be made across racial and ethnic groups. Conceptual equivalence can be assumed when a psychological concept as perceived by individuals in one racial or ethnic group has an equivalent for people in another group (van de Vijver 2001). Qualitative research designed to explore what it means to have a happy life in different racial groups could help to establish evidence for conceptual equivalence of well-being constructs. Furthermore, measurement equivalence is present when instruments are measuring a well-being construct in an equivalent manner across groups, and this can be tested via multiple-group confirmatory factor analysis. Both qualitative inquiry and quantitative scrutiny on the meaning of the construct and psychometric properties of well-being measures are needed to ensure that we are comparing "apples" with "apples" when making conclusions about well-being of individuals with different racial and ethnic backgrounds. A thorough discussion on these issues is beyond the scope of this chapter. Those who are interested in these topics may see Chaps. 3 and 4 of this volume or Miller and Sheu (2008) and Sheu and Sedlacek (2009).

Another methodological issue pertains to unequal and relatively small sample sizes of racial and ethnic groups in well-being research (Rankin et al. 2009; Thomas and Holmes 1992). Different sample sizes will lead to differential statistical power in detecting differences between groups, and small sample sizes often produce unreliable results. Future research should strive for larger and compatible sample sizes to generate reliable and valid cross-racial comparisons on well-being outcomes. Researchers should also keep in mind that individuals with different racial and ethnic backgrounds may exhibit different response patterns to a Likert-type scale. For example, Chinese and Japanese Americans tend to choose mid-point of the metric when responding to items on positive emotions while White Americans may be more likely to use "often" response category for the same items (Lee et al. 2002). Finally, to complement existing cross-sectional findings, longitudinal designs can be used to establish temporal order of well-being predictor and outcome variables, and experimental research can be utilized to test causal relationships between these variables.

In addition to the inclusion of cultural variables as recommended by Sheu and Lent (2009), future empirical efforts should also focus on theory-based research. In recent years, different theoretical frameworks, such as social cognitive perspective and self-determination theory, have been developed for well-being research (Lent 2004; Ryan and Deci 2000). Researchers have adopted these theories in predicting well-being of different racial, ethnic, or cultural groups, including Mexican Americans (Ojeda et al. 2011), African Americans (Yap et al. 2011), Asian American (Sheu et al. 2011), and Portuguese college students (Lent et al. 2009). More research should be devoted to applying the same theoretical model to different racial and ethnic groups to improve our understanding of how the same set of theory-derived predictors function differently (or similarly) as predictors of well-being for individuals in each group. Findings from this line of research will provide relevant guidelines to practitioners on how to adjust intervention strategies to fit the needs of individuals with different racial and ethnic backgrounds.

5.7 An Exemplar of Testing Racial and Ethnic Differences in Well-Being Outcomes

An empirical investigation is presented here as an exemplar to address some of the methodological issues discussed in the previous section. Specifically, it tested measurement equivalence before comparing positive emotions and life satisfaction among Asian American, Latino/a American, and White American college students. The exemplar utilized data of 150 participants from each of these groups, which were randomly drawn from a data set collected at a large public university in the U.S. Other findings derived from this data set have been reported elsewhere (e.g., Sheu 2012).

The current sample (n = 450) consisted of college students who had a mean age of 20.31 years and a mean GPA of 3.27 on a 0–4 scale. Participants were 49 % male and 51 % female with similar gender breakdown within each racial and ethnic group. Following the procedure used by Kitayama et al. (2000), four pairs of adjectives were selected to assess positive emotions: angry-calm, tense-relaxed, nervous-at ease, and discontented-contented. Participants rated these items on a 1–9 scale with higher average scores indicating higher positive emotions. Reliability estimates were .75 to .83 across Asian American, Latino/a American, and White American groups. Life satisfaction was assessed by the 5-item Satisfaction with Life Scale (SWLS; Diener et al. 1985). A sample item is "The conditions of my life are excellent." Higher average scores represent greater satisfaction with life. Reliability estimates derived from the current sample ranged from .80 to .87 across the three groups.

Measurement equivalence concerns the extent to which the psychometric properties of the item scores are generalizable across groups/conditions or over time. It allows us to infer that the instrument is measuring the same construct in the same way across different groups, and the differences among groups are caused by the construct of our interest rather than measurement artifacts. In this exemplar, three different types of measurement equivalence (i.e., configural invariance, metric invariance, and scalar invariance) were tested for the purpose of making cross-racial and ethnic comparisons on positive emotions and life satisfaction. Configural invariance assesses whether the same factor configuration is applicable to different groups separately, whereas metric invariance and scalar invariance evaluate the degree to which the magnitudes of factor loadings and item intercepts (i.e., the value of the measured item when the value of the common factor is zero) are equivalent across groups (see Miller and Sheu 2008; Vandenberg and Lance 2000 for reviews). Using various structural equation modeling (SEM) techniques in EQS 6.1 (Bentler and Wu 2005), the three types of measurement equivalence were tested sequentially in the order they are introduced here. The criteria of Comparative Fit Index (CFI) $\geq .95$ and Standardized Root Mean Square Residual (SRMR) $\leq .08$ (Hu and Bentler 1999) were used to evaluate data model fit, and the alpha level of .01 was adopted to accommodate the number of analyses when comparing models and testing racial and ethnic differences.

For the four items used to measure positive emotions, confirmatory factor analysis was used in the first step to test configural invariance, in which the same 1-factor structure was imposed separately on the data of Asian Americans ($\chi^2 = 1.24$, $df = 2$, $p = .54$; CFI = 1.00, SRMR = .02), Latino/a Americans ($\chi^2 = 4.55$, $df = 2$, $p = .10$; CFI = .99, SRMR = .03), and White Americans ($\chi^2 = 16.82$, $df = 2$, $p < .001$; CFI = .93, SRMR = .05). These findings indicated that the 1-factor structure was appropriate for all three groups in assessing positive emotions. Using multi-group SEM techniques, the second step involved constraining the factor loading on each item to be equal across groups, and comparing this model with the model without any constraints. Metric invariance was supported by a non-significant result in comparing these two models; that is, factor loadings of each of the four items were compatible across the three groups. Scalar invariance was tested in the third step, in which the intercept of each item was assumed to be equal across groups. The result showed evidence for partial scalar invariance because three out of four items had statistically compatible intercepts across the three racial and ethnic groups.

Together, these findings offered strong evidence for measurement equivalence and indicated that the four items were measuring positive emotions in the same way across the three groups. The next step was to test group differences in latent means of positive emotions, which controls for measurement imprecision and therefore paints a more accurate picture about racial and ethnic differences. With the presence of fully constrained factor loadings and partially constrained intercepts derived from previous steps, the results of a Latent Means analysis showed that Latino/a Americans had higher positive emotions than Asian Americans ($b = .41$, $z = 2.74$, $p = .006$), and the effect size ($\hat{d}$) was .35. The differences between White Americans and Asian Americans and between White Americans and Latino/a Americans did not reach the predetermined significance level.

The same procedure was carried out to examine measurement equivalence of the SWLS for assessing life satisfaction. The robust maximum likelihood estimation was used due to the violence of the multivariate normality assumption. The first step showed that the same 1-factor structure fit the data well for Asian Americans (S-B $\chi^2 = 4.33$, $df = 5$, $p = .50$; CFI = 1.00, SRMR = .03), Latino/a Americans (S-B $\chi^2 = 10.14$, $df = 5$, $p = .07$; CFI = .98, SRMR = .04), and White Americans (S-B $\chi^2 = 11.51$, $df = 5$, $p < .01$; CFI = .97, SRMR = .04). While results of the second step supported metric invariance with compatible factor loadings across groups, those of the third step indicated the lack of scalar invariance. Intercepts of all five SWLS items varied significantly as the function of group membership. The lack of scalar invariance suggested that meaningful mean comparisons in life satisfaction among the three groups could not be made because measurement artifacts, instead of the construct itself, might account for differences among Asian Americans, Latino/a Americans, and White Americans. In spite of this limitation, it should be noted that the presence of configural and metric invariance allows for examining the relations of SWLS scores to other variables among these three groups.

In cross-cultural or cross-racial research, measurement equivalence is often assumed, not tested. The exemplar demonstrated the procedure for testing this important assumption before making cross-racial comparisons in positive emotions and life satisfaction. Results supported measurement equivalence for the four items on positive emotions and showed that Latino/a Americans had higher positive emotions than Asian Americans. This cross-racial difference is consistent with previous research (Jang et al. 2010). On the other hand, while the factor structure and factor loadings of the SWLS were invariant, the lack of scalar invariance suggested that it was not appropriate to use the SWLS to compare means of life satisfaction among Asian American, Latino/a American, and White American college students from this sample.

5.8 Conclusions

In this chapter, research relevant to racial and ethnic differences in happiness and positive/negative emotions were reviewed. White Americans and Latino/a Americans tended to report higher affective well-being than other racial groups. Variables, such as acculturation and ethnic identity, were also found to be associated with well-being. These findings should be interpreted with caution because of methodological flaws in existing literatures. Included to address some of the methodological issues, an exemplar showed that the items used to assess positive emotions were equivalent across three racial and ethnic groups, and that Latino/a Americans reported higher positive emotions than Asian Americans. However, the lack of scalar invariance precluded the possibility of using the SWLS to compare life satisfaction across groups. Future research should employ psychometrically sound measures to assess the affective component of well-being cross-racially and should be based on theories that include relevant cultural factors to account for racial and ethnic differences.

References

Aune, K. S., & Aune, R. K. (1996). Cultural differences in the self-report experience and expression of emotions in relationships. *Journal of Cross-Cultural Psychology, 29*, 67–81. doi:10.1177/0022022196271005.

Bentler, P. M., & Wu, E. J. C. (2005). *EQS 6.1 for Windows user's guide*. Encino: Multivariate Software.

Bradburn, N. M. (1969). *The structure of psychological well-being*. Chicago: Aldine.

Brown, T. N., Wallace, J. M., & Williams, D. R. (2001). Race-related correlates of young adults' subjective well-being. *Social Indicators Research, 53*, 97–116. doi:10.1023/A:1007190226538.

Burton, R. P. D., Rushing, B., Ritter, C., & Rakocy, A. (1993). Roles, race and subjective well-being: A longitudinal analysis of elderly men. *Social Indicators Research, 28*, 137–156. doi:10.1007/BF01079655.

Bushman, B. B., & Crowley, S. L. (2010). Is the structure of affect similar for younger and older children? Cross-sectional differences in negative and positive affectivity. *Journal of Psychoeducational Assessment, 28*, 31–39. doi:10.1177/0734282909337584.

Collins, J. W., David, R. J., Handler, A., Wall, S., & Andes, S. (2004). Very low birthweight in African American infants: The role of maternal exposure to interpersonal racial discrimination. *American Journal of Public Health, 94*, 2132–2138. doi:10.2105/AJPH.94.12.2132.

Compton, W. C., Smith, M. L., Cornish, K. A., & Qualls, D. L. (1996). Factor structure of mental health measures. *Journal of Personality and Social Psychology, 71*, 406–413. doi:10.1037/0022-3514.71.2.406.

Diener, E. (1984). Subjective well-being. *Psychological Bulletin, 95*, 542–575. doi:10.1037/0033-2909.95.3.542.

Diener, E., & Suh, E. M. (Eds.). (2000). *Culture and subjective well-being*. Cambridge, MA: The MIT Press.

Diener, E., Emmons, A., Larsen, R. J., & Griffin, S. (1985). The Satisfaction with Life Scale. *Journal of Personality Assessment, 49*, 71–75. doi:10.1207/s15327752jpa4901_13.

Diener, E., Diener, M., & Diener, C. (1995). Factors predicting the subjective well-being of nations. *Journal of Personality and Social Psychology, 69*, 851–864. doi:10.1037/0022-3514.69.5.851.

Diener, E., Lucas, R. E., & Oishi, S. (2002). Subjective well-being: The science of happiness and life satisfaction. In C. R. Snyder & S. J. Lopez (Eds.), *Handbook of positive psychology* (pp. 63–73). New York: Oxford University Press.

Hills, P., & Argyle, M. (2002). The Oxford happiness questionnaire: A compact scale for the measurement of psychological well-being. *Personality and Individual Differences, 33*, 1073–1082. doi:10.1016/S0191-8869(01)00213-6.

Hu, L. T., & Bentler, P. M. (1999). Cutoff criteria for fit indexes in covariance structure analysis: Conventional criteria versus new alternatives. *Structural Equation Modeling: A Multidisciplinary Journal, 6*, 1–55. doi:10.1080/10705519909540118.

Huebner, E. S. (1995). The Students' Life Satisfaction Scale: An assessment of psychometric properties with Black and White elementary school students. *Social Indicators Research, 34*, 315–323. doi:10.1007/BF01078690.

Huebner, E. S., Suldo, S., Valois, R. F., Drane, J. W., & Zullig, K. (2004). Brief Multidimensional Students' Life Satisfaction Scale: Sex, race, and grade effects for a high school sample. *Psychological Reports, 94*, 351–356. doi:10.2466/pr0.94.1.351-356.

Hughes, M., & Thomas, M. E. (1998). The continuing significance of race revisited: A study of race, class, and quality of life in America, 1972 to 1996. *American Sociological Review, 63*, 785–795. doi:10.2307/2657501.

Jang, Y., Kwag, K. H., & Chiriboga, D. A. (2010). Not saying I am happy does not mean I am not: Cultural influences on responses to positive affect items in the CES-D. *Journal of Gerontology: Psychological Sciences, 65B*, 684–690. doi:10.1093/geronb/gbq052.

Kashdan, T. B., Biswas-Diener, R., & King, L. A. (2008). Reconsidering happiness: The costs of distinguishing between hedonics and eudaimonia. *Journal of Positive Psychology, 3*, 219–233. doi:10.1080/17439760802303044.

Keyes, C. L. M., & Annas, J. (2009). Feeling good and functioning well: Distinctive concepts in ancient philosophy and contemporary science. *Journal of Positive Psychology, 4*, 197–201. doi:10.1080/17439760902844228.

Kitayama, S., Markus, H. R., & Kurokawa, M. (2000). Culture, emotion, and well-being: Good feelings in Japan and the United States. *Cognitive and Emotion, 14*, 93–124. doi:10.1080/026999300379003.

Kitayama, S., Markus, H. R., & Matsumoto, H. (1995). Culture, self, and emotion: A cultural perspective on "self-conscious" emotions'. In J. P. Tangney & K. W. Fischer (Eds.), *Self-conscious emotions: The psychology of shame, guilt, embarrassment, and pride* (pp. 439–464). New York: Guilford Press.

Laurent, J., Catanzaro, S. J., Joiner, T. E., Rudolph, K. D., Potter, K. I., Lambert, S., Osborne, L., & Gathright, T. (1999). A measure of positive and negative affect for children: Scale development and preliminary validation. *Psychologist Assessment, 11*, 326–338. doi:10.1037/1040-3590.11.3.326.

Lawrence, R. H., & Liang, J. (1988). Structural integration of the Affect Balance Scale and the Life Satisfaction Index A: Race, sex, and age differences. *Psychology and Aging, 3*, 375–384. doi:10.1037/0882-7974.3.4.375.

Le, T. N., Lai, M. H., & Wallen, J. (2009). Multiculturalism and subjective happiness as mediated by cultural and relational variables. *Cultural Diversity and Ethnic Minority Psychology, 15*, 303–313. doi:10.1037/a0015507.

Lee, J. W., Jones, P. S., Mineyama, Y., & Zhang, X. E. (2002). Cultural differences in response to a Likert scale. *Research in Nursing & Health, 25*, 295–306. doi:10.1002/nur.10041.

Lent, R. W. (2004). Toward a unifying theoretical and practical perspective on well-being and psychosocial adjustment. *Journal of Counseling Psychology, 51*, 482–509. doi:10.1037/0022-0167.51.4.482.

Lent, R. W., Taveira, M., Sheu, H., & Singley, D. (2009). Social cognitive predictors of academic adjustment and life satisfaction in Portuguese college students: A longitudinal analysis. *Journal of Vocational Behavior, 74*, 190–198. doi:10.1016/j.jvb.2008.12.006.

Leu, J., Wang, J., & Koo, K. (2011). Are positive emotions just as "positive" across cultures? *Emotion, 11*, 994–999. doi:10.1037/a0021332.

Linley, P. A., Harrington, S., & Garcea, N. (Eds.). (2010). *Oxford handbook of positive psychology and work*. New York: Oxford University Press.

Lu, L., & Gilmour, R. (2004). Culture and conceptions of happiness: Individual oriented and social oriented SWB. *Journal of Happiness Studies, 5*, 269–291. doi:10.1007/s10902-004-8789-5.

Lyubomirsky, S., & Lepper, H. S. (1999). A measure of subjective happiness: Preliminary reliability and construct validation. *Social Indicators Research, 46*, 137–155. doi:10.1023/A:1006824100041.

Maitland, S. B., Dixon, R. A., Hultsch, D. F., & Hertzog, C. (2001). Well-being as a moving target: Measurement equivalence of the Bradburn Affect Balance Scale. *Journal of Gerontology: Psychological Sciences, 56B*, 69–77. doi:10.1093/geronb/56.2.P69.

Miller, M., & Sheu, H. (2008). Measurement and research issues in multicultural psychology. In S. D. Brown & R. W. Lent (Eds.), *Handbook of counseling psychology* (4th ed., pp. 103–120). New York: Wiley.

Molix, L., & Bettencourt, B. A. (2010). Predicting well-being among ethnic minorities: Psychological empowerment and group identity. *Journal of Applied Social Psychology, 40*, 513–533. doi:10.1111/j.1559-1816.2010.00585.x.

Ojeda, L., Flores, L. Y., & Navarro, R. L. (2011). Social cognitive predictors of Mexican American college students' academic and life satisfaction. *Journal of Counseling Psychology, 58*, 61–71. doi:10.1037/a0021687.

Okazaki, S. (1997). Sources of ethnic differences between Asian American and White American college students on measures of depression and social anxiety. *Journal of Abnormal Psychology, 106*, 52–60. doi:10.1037/0021-843X.106.1.52.

Okazaki, S. (2000). Asian American and White American differences on affective distress symptoms: Do symptom reports differ across reporting methods? *Journal of Cross-Cultural Psychology, 31*, 603–625. doi:10.1177/0022022100031005004.

Ram, R. (2010). Social capital and happiness: Additional cross-country evidence. *Journal of Happiness Studies, 11*, 409–418. doi:10.1007/s10902-009-9148-3.

Rankin, L. E., Jost, J. T., & Wakslak, C. J. (2009). System justification and the meaning of life: Are the existential benefits of ideology distributed unequally across racial groups? *Social Justice Research, 22*, 312–333. doi:10.1007/s11211-009-0100-9.

Ryan, R. M., & Deci, E. L. (2000). Self-determination theory and the facilitation of intrinsic motivation, social development, and well-being. *American Psychologist, 55*, 68–78. doi:10.1037/0003-066X.55.1.68.

Ryff, C. D. (1989). Happiness is everything, or is it? Explorations on the meaning of psychological well-being. *Journal of Personality and Social Psychology, 57*, 1069–1081. doi:10.1037/0022-3514.57.6.1069.

Scollon, C. N., Diener, E., Oishi, S., & Biswas-Diener, R. (2009). Emotions across cultures and methods. In E. Diener (Ed.), *Culture and well-being: The collected works of Ed Diener* (pp. 203–228). New York: Springer.

Sheldon, K. M., & Hoon, T. H. (2007). The multiple determination of well-being: Independent effects of positive traits, needs, goals, selves, social supports, and cultural contexts. *Journal of Happiness Studies, 8*, 565–592.

Sheu, H. (Chair). (2012, July). *Using self-determination theory to predict well-being of college students of Asian descent in Singapore, Taiwan, and the U.S.* Symposium presented at the 30th International Congress of Psychology, Cape Town.

Sheu, H., & Lent, R. W. (2009). A social cognitive perspective on well-being in educational and work settings: Cross-cultural consideration. *International Journal for Educational and Vocational Guidance, 9*, 45–60. doi:10.1007/s10775-008-9147-7.

Sheu, H., & Sedlacek, W. E. (2009). Cross-cultural issues in counseling research. In C. C. Lee, D. A. Burnhill, A. L. Butler, C. P. Hipolito-Delgado, M. Humphrey, O. Muñoz, et al. (Eds.), *Elements of culture in counseling* (pp. 226–241). Boston: Allyn & Bacon.

Sheu, H., Chong, S. S., Lin, W., & Chen, H. (2011, August). *Well-being of Asian American students: A self-determination perspective*. Poster presented at the 2011 annual convention of the Asian American Psychological Association, Washington, DC.

Thomas, M. E., & Holmes, B. J. (1992). Determinants of satisfaction for blacks and whites. *The Sociological Quarterly, 33*, 459–472. doi:10.1111/j.1533-8525.1992.tb00385.x.

Tsai, J. L., Knutson, B., & Fung, H. H. (2006). Cultural variation in affect valuation. *Journal of Personality and Social Psychology, 90*, 288–307. doi:10.1037/0022-3514.90.2.288.

Uchida, Y., & Kitayama, S. (2009). Happiness and unhappiness in east and west: Themes and variations. *Emotion, 9*, 441–456. doi:10.1037/a0015634.

Uchida, Y., Norasakkunkit, V., & Kitayama, S. (2004). Cultural constructions of happiness: Theory and empirical evidence. *Journal of Happiness Studies, 5*, 223–239. doi:10.1007/s10902-004-8785-9.

van de Vijver, F. J. R. (2001). The evolution of cross-cultural research methods. In D. Matsumoto (Ed.), *The handbook of culture and psychology*. New York: Oxford University Press.

Vandenberg, R. J., & Lance, C. E. (2000). A review and synthesis of the measurement invariance literature: Suggestions, practices, and recommendations for organizational research. *Organizational Research Methods, 3*, 4–70. doi:10.1177/109442810031002.

Watson, D., & Clark, L. A. (1994). *PANAS-X: Manual for the positive and negative affect schedule – Expanded form*. Unpublished manuscript, The University of Iowa.

Watson, D., Clark, L. A., & Tellegen, A. (1988). Development and validation of brief measures of positive and negative affect: The PANAS Scales. *Journal of Personality and Social Psychology, 54*, 1063–1070. doi:10.1037/0022-3514.54.6.1063.

Yang, Y. (2008). Social inequalities in happiness in the United States, 1972 to 2004: An age-period-cohort analysis. *American Psychological Review, 73*, 204–226.

Yap, S. C. Y., Settles, I. H., & Pratt-Hyatt, J. S. (2011). Mediators of the relationship between racial identity and life satisfaction in a community sample of African American women and men. *Cultural Diversity and Ethnic Minority Psychology, 17*, 89–97. doi:10.1037/a0022535.

Chapter 6
Cognitive Constructs in the Context of Positive Psychology

Christine Robitschek, Danielle Sirles, and Erin E. Hardin

How we think matters. For example, our abilities to process information will have obvious impact on how well we succeed in the educational system. *What* we think also matters. Cognitive theories (e.g., Barutta et al. 2011; Beck 1976) tell us that if we think of ourselves, our environment, and the future as positive we are more likely not to be depressed than people who think of these things as negative. Our cognitive processes and content affect every domain of our lives, including school, work, and interpersonal relationships, and influence multiple aspects of these domains, including functioning and satisfaction.

The topic of this chapter is positive cognitive constructs, with a focus on diversity defined by race, ethnicity, and/or national heritage. The majority of our attention will be given to constructs that are primarily cognitive. In addition, limited attention will be given to other more complex psychological constructs with important cognitive components (i.e., that also contain other important components). Relevant constructs exist in two well-known taxonomies of positive human traits, the Clifton StrengthsFinder 2.0 (Rath 2007) and the Values in Action – Inventory of Strengths (VIA-IS: Peterson et al. 2005), and identified additional relevant constructs not included in these taxonomies that are prominent or gaining prominence in the literature. We will begin with an overview of the current state of the literature on these constructs, including a summary of the extent to which culture has been addressed across the identified constructs as well as information from large scale studies. This is followed by a description of the Cultural Lens Approach (CLA; Hardin 2007), which provides the theoretical perspective through which we

C. Robitschek, Ph.D. (✉) • D. Sirles
Department of Psychology, Texas Tech University, 18th and Boston,
Lubbock, TX 79409-2051, USA
e-mail: chris.robitschek@ttu.edu

E.E. Hardin
Department of Psychology, University of Tennessee – Knoxville, Austin Peay Building,
University of Tennessee, Knoxville, TN 37996, USA

J. Teramoto Pedrotti and L.M. Edwards (eds.), *Perspectives on the Intersection of Multiculturalism and Positive Psychology*, Cross-Cultural Advancements in Positive Psychology 7, DOI 10.1007/978-94-017-8654-6_6,

evaluated the literature for this chapter. Briefly, the CLA applies a deeper cultural perspective on theory than is typical of most multicultural perspectives, requiring practitioners and scholars to view constructs through a cultural lens. The main body of the chapter provides examples of constructs that are covered well versus poorly in the literature, all viewed through the CLA, to provide readers with a vision of *what is* and *what could be* regarding multicultural research on positive cognitive constructs.

6.1 Current State of the Literature

Table 6.1 lists the positive cognitive constructs covered here along with their definitions. Ten primarily cognitive strengths can be found in the StrengthsFinder 2.0 (Rath 2007). In the VIA-IS (Peterson et al. 2005), the five strengths in the wisdom and knowledge category are primarily cognitive, as are four additional strengths categorized elsewhere in the measure. We identified six important primarily cognitive constructs found outside these taxonomies. Of these, self-efficacy (Bandura 1977) and life satisfaction (Diener et al. 1985) will be examined in greater detail. There also are relevant constructs within the two taxonomies that seemed to contain a blend of cognitive and other important components (such as emotional or relational; see Table 6.1). In StrengthsFinder 2.0 we found eight such constructs; from the VIA-IS, we identified two. Outside these taxonomies we identified personal growth initiative (Robitschek 1998; Robitschek et al. 2012), which will be discussed below.

The quantity and quality of multicultural and cross-cultural research involving these positive cognitive constructs is quite varied. For example, a strength of this literature is the large-scale cross-national research used in development of the VIA-IS and StrengthsFinder (e.g., Peterson et al. 2005; Rath 2007). This research recognized there may be important differences between cultures in the perceptions of strengths but also looked for possible commonalities in these perceptions (Lopez et al. 2005; Niemiec 2011). Little research has examined within group differences for any of the constructs. Of course, this is a limitation for much of the multicultural psychology research at this time. We were able to locate considerable multicultural and cross-cultural research for some constructs (e.g., self-efficacy and satisfaction with life), and little relevant research outside of the large-scale cross-national research used for instrument development for other constructs such as the StrengthsFinder aspects of belief and ideation. Attempts to establish conceptual equivalence vary in these studies as well. Sections that follow describe the quality and quantity of the literature in more detail.

6.1.1 *What Do Large Scale Studies Tell Us?*

Large-scale, cross-national research provides evidence for pan-cultural positive cognitive constructs. Research on the StrengthsFinder supports the universality of the 34 character strengths, with relatively similar structure across many different cultures (Lopez et al. 2005). Regardless of an individual's language or country of

Table 6.1 Primarily and partially cognitive constructs and their definitions

Construct	Definition
Primarily cognitive constructs	
StrengthsFinder 2.0[a]	
Analytical	Searching for and considering causes and effects
Belief	Possessing enduring values that are expressed across life domains
Context	Utilizing historical information and perspectives to formulate visions of the present and future
Futuristic	Focus on future possibilities that one applies across situations
Ideation	Captivated by the content of ideas and connections among phenomena that they bring
Intellection	Captivated by one's own process of thinking
Relator	Attitude toward existing relationships that leads to strengthening bonds
Responsibility	Attitude of an ethical/moral obligation to fulfill one's commitments
Self-assurance	Confidence in our own decisions and judgments
Strategic	Ability to think ahead and formulate a plan of action taking into account the "what-ifs"
VIA-IS[b]	
Creativity	Generating/using ideas for artistic, problem-solving, or communication purposes
Judgment and open-mindedness	Ability to critically evaluate information; base decisions on this information
Love of learning	Strong desire to add knowledge, in many areas by multiple methods
Perspective	Viewpoints of life and the world that are helpful to self and others
Social intelligence	Accurately perceiving internal experiences of others and knowing how to become part of multiple social groups
Appreciation of beauty and excellence	Valuing/experiencing wonder when encountering beauty or talent in any area of life
Hope	Anticipating a positive future and working to bring it to fruition
Religiousness and spirituality	Possessing thoughtful beliefs about purpose and meaning in life
Constructs outside the taxonomies	
Self-efficacy[c]	Confidence in one's abilities to perform specific behaviors
Collective efficacy[d]	Beliefs about group's ability to plan and carry out activities and tasks
Vocational interests[e]	Extent to which we like or dislike specific activities that can be related to the world of work
Self-acceptance[f]	A positive perspective on all components of the self
Hypo-egoic states[g]	Weighing one's own needs and wants as equal to other people's needs and wants and other external considerations
Life satisfaction[h]	Cognitive assessment of one's overall quality of life
Mindfulness[i]	Awareness of an immersion in the present moment
Partially cognitive constructs	
StrengthsFinder 2.0	
Arranger	Flexible and effective organization
Connectedness	Belief in the interconnectedness of all things; everything happens for a reason

(continued)

Table 6.1 (continued)

Construct	Definition
Deliberative	Carefully considering all aspects and potential risks in any situation; also applying this care in one's actions
Individualization	Being knowledgeable about the unique qualities of other people
Input	Amassing large quantities of information
Learner	Seeking out opportunities to learn
Positivity	Taking an optimistic view of life
Restorative	Problem-solving capabilities
VIA-IS	
Curiosity	Engaging in experiences to satisfy desires for discovery/exploration
Self-regulation	Exercising control over one's thoughts, feelings, and behaviors
Constructs outside the taxonomies	
Personal growth initiative[j]	Intentional engagement in the self-improvement process

[a]Rath (2007)
[b]Peterson et al. (2005)
[c]Bandura (1977)
[d]Bandura (2000, 2002)
[e]Hansen (2005)
[f]Ryff (1989)
[g]Leary and Guadagno (2011)
[h]Diener et al. (1985)
[i]Schuster (1979)
[j]Robitschek (1998)

residence, some researchers state that the StrengthsFinder is capable of revealing personal assets that, if nurtured and fully developed, can lead to educational and vocational success (Lopez et al. 2005).

Much like the StrengthsFinder, developers of the VIA-IS maintain that similar cognitive constructs can be found across the globe (Dahlsgaard et al. 2005; Park et al. 2006). These positive traits are seen as not only important to individual success but also essential to the health of general society (Park et al. 2006). Multinational research suggests that VIA-IS character strengths follow the same maturation process, are defined similarly, and have the same amount of social appeal in both highly developed and developing societies (Biswas-Diener 2006; Niemiec 2011; Park et al. 2006), suggesting that the identified positive cognitive constructs do not differ across cultures or national boundaries. This said, methodological issues may make comparisons difficult when using measures designed primarily in the West (Diener and Suh 2000). Thus, an alternate perspective, suggests that at least some constructs cannot be understood outside specific cultural contexts (e.g., Constantine and Sue 2006; Helms 1992; Sue and Sue 2013). Researchers espousing this perspective argue that constructs must be considered within their unique contexts to determine the extent to which they are or are not universal. Building upon this literature, we propose an approach for viewing cognitive cultural constructs, the CLA (Hardin 2007, 2010).

6.2 The Cultural Lens Approach

Most multicultural approaches focus on distinguishing between (e.g., Leong and Brown 1995) or integrating (Cheung et al. 2011) etic (universal) and emic (culturally specific) theoretical propositions, thereby using the multicultural approach in a primarily evaluative function. Similarly, most of what has been written about cultural equivalence has focused on evaluating characteristics of assessment instruments (e.g., Hui and Triandis 1989), specifically either conceptual (Lonner 1985) or methodological/statistical (e.g., Ægisdottir et al. 2008) types of equivalence in assessment instruments (see Chaps. 3 and 4 in this volume for a more full description of equivalence). In other words, existing perspectives in cross-cultural and multicultural research focus on evaluating and determining *the extent to which* concepts, theory, and measures are equivalent across cultures. And then based on this evaluation, researchers and practitioners should make decisions about *whether or not to use* the existing measures and constructs with specific populations. In a sense, these approaches are using a process similar to summative evaluation that is, focusing on *bottom line* questions regarding use (c.f., McDavid and Hawthorn 2006; Weiss 1998). In this example, *use* is operationalized as use of the construct based on assessed cultural equivalence.

In contrast, the Cultural Lens Approach (Hardin 2007, 2010; Hardin et al. in press) takes a formative evaluation perspective (c.f. McDavid and Hawthorn 2006; Weiss 1998) meaning that the intended use of the approach is to enhance the object of the evaluation, in this case the cultural utility of constructs and theory. This approach goes deeper than the summative evaluative functions that yield use/do not use or relevant/not relevant decisions. Instead of asking only "Is this construct or theoretical proposition equivalent across cultures?" the CLA asks "In what ways might this construct or theoretical proposition be operationalized in culturally relevant ways so that it is applicable or useful in this culture?" The emphasis in the CLA is on experimental and behavioral operationalization and utility of constructs and theoretical propositions, more so than equivalence in measurement. This approach broadens not only the cultural validity, but importantly also the utility of existing and new theories. The CLA offers a systematic multi-step approach to examining the impact of functional and conceptual equivalence on theoretical propositions and actual behavior *and then using this knowledge to apply theoretical propositions and constructs in culturally appropriate ways in research.* This approach generates testable hypotheses to stimulate future research that broadens our understanding not only of cultural differences in the expression of theoretical constructs, but also of the implications of these differences for theory development and implementation, and people's real-life experiences. Whereas traditional approaches focus on questions of the conceptual or functional equivalence of measures (e.g., "Is this measure of self-esteem valid with different cultural groups?"), the CLA uses the answer to such questions to focus on broader questions about the cultural validity of theoretical propositions (e.g., "Is the proposition that higher self-esteem is associated with positive outcomes valid with different cultural groups?").

The CLA comprises five steps (Hardin et al. in press), beginning with steps similar to conceptual equivalence and then moving beyond this limited perspective.

1. "*Articulate how central constructs have been defined (implicitly or explicitly) and thus operationalized in past research*" (p. 9).
   - In the example of the theoretical proposition that *Higher self-esteem is associated with positive outcomes*, one central construct is *self-esteem*, which has been defined as a positive attitude toward or evaluation of the self (Rosenberg 1965). Note that implicit in the definition of self-esteem and explicit in the measurement tool is the assumption of an *individual* or *personal* self. This step is similar to elements of traditional assessment for conceptual equivalence.
2. "*Identify the groups (a) from which the constructs have been derived and (b) to which the constructs have either not been applied or with which surprising results have been found*" (p. 10).
   - This is the part of the approach in which culture begins to play a role. In the case of self-esteem, before 1990, almost all of the outcome research linking self-esteem to positive outcomes such as greater satisfaction with life (see Diener 1984) was done with White North Americans; although a few studies did examine self-esteem among racial and ethnic minorities in the U.S. (e.g., Martinez and Dukes 1987) or elsewhere (e.g., Verkuyten 1989), these studies tended to focus on between-groups differences in mean levels of self-esteem.
3. "*Identify relevant dimensions underlying cultural variability: What do we know about the cultural contexts of groups A and B?*" (p. 10).
   - In this step the researcher assembles cultural knowledge needed to understand why inter- and intra-group differences noted in Step 2 might exist. Consideration of ethnic and other (e.g., social class) cultural factors is important. Questions in this step include: *What are salient cultural differences between the groups in question and how might they be relevant?* In the example of self-esteem, Luhtanen and Crocker (1992) recognized that the *individual or private self* is one of several possible selves; although this self is indeed likely to be most salient to White North Americans, the *collective* self is likely to be more salient among those from more collectivist cultures. At this step it is incumbent upon the researcher to fully explore multiple ways in which the groups might differ that have potential to be relevant.
4. "*Evaluate the definitions/operationalizations of the central constructs (from Step 1) in the context of broader cultural knowledge about those groups (from Step 3): What do we know about construct X within the cultural context of group B*" (p. 11).
   - This is the step that distinguishes the CLA from other approaches. It involves the integration of cultural knowledge from Step 3 with knowledge from Step 1 about how constructs and propositions have been operationalized previously. Researchers consider if existing conceptualizations are culturally limited. Regarding self-esteem, traditional approaches to equivalence would

stop after Step 3, concluding that existing measures of self-esteem are not culturally valid because of their exclusive focus on the individual self or that new measures of collective self-esteem are needed. However, the CLA goes one step further and considers the implications of these conclusions for the larger theoretical propositions. Possible questions at this step include: *How might we operationalize the constructs differently? How might the cultural factors we have identified impact how people experience this experimental manipulation?*

5. "*Derive research questions and specific hypotheses based on the questions and answers from Step 4*" (p. 12).
   - For example, returning to the larger theoretical proposition that *higher self-esteem is associated with positive outcomes*, we would here consider questions such as whether higher collective self-esteem is more likely to be associated with positive outcomes for some racial and ethnic minorities, whereas higher personal self-esteem is more likely to be associated with positive outcomes for White North Americans. This step goes beyond the summative evaluation nature of establishing or discrediting equivalence across cultures in measurement tools. Instead, this step compels us to integrate the knowledge of cultural context with the existing theoretical propositions to suggest testable hypotheses.

In this chapter, we will focus on Steps 4 and 5 of the CLA in order to evaluate the existing multicultural literature on positive cognitive constructs and to make recommendations for future research in this area.

6.3 Primarily Cognitive Constructs

Intellection (Rath 2007) provides an example of a positive cognitive construct that, although it may have similarities in mean scores across cultures, might be importantly different across cultures. When viewed through a Cultural Lens these differences might have implications for theory and behavior. Intellection refers to being captivated by one's own process of thinking (Buckingham and Clifton 2001). It is content-free, focused on the process of thinking itself. The summative evaluative nature of conceptual equivalence approaches would lead us to determine if there is equivalence across cultures in the measured operationalization of intellection. Then, based on this determination, researchers and practitioners would decide if it was appropriate to use established measures of intellection with specific cultural groups. In contrast, the CLA asks us to use this evaluative knowledge in a formative way, e.g., to adapt our behavioral operationalizations of intellection and relevant theoretical propositions within our research to accommodate cultural differences.

Consider the differences we might encounter if we group people who think about things (i.e., objects) with people who think about emotions as well as with people who think about data. Other taxonomies or theories would identify these as quite different from each other. For example, the Myers-Briggs Type Indicator identifies Thinking and Feeling as two different preferences for sources of information (Thinking or Feeling, n.d.). Yet if Feelings are a source of information, then surely we are processing the feelings in some way, which could be considered *thinking about feelings*. So does it matter if people from different cultures like to think about different things? Our answer is yes. In one culture the people identified as thinkers might be the scientists and scholars; driven by cultural values of rational thought, they might be skilled at thinking about how to solve problems and understand the world in a rational way. Elsewhere, the thinkers might be business executives; driven by cultural values of profit and prestige; they might be skilled at thinking about financial and marketing issues. In another culture the thinkers might be holy people; driven by cultural values of spirituality and connection to a higher power, they might be skilled at thinking about life meaning and purpose. And in yet another culture the thinkers might be the elderly; driven by cultural values of respect for elders, they might be skilled in wisdom and perspective. A conceptual equivalence approach would stop at decisions of whether or not to use existing measures of intellection. For example, the dominant culture in the U.S. might operationalize intellection as general intelligence, which is known to be a strong predictor of individual success (e.g., Ridgell and Lounsbury 2004). Inherent in this statement are culturally bound operationalizations of not only intellection but also of success. If we were to find that for another culture, intellection did not predict this type of success, we might assume that intellection was not a culturally valid construct. The CLA takes us beyond this, instead leading us to formulate specific testable hypotheses that take into account cultural operationalizations of constructs such as thinking and success. We might hypothesize that the theoretical proposition that intellection predicts success would be supported if the relevant constructs were operationalized in culturally appropriate ways. It also could be hypothesized that it is the culture-specific manifestation of intellection that is yielding importantly different relations with other constructs, such as culturally defined success. Further, if we operationalize intellection and success in ways consistent with the cultures we are studying, then this relation might be found across cultures. Unfortunately, we found little multicultural research on intellection or related constructs, and so view intellection as a fruitful avenue for future research from within the CLA.

Several of the positive cognitive constructs we identified have considerable multicultural research. These include hope, self-efficacy, optimism, responsibility, life satisfaction, wisdom, and knowledge. We focus on two of these constructs, *satisfaction with life* and *self-efficacy*, to provide examples of research being conducted and to evaluate the literature using the CLA.

6.3.1 Satisfaction with Life

Relevant multicultural research suggests that meeting basic needs, such as having sufficient resources for food, shelter, and education, is a more fundamental determinant of *satisfaction with life* than cultural factors (e.g., Oishi et al. 1999a). For example, Blacks and Latina/os in the U.S. report lower levels of satisfaction with life than do White Americans, and these differences appear to be accounted for largely by disparities in socioeconomic status, health, and social relationships in the samples studied (Barger, Donoho, and Wayment 2009). When basic needs are met, however, variability between having sufficient resources and having more than sufficient resources (i.e., wealth) matters little in predicting satisfaction with life (Pavot and Diener 2009). It is in these circumstances that culture has a more influential role in determining satisfaction with life (Oishi et al. 1999a). Interestingly, when members of racial or ethnic minority groups experience discrimination, this can have negative and positive effects on satisfaction with life. The negative effects are easy to understand, although the relationship can be mediated by dissatisfaction with the majority culture (Verkuyten 2008). The positive effects are less obvious. It seems that experiencing discrimination, particularly systematic discrimination embedded in the structure of the majority society, can increase ethnic identification in some individuals, which in turn can predict higher levels of satisfaction with life (Verkuyten 2008).

With the CLA we might first consider culturally diverse definitions of the terms *life* and *satisfaction*. This is similar to an examination of cultural/conceptual equivalence. Consider the wide range of answers that might be given in response to the statement "Tell me about your life." Similar to Super's (Super et al. 1996) conceptualization of the life-space, cultural factors may determine which life roles or domains are sufficiently salient to comprise one's life. If researchers do not stop to ask how one's life is operationalized, science might miss importantly different categories of potential predictors of satisfaction with life. Importantly, the CLA goes beyond this to formulate testable hypotheses regarding how these differing definitions of one's life might serve as mechanisms for enhancing satisfaction with life. For example, will satisfaction with culturally valued life roles predict satisfaction with life more strongly than prediction by satisfaction with culturally devalued life roles? The CLA also might suggest exploration of culturally-specific definitions of life domains. For example, much research has addressed the importance of interpersonal relationships in predicting and promoting satisfaction with life (e.g., Diener and Seligman 2002). However, virtually all of this research has operationalized *interpersonal relationships* in terms of dyadic relationships with family and close friends. We know, however, that the range of interpersonal relationships is often much broader for members of collectivist versus individualist cultures (Kang et al. 2003), and that it is important to distinguish between dyadic relations with important individuals (i.e., relational interdependence; Cross and Madson 1997) and collective relations with important groups (i.e., collective interdependence; Gabriel and Gardner 1999).

A final category of multicultural literature has additional similarities to the CLA. This type of research explores potential cultural moderators of the relations between predictors and satisfaction with life. The values-as-moderator model (Oishi et al. 1999b) identifies the importance of cultural values in moderating the relations of specific life domains with satisfaction with life and recognizes that the salience of these domains may vary across developmental stages. When a life domain is highly valued in a culture (and at a particular life-stage) that domain will be a stronger predictor of overall satisfaction with life. Initial support for this model (Oishi et al. 1999b) was found with a predominantly White American group of college students in the U.S. Subsequent research has extended to more diverse samples, including cross-national samples. For example, in a comparison of Korean and U.S. adolescents, Park and Huebner (2005) note the importance of cultural value differences. Most Korean students in this sample viewed educational pursuits and attainment as the most important aspect of their lives, compared with the Western emphasis on personal self-related concepts, such as self-esteem, independence, and personal interests (Park and Huebner 2005). This research supported the values-as-moderator model, in that satisfaction with school was a significant predictor of satisfaction with life only for Korean students and satisfaction with self was a significantly stronger predictor of satisfaction with life for US students than for Korean students. The CLA expands the values-as-moderator model in two ways. First, the CLA is not limited to cultural values, instead including other important cultural constructs, such as behaviors and identity. Second, the CLA follows up research such as the Park and Huebner (2005) study by generating testable hypotheses regarding the impact of varying the operationalization of all variables to improve cultural relevance. The values-as-moderator model appears to draw conclusions when moderation is found, rather than formulating hypotheses.

As this limited review indicates, there is both progress and potential in examining the cultural nuances of satisfaction with life from the CLA. Likely due to the highly generative nature of this construct, multicultural research on satisfaction with life has moved beyond simple questions about differences in mean levels of satisfaction with life to more sophisticated questions about cultural moderators (i.e., what predicts satisfaction with life for whom). We contend that researchers also need to carefully consider how life is operationalized when measuring satisfaction with life, as well as to consider how important predictors, such as interpersonal relationships, are defined. Such considerations raise important new questions about the cultural manifestations and predictors of satisfaction with life.

6.3.2 Self-Efficacy

The *self-efficacy* literature is vast. An online search in PsycInfo and MedLine using the term self-efficacy yielded almost 34,000 hits. Adding the term *culture* still yielded over 1,000 hits. Our discussion of self-efficacy will summarize briefly key findings in the multicultural research on this topic, describe the contributions of traditional approaches to equivalence, and apply the CLA to extend research in this area.

Literature reviews (e.g., Klassen 2004; Lindley 2006) indicate several general conclusions about the application of self-efficacy in diverse ethnic and cultural groups. First, self-efficacy tends to be higher in Western, individualistic societies and European American cultures than in Eastern, collectivist societies and ethnic minority cultures within the U.S. (e.g., Eaton and Dembo 1997; Salili et al. 2001). Second, self-efficacy generally is at least as good if not a better predictor of performance in Eastern, collectivist cultures than in Western, individualistic cultures (e.g., Leung 2001; Salili et al. 2001). Many factors could be contributing to these group differences. For example, perhaps greater average access to material and power resources contributes to realistically higher levels of efficacy in many domains. It also is possible that cultural factors create variability in people's perceptions of the relative importance of factors impacting the outcomes of one's efforts, perhaps leading to a devaluing of *self*-efficacy in more highly interdependent-cultures as other factors take on more relevance. And finally, some research suggests that members of collectivist cultures have more realistic self-efficacy than do their independent-oriented counterparts (c.f., Klassen 2004). This may account for the stronger correlations between efficacy estimates and outcome measures. These possible explanations can be derived from traditional approaches to conceptual equivalence, for example, incorporating contextual factors in understanding group differences.

Also, from within a traditional approach, scholars have compared and contrasted variable definitions of the self (e.g., Individualist and Collectivist perspectives) and their manifestations in importantly different operationalizations of self-efficacy. For example, scholars have examined *collective efficacy* (i.e., beliefs about the group's ability to plan and carry out activities and tasks; Bandura 2000) as a viable alternative to self-efficacy in interdependent cultures (e.g., Alavi and McCormick 2008). And this is where traditional approaches typically stop, having assessed the extent to which self-efficacy and collective efficacy are equivalent across cultures. In contrast, the CLA incorporates this evaluative step and then goes beyond it to consider the application of these concepts (i.e., the two types of efficacy) within the existing theory (in this case, Bandura's theory), by formulating specific testable hypotheses derived from the theory by incorporating culturally-based manifestations of the relevant concepts.

For example, although Bandura (2002) acknowledges the existence and relevance of a collective efficacy, he disputes the idea that it might replace the central importance of self-efficacy in predicting behavior; instead positing that collective efficacy develops from self-efficacy even in collectivist cultures. Drawing on theoretical and empirical evidence that all individuals have multiple selves (e.g., Triandis 1989), Bandura notes that individualism and collectivism are not diametrically opposed cultural values; instead, each person has some individualistic and some collective beliefs and values. Thus, he contends that self-efficacy is relevant cross-culturally. Moreover, instead of classifying people as one or the other, it is more appropriate to describe people in terms of their balance of individualism and collectivism.

However, Bandura's contention that collective efficacy always develops from self-efficacy seems to assume a centrality and pre-eminence of the individual self that is questionable. Considerable research has been conducted on the cultural basis for definitions of the self and the implications of these culturally-derived definitions (e.g., Heine 2001; Markus and Kitayama 1991; Oyserman and Lee 2008), much of which suggests that culture determines which selves are chronically more accessible and thus influential on behavior. In other words, for individuals for whom their interdependent (Markus and Kitayama 1991) or collective (Triandis 1989) selves are most salient, self-efficacy may well develop from collective efficacy. Testable hypotheses based on the CLA might include: (a) collective efficacy leads to self-efficacy in highly interdependent cultures; and (b) the difference in levels of self-efficacy for people from interdependent versus independent cultures is reduced (or even reversed) if the scope of domain-specific self-efficacy is broadened to include domains that are particularly relevant for members of Eastern, collectivist cultures, such as fulfilling one's role in a group.

As with satisfaction with life, we see both progress and much potential in terms of multicultural research on self-efficacy using the CLA. Developing the construct of collective efficacy is an important step in increasing the cultural validity of self-efficacy, by broadening the definition of self from the individual to the group. Just as research on self-esteem was advanced by the introduction of collective self-esteem (Luhtanen and Crocker 1992) to augment measures of personal self-esteem, research that integrates collective efficacy with individual self-efficacy will likely advance our understanding of the predictors and outcomes of efficacy. The CLA can strengthen this research by examining not only cultural manifestations of the constructs, themselves, but also the theoretical propositions involving these constructs. Moreover, research that broadens the specific domains for which one might develop efficacy, such as efficacy for acculturative processes (cf. Rodriguez-Siuts 2011) or for coping with discrimination, also has tremendous potential. Again, the CLA can add to the literature by encouraging broad theoretical models that allow for varied operationalizations of the specific constructs in the model.

6.4 Constructs with Important Cognitive Components

Not all positive cognitive constructs are exclusively cognitive. Many contain additional components to create a more complex overall construct. Due to space limitations, only one example is given here; it was chosen because of how it illustrates the integration of the CLA. This construct is *personal growth initiative* (PGI). As noted above, PGI is defined as cognitive and behavioral actions, intentionally directed toward improving the self (Robitschek 1998; Robitschek et al. 2012). Recalling that *how* and *what* we think matters, PGI theory clearly speaks to how we think. The theory informs how to cognitively approach life situations as growth experiences (Robitschek and Kashubeck 1999), how to determine if and when we are ready to make changes in ourselves (i.e., *readiness for change*; Robitschek et al. 2012), how to plan steps to reach specific personal growth goals (i.e., *planfulness*; Robitschek 1998; Whittaker and Robitschek 2001), and knowledge of resources useful in the personal growth process (i.e., *using resources*; Robitschek et al. 2012). PGI theory states that PGI develops from being taught the process of intentional personal growth and experiencing environmental encouragement to engage in this process.

The theory predicts that higher levels of PGI will enhance mental health and protect against or reduce psychological distress. Support for these propositions has been found in samples of predominantly White American college students in the U.S. (e.g., Robitschek and Keyes 2009; Robitschek and Kashubeck 1999) and internationally (e.g., Ayub and Iqbal 2012; Joshanloo and Ghaedi 2009; Ogunyemi and Mabekoje 2007).

Taking a traditional approach to equivalence, the first multicultural study of PGI (Robitschek 2003) examined mean scores and the structure of PGI. This research found support for the structural and cultural validity of the original Personal Growth Initiative Scale (Robitschek 1998) in a sample of Mexican American college students. An important area of concern was the extent to which the personal focus of the construct was a manifestation of the White American, independent self-construal of the theorist and majority of the research participants to date. Although predating the development of the CLA, Robitschek (2003) took a similar approach by suggesting that the internal desire to grow and develop likely is pan-cultural, but that culture plays an important role not in determining the *level* of that desire, but rather in determining the domains in which people will choose to grow. In other words, culture (among other factors) tells us what to think about changing about ourselves and PGI tells us how to think about making those changes. This perspective on internal drives and desires is reflected in the concepts of *agency* and *autonomy*. Kagitcibasi (2005) argued that agency and autonomy are pan-cultural, reflecting motivated action (Bandura 1989) and volition. Applying Step 5 of the CLA, we would formulate hypotheses to test the ways in which these cultural manifestations of intentional personal growth supported (or challenged) propositions in PGI theory. For example, when we operationalize environmental support for engagement in the process of intentional personal growth in culturally appropriate ways, do we find that this support leads to the development of PGI in the youth of specific cultures?

6.5 Conclusion

Exploring cognitive constructs in positive psychology is a relatively new field. Despite its young age, this field is more advanced in terms of cultural considerations than many young areas of psychology because, at least for the VIA-IS (Peterson et al. 2005) and StrengthsFinder (Rath 2007), the constructs grew out of multicultural research. This area still has far to go, however. We still know little about the wide variety of cultural manifestations of most of our positive cognitive constructs. We also know little about positive cognitive constructs that may be unique to particular cultures or subgroups of cultures. We offer the CLA as a perspective from which to evaluate the cultural validity of known positive cognitive constructs as well as to enrich our understanding of positive aspects of functioning across and within specific cultures.

References

Ægisdottir, S., Gerstein, L. H., & Çinarbaş, D. C. (2008). Methodological issues in cross-cultural counseling research: Equivalence, bias, and translations. *The Counseling Psychologist, 36*, 188–219. doi:10.1177/0011000007305384.

Alavi, S. B., & McCormick, J. (2008). The roles of perceived task interdependence and group members' interdependence in the development of collective efficacy in university student group contexts. *British Journal of Educational Psychology, 78*, 375–393. doi:10.1348/000709907X240471.

Ayub, N., & Iqbal, S. (2012). The relationship of personal growth initiative, psychological well-being, and psychological distress among adolescents. *Journal of Teaching and Education, 1*(6), 101–107.

Bandura, A. (1977). Self-efficacy: Toward a unifying theory of behavioral change. *Psychological Review, 84*, 191–215. doi:10.1037/0033-295X.84.2.191.

Bandura, A. (1989). Human agency in social cognitive theory. *American Psychologist, 44*, 1175–1184. doi:10.1037/0003-066X.44.9.1175.

Bandura, A. (2000). Exercise of human agency through collective agency. *Current Directions in Psychological Science, 9*, 75–78. doi:10.1111/1467-8721.00064.

Bandura, A. (2002). Social cognitive theory in cultural context. *Applied Psychology: An International Review, 51*, 269–290. doi:10.1111/1464-0597.00092.

Barger, S. D., Donoho, C. J., & Wayment, H. A. (2009). The relative contributions of race/ethnicity, socioeconomic status, health, and social relationships to life satisfaction in the United States. *Quality of Life Research: An International Journal of Quality of Life Aspects of Treatment, Care & Rehabilitation, 18*, 179–189. doi:10.1007/s11136-008-9426-2.

Barutta, J., Cornejo, C., & Ibáñez, A. (2011). Theories and theorizers: A contextual approach to theories of cognition. *Integrative Psychological & Behavioral Science, 45*, 223–246. doi:10.1007/s12124-011-9156-9.

Beck, A. T. (1976). *Cognitive therapy and the emotional disorders*. New York: International Universities Press.

Biswas-Diener, R. (2006). From the equator to the North Pole: A study of character strengths. *Journal of Happiness Studies, 7*, 293–310. doi:10.1007/s10902-005-3646-8.

Buckingham, M., & Clifton, D. O. (2001). *Now, discover your strengths*. New York: Free Press.

Cheung, F., van de Vijver, F. J. R., & Leong, F. T. L. (2011). Toward a new approach to the study of personality in culture. *American Psychologist, 66*, 593–603. doi:10.1037/a0022389.

Constantine, M. G., & Sue, D. W. (2006). Factors contributing to optimal human functioning in people of color in the United States. *The Counseling Psychologist, 34*, 228–244. doi:10.1177/0011000005281318.

Cross, S. E., & Madson, L. (1997). Models of the self: Self-construals and gender. *Psychological Bulletin, 122*, 5–37. doi:10.1037/0033-2909.122.1.5.

Dahlsgaard, K., Peterson, C., & Seligman, M. E. P. (2005). Shared virtue: The convergence of valued human strengths across culture and history. *Review of General Psychology, 9*, 203–213. doi:10.1037/1089-2680.9.3.203.

Diener, E. (1984). Subjective well-being. *Psychological Bulletin, 95*, 542–575. doi:10.1037/0033-2909.95.3.542.

Diener, E., & Seligman, M. E. P. (2002). Very happy people. *Psychological Science, 13*, 81–84. doi:10.1111/1467-9280.00415.

Diener, E., & Suh, E. M. (2000). Measuring subjective well-being to compare the quality of life of cultures. In E. Diener & E. M. Suh (Eds.), *Culture and subjective well-being*. Cambridge, MA: MIT Press.

Diener, E., Emmons, R. A., Larsen, R. J., & Griffin, S. (1985). The Satisfaction with Life Scale. *Journal of Personality Assessment, 49*, 71–75. doi:10.1207/s15327752jpa4901_13.

Eaton, M. J., & Dembo, M. H. (1997). Differences in the motivation beliefs of Asian Americans and non-Asian students. *Journal of Educational Psychology, 89*, 433–440. doi:10.1037/0022-0663.89.3.433.
Gabriel, S., & Gardner, W. L. (1999). Are there "his" and "hers" types of interdependence? The implications of gender differences in collective versus relational interdependence for affect, behavior, and cognition. *Journal of Personality and Social Psychology, 77*, 642–655. doi:10.1037/0022-3514.77.3.642.
Hansen, J. C. (2005). Assessment of interests. In S. D. Brown & R. W. Lent (Eds.), *Career development and counseling: Putting theory and research to work* (pp. 281–304). Hoboken: Wiley.
Hardin, E. E. (2007, August). Cultural validity of career theories: A new perspective. In E. E. Hardin (Chair), *Cultural validity of career theories: A new perspective*. Symposium presented at the annual meeting of the American Psychological Association, San Francisco.
Hardin, E. (2010, August). The next big question about the cultural validity of vocational theories: The Cultural Lens approach. In W. B. Walsh (Chair), *The next big questions in vocational psychology*. Symposium presented at the American Psychological Association National Convention, San Diego
Hardin, E. E., Robitschek, C., Flores, L. Y., Navarro, R. L., & Ashton, M. W. (in press). The cultural lens approach to evaluating cultural validity of psychological theory. *American Psychologist.*
Heine, S. J. (2001). Self as a cultural product: An examination of East Asian and North American selves. *Journal of Personality, 69*, 881–906. doi:10.1111/1467-6494.696168.
Helms, J. E. (1992). Why is there no study of cultural equivalence in standardized cognitive ability testing? *American Psychologist, 47*, 1083–1101. doi:10.1037/0003-066X.47.9.1083.
Hui, C. H., & Triandis, H. C. (1989). Effects of culture and response format on extreme response style. *Journal of Cross-Cultural Psychology, 20*, 296–309. doi:10.1177/0022022189203004.
Joshanloo, M., & Ghaedi, G. (2009). Psychometric characteristics of "Personal Growth Initiative" scale in university students. *Journal of Behavioral Sciences (Iran), 3*, 121–125.
Kagitcibasi, C. (2005). Autonomy and relatedness in cultural context: Implications for self and family. *Journal of Cross-Cultural Psychology, 36*, 403–422. doi:10.1177/0022022105275959.
Kang, S., Shaver, P., Sue, S., Min, K., & Jing, H. (2003). Culture-specific patterns in the prediction of life satisfaction: Roles of emotion, relationship quality, and self-esteem. *Personality and Social Psychology Bulletin, 29*, 1596–1608. doi:10.1177/0146167203255986.
Klassen, R. M. (2004). Optimism and realism: A review of self-efficacy from a cross-cultural perspective. *International Journal of Psychology, 39*, 205–530. doi:10.1080/00207590344000330.
Leary, M. R., & Guadagno, J. (2011). The role of hypo-egoic self-processes in optimal functioning and subjective well-being. In K. M. Sheldon, T. B. Kashdan, & M. F. Steger (Eds.), *Designing positive psychology: Taking stock and moving forward* (pp. 135–146). Oxford: Oxford University Press.
Leong, F. T. L., & Brown, M. T. (1995). Theoretical issues in cross-cultural career development: Cultural validity and cultural specificity. In W. B. Walsh & S. H. Osipow (Eds.), *Handbook of vocational psychology: Theory, research, and practice* (2nd ed., pp. 143–180). Mahwah: Erlbaum.
Leung, C. (2001). The psychological adaptation of overseas and migrant students in Australia. *International Journal of Psychology, 36*, 251–259. doi:10.1080/00207590143000018.
Lindley, L. D. (2006). The paradox of self-efficacy: Research with diverse populations. *Journal of Career Assessment, 14*, 143–160. doi:10.1177/1069072705281371.
Lonner, W. J. (1985). Issues in testing and assessment in cross-cultural counseling. *The Counseling Psychologist, 13*, 599–614. doi:10.1177/0011000085134004.
Lopez, S., Hodges, T., & Harter, J. (2005). *The Clifton StrengthsFinder ® technical report: Development and validation.* Retrieved from Clifton Strengths School™ website: http://strengths.org/docs/CSFTechnicalReport.pdf
Luhtanen, R., & Crocker, J. (1992). A collective self-esteem scale: Self-evaluation of one's social identity. *Personality and Social Psychology Bulletin, 18*, 302–318. doi:10.1177/0146167292183006.
Markus, H. R., & Kitayama, S. (1991). Culture and the self: Implications for cognition, emotion, and motivation. *Psychological Review, 98*, 224–253. doi:10.1037/0033-295X.98.2.224.

Martinez, R., & Dukes, R. L. (1987). Race, gender and self-esteem among youth. *Hispanic Journal of Behavioral Sciences, 9*, 427–443. doi:10.1177/07399863870094005.
McDavid, J. C., & Hawthorn, L. R. L. (2006). *Program evaluation and performance measurement: An introduction to practice*. Thousand Oaks: Sage.
Niemiec, R. (2011). *Character strength summaries*. VIA Institute on Character website: http://viacharacter.org/www/en-us/research/summaries.aspx
Ogunyemi, A. O., & Mabekoje, S. O. (2007). Self-efficacy, risk-taking behavior and mental health as predictors of personal growth initiative among university undergraduates. *Electronic Journal of Research in Educational Psychology, 5*, 349–362.
Oishi, S., Diener, E., Lucas, R. E., & Suh, E. (1999a). Cross-cultural variations in the prediction of life-satisfaction: Perspectives from needs and values. *Personality and Social Psychology Bulletin, 25*, 980–990. doi:10.1177/01461672992511006.
Oishi, S., Diener, E., Suh, E., & Lucas, R. E. (1999b). Value as a moderator in subjective well-being. *Journal of Personality, 67*, 157–184. doi:10.1111/1467-6494.00051.
Oyserman, D., & Lee, S. W. S. (2008). Does culture influence what and how we think? Effects of priming individualism and collectivism. *Psychological Bulletin, 134*, 311–342. doi:10.1037/0033-2909.134.2.311.
Park, N., & Huebner, E. S. (2005). A cross-cultural study of the levels and correlates of life satisfaction among adolescents. *Journal of Cross-Cultural Psychology, 36*, 444–456. doi:10.1177/0022022105275961.
Park, N., Peterson, C., & Seligman, M. E. P. (2006). Character strengths in fifty-four nations and the fifty US states. *The Journal of Positive Psychology, 1*, 118–129. doi:10.1080/17439760600619567.
Pavot, W., & Diener, E. (2009). Review of the Satisfaction with Life Scale. In E. Diener & E. Diener (Eds.), *Assessing well-being: The collected works of Ed Diener* (pp. 101–117). New York: Springer.
Peterson, C., Park, N., & Seligman, M. E. P. (2005). Assessment of character strengths. In G. P. Koocher, J. C. Norcross, & S. S. Hill III (Eds.), *Psychologists' desk reference* (2nd ed., pp. 93–98). New York: Oxford University Press.
Rath, T. (2007). *Strengths Finder 2.0*. New York: Gallup Press.
Ridgell, S. D., & Lounsbury, J. W. (2004). Predicting academic success: General intelligence, "Big Five" personality traits, and work drive. *College Student Journal, 38*, 607–619.
Robitschek, C. (1998). Personal growth initiative: The construct and its measure. *Measurement and Evaluation in Counseling and Development, 30*, 183–198.
Robitschek, C. (2003). Validity of Personal Growth Initiative Scale scores with a Mexican American college student population. *Journal of Counseling Psychology, 50*, 496–502. doi:10.1037/0022-0167.50.4.496.
Robitschek, C., & Kashubeck, S. (1999). A structural model of parental alcoholism, family functioning, and psychological health: The mediating effects of hardiness and personal growth orientation. *Journal of Counseling Psychology, 46*, 159–172. doi:10.1037/0022-0167.46.2.159.
Robitschek, C., & Keyes, C. L. M. (2009). Keyes' model of mental health with personal growth initiative as a parsimonious predictor. *Journal of Counseling Psychology, 56*, 321–329. doi:10.1037/a0013954.
Robitschek, C., Ashton, M. W., Spering, C. C., Geiger, N., Byers, D., Schotts, G. C., & Thoen, M. (2012). Development and psychometric properties of the Personal Growth Initiative Scale – II. *Journal of Counseling Psychology, 59*, 274–287. doi:10.1037/a0027310.
Rodriguez-Siuts, S. (2011). *Acculturative Self-Efficacy: A new view on the acculturation process for individuals of Mexican descent* (Unpublished doctoral dissertation). Texas Tech University, Lubbock.
Rosenberg, M. (1965). *Society and the adolescent self-image*. Princeton: Princeton University Press.
Ryff, C. D. (1989). Happiness is everything, or is it? Explorations on the meaning of psychological well-being. *Journal of Personality and Social Psychology, 57*, 1069–1081. doi:10.1037/0022-3514.57.6.1069.

Salili, F., Chiu, C. Y., & Lai, S. (2001). The influence of culture and context on students' motivational orientation and performance. In F. Salili, C. Y. Chie, & Y. Y. Hong (Eds.), *Student motivation: The culture and context of learning* (pp. 221–247). New York: Kluwer.

Schuster, R. (1979). Empathy and mindfulness. *Journal of Humanistic Psychology, 19*(1), 71–77.

Sue, D. W., & Sue, D. (2013). *Counseling the culturally diverse: Theory and practice* (6th ed.). Hoboken: Wiley.

Super, D. E., Savickas, M. L., & Super, C. M. (1996). The life-span, life-space approach to careers. In D. Brown & L. Brooks (Eds.), *Career choice and development* (3rd ed., pp. 121–178). San Francisco: Jossey-Bass.

Thinking or Feeling. (n.d.). *The Myers-Briggs Foundation.* Retrieved from http://www.apastyle.org/learn/faqs/cite-website-material.aspx

Triandis, H. C. (1989). The self and social behavior in differing cultural contexts. *Psychological Review, 96*, 506–520. doi:10.1037/0033-295X.96.3.506.

Verkuyten, M. (1989). Self-esteem among Dutch and Turkish children in the Netherlands. *The Journal of Social Psychology, 129*, 269–271. doi:10.1080/00224545.1989.9711727.

Verkuyten, M. (2008). Life satisfaction among ethnic minorities: The role of discrimination and group identification. *Social Indicators Research, 89*, 391–404. doi:10.1007/s11205-008-9239-2.

Weiss, C. H. (1998). Have we learned anything new about the use of evaluation? *American Journal of Evaluation, 19*, 21–23. doi:10.1177/109821409801900103.

Whittaker, A. E., & Robitschek, C. (2001). Multidimensional family functioning: Predicting personal growth initiative. *Journal of Counseling Psychology, 48*, 420–427. doi:10.1037/0022-0167.48.4.420.

Chapter 7
Relationships in Multicultural Contexts

Belinda Campos and Sharon Shenhav

Like everything else, relationships are embedded in culture. In the United States, one of many societies characterized by ever increasing cultural heterogeneity, relationships are further embedded in multicultural contexts where people have regular interaction with others who may approach relationships in a variety of ways. All too often, these experiences highlight difference in the negative light of the unfamiliar. A positive psychology lens on relationships in a multicultural context thus provides an important opportunity to meet one of positive psychology's primary goals – to shift away from a focus on deficits in favor of a more balanced focus that also includes strengths. In this chapter, we focus on examining family and couple relationships in three U.S. groups – European, East Asian, and Latino cultural heritage – that share the universal need to belong to valued social relationships, but differ in their approaches to achieving this need. In the pages that follow, we define culture in a multicultural environment, describe how culture has been shown to shape family and couple relationships in people of European, East Asian, and Latino heritage in the U.S., and consider the possibilities of multicultural settings for offering people multiple routes to positive relationship outcomes. We conclude by offering suggestions for future directions that can move forward theory and generate new possibilities for application that benefits people across groups and circumstances.

B. Campos, Ph.D. (✉)
Department of Chicano/Latino Studies, University of California,
3151 Social Science Plaza A, Irvine, CA 92697-5100, USA
e-mail: bcampos@uci.edu

S. Shenhav
Department of Psychology and Social Behavior, University of California,
4201 Social & Behavioral Sciences Gateway, Irvine, CA 92697-7085, USA

J. Teramoto Pedrotti and L.M. Edwards (eds.), *Perspectives on the Intersection of Multiculturalism and Positive Psychology*, Cross-Cultural Advancements in Positive Psychology 7, DOI 10.1007/978-94-017-8654-6_7,

7.1 What Is Culture in a Multicultural Environment?

Humans are a social species; we have a need to belong and a need for social connections (Baumeister and Leary 1995). As such, relationships play a crucial role in life – they can bring happiness, health and meaning or compromise happiness, health and meaning (Berscheid and Reis 1998; Diener and Diener 1996). For all people, culture provides a map of socially accepted routes for reaching the universal goal of belonging and social connection. To understand these various routes, it is important to first define culture. Culture is "any kind of information that is acquired from other members of one's species through social learning that is capable of affecting an individual's behaviors" (Heine 2011, p. 3) or "the knowledge that one must possess to function adequately in society" (Dressler 2004, p. 24). Both definitions emphasize the social nature of culture in shaping people's thoughts and behaviors. Culture is learned from the shared beliefs and behavior norms that we see around us; behaviors that are normative and approved are those that are consistent with cultural ideals about how people *should* be.

In a multicultural society, three additional issues must be considered. First, and perhaps most important, is recognizing that *everyone* has culture (e.g., Heine 2011). Each and every one of us is socialized to organize our relationships according to culture-based rules. When we are surrounded by others who share our culture, culture can become as unnoticeable and taken for granted as the air we breathe. In multicultural settings where one culture predominates over others, the invisible air of the majority culture can lead to the misconception that culture is the domain of "others" who are often viewed from a deficit perspective where difference is inferior (e.g., Gaines et al. 1997). Positive psychology's emphasis on the strengths of multiple cultures offers the opportunity to redress imbalances wrought by deficit models and generate a better understanding of the multiple routes through which strong relationships can be obtained. Second, people vary in the extent to which personal values align with cultural values (e.g., Dressler et al. 2007). Cultures that value open expressions of affection have people who are reserved and, conversely, cultures that value private expressions of affection have people who prefer to openly express affection. We would be remiss to assume that knowledge of a specific culture is sufficient to describe any particular individual's experience and preferences. Third, culture is dynamic and changing; what is true today may not be true in 50 years and change may be accelerated in multicultural settings characterized by easy access to various cultural ideals (e.g. Farver et al. 2007).

7.2 Culture and Relationships in Broad Strokes

We chose to focus on European, East Asian, and Latino heritage groups in the U.S. because they are examples of distinct cultural approaches to relationships. Most broadly, the three vary in the extent to which they regard the self as separate or interconnected from their social relations (Markus and Kitayama 1991). People of

European heritage in the U.S. typically view the self as inherently independent from others whereas people of East Asian and Latino heritage in the U.S. typically view the self as inherently interdependent with important others. There is also variation within interdependent contexts. People of East Asian heritage in the U.S. often place emphasis on maintaining relationships through moderated positive emotion and implicitly communicated social support (Kim et al. 2008; Tsai et al. 2006), whereas people of Latino heritage in the U.S. commonly place emphasis on maintaining relationships through openly expressed positive emotion and social support (Holloway et al. 2009; Ruby et al. 2012).

A few examples highlight these relative priorities. For people of European-heritage, relationships are voluntarily chosen and individuals may choose to allow family and/or partners to influence personal decisions or to eschew these influences (e.g., Cheng and Landale 2011; Cross et al. 2000). For people of East Asian and Latino heritage, the needs and goals of family and/or partners overlap with the self on a more assumed basis, and the preferences of important others are factored into personal decisions. Young adults of East Asian and Latino heritage, for example, are more likely to pursue careers that reflect parent preference in part because they want to be able to meet shared expectations of providing assistance to family members (Fuligni 2007). Similarly, Latinos, whose culture values physical proximity and frequent positive social interaction with family members, often attend colleges and universities whose physical proximity to home allows for regular visits with family (Desmond and Lopez Turley 2009). As evidence of the cultural appropriateness of this latter choice, family support is uniquely linked to positive academic adjustment in Latinos (Schneider and Ward 2003).

In sum, a culturally independent person tends to view their life in terms of enacting choices that best suit personal needs and preferences whereas a culturally interdependent person tends to view their life as naturally incorporating the needs and preferences of the people in one's important relationships.

7.3 Family Relationships

Family relationships typically begin at birth and endure across the life-span. The centrality of family in early life gives these relationships a principal role in socializing children into culture via language, social referencing, interaction, and observation (Bandura 1976; Campos 1980–1981; Schiefflin and Ochs 1986). Language teaches and reinforces the relative importance of "I" versus "we," observing the emotional responses of important others lets us develop similar responses, and participating in social interaction trains us to be active members of our own culture. These processes, over time, shape an individual's worldviews and behaviors and have consequences for psychological functioning and physical health throughout the life course (e.g., Bowlby 1969; Repetti et al. 2002).

As evidenced by the high levels of cooperation and affiliation that are universally observed among kin (Hamilton 1964; Hrdy 1999), all cultures value family. The people who are counted in the family category and the behaviors that are considered desirable ways to express value for family, however, do show cultural variation. *Familism*, broadly defined as a strong identification and attachment with nuclear and extended family, is a construct developed by family scholars to capture cultural variation in approaches to family relationships (Bardis 1959; Keefe et al. 1979; Sabogal et al. 1987). At the lower end of familism are members of independent cultures whose separation from family of origin is enacted via preference for nuclear family households, time spent with peers rather than family, and a focus on "launching" children from the family home upon young adulthood (Fuligni et al. 1999; Magaña and Smith 2006; Smith 1993).[1] At the higher end of familism are members of interdependent cultures who are likely to live in close proximity or share households with nuclear and extended family members, readily contribute to family financial well-being through work or career choices, and divide time equitably between peers and family (e.g., Fuligni et al. 1999; Updegraff et al. 2005). Here again, we see variation within the interdependence of East Asians and Latinos. *Asian familism*, termed *filial piety*, places more emphasis on displays of respect stemming from hierarchical obedience (Yeh and Bedford 2004; Ho 1994) whereas *Latino familism*, or *familismo*, places more emphasis on positive emotional tone and readily accessible social support (Campos et al. 2008; Sabogal et al. 1987; Updegraff et al. 2005).

These culture-based rules for desirable family relationships each offer unique routes to well-being. For people of European heritage, choice and freedom from parental control are associated with positive feelings and well-being. For example, in one self-report study that measured parental control and anger responses to parental control among adolescents of East Asian and European heritage in the U.S., European heritage adolescents reported less parent control but more anger in response to parental control than their East Asian heritage counterparts (Chao and Aque 2009). Rather than responding to parental control with anger, there is some evidence that parental control is linked to relatively greater feelings of being loved and cared for in adolescents whose cultures place greater emphasis on family primacy than independence. For example, a self-report study that asked adolescents to rate their feelings towards parental control behavior (guilt, general control, enforcement, and intrusiveness) found that control though guilt was more associated with feeling loved and cared for than feeling hurt, angry, or manipulated in the Latino heritage sample (Mason et al. 2004). Among European heritage adolescents, however, control through guilt was associated with feeling loved and cared for but also with feeling manipulated (Mason et al. 2004).

It is interesting to note that explanations for behaviors show cultural shaping even when the behaviors themselves are the same. For example, when asked about parent-child conflict situations (e.g., family dinner, chores, dating partner), European, East Asian, and Latino adolescents and young adults in the United States all cited respect as a reason for complying with parents (Phinney et al. 2005). A closer

[1]Some studies, however, have found that familism is also high in European heritage samples (e.g., Schwartz 2007; Vega et al. 1986).

examination of their reasons, however, revealed the expected cultural variation. European heritage adolescents and young adults tended to report complying with parents' wishes either because they felt their parents must have good reason for expressing disagreement or for self-oriented reasons such as wishing to obtain parent approval for future rewards or privileges. In contrast, East Asian heritage adolescents and young adults tended to report that they complied due to the importance of obeying and honoring parents. Finally, Latino heritage adolescents and young adults tended to report that they complied due to care and concern for family members (Phinney et al. 2005).

As people move into adulthood and start their own families, culture continues to shape experience. People in high familism contexts tend to have highly positive attitudes toward motherhood and childbearing. For example, pregnant Latinas report positive attitudes toward pregnancy and motherhood (e.g., Zambrana et al. 1999) and their sense of familism is tightly linked with perceptions of being socially supported (Campos et al. 2008). People also benefit from coping in culturally appropriate ways. For example, pregnant women of European heritage in the U.S. have been found to benefit from coping with pregnancy via a more culturally appropriate self-focused approach that emphasized accepting the stresses of the situation whereas pregnant women of East Asian heritage (Japan) were found to benefit from coping with pregnancy via social support (Morling et al. 2003).

In sum, familism captures important variation in the routes that cultures offer for obtaining good family relationships.

7.4 Couple Relationships

Couple relationships, or pair bonds, are typically first formed at some point in late adolescence or young adulthood but thereafter can be formed and dissolved throughout life. Couple relationships are a domain of historically great cultural variability, but may be becoming more similar as part of the worldwide shift to committed couple relationships that are based on love and mutual regard rather than social, economic, or political considerations (Coontz 2005). In multicultural settings such as the U.S., these relationships are particularly interesting because of the increased opportunity to couple with someone of another cultural heritage background. In this section, we will focus on the cultural shaping of processes that relate to (a) couple relationship formation and (b) couple relationship maintenance. We will also note the influence of gender variation in these processes where data are available.

For couple formation, we start with the constructs of attraction and courtship. For attraction, defined broadly as characteristics that invite approach, there is strong empirical evidence that all people are attracted to beauty and there is wide agreement across human societies about certain facets of beauty such as facial symmetry, waist-to-hip ratios in women, and shoulder-to waist ratios in men (Miller et al. 2007). Importantly, however, attraction also includes desirable personality characteristics, shared interests, familiarity, perceived similarity, and perhaps most critically, reciprocal liking (Miller et al. 2007; Riela et al. 2010; Montoya et al. 2008).

The experience of mutual attraction appears to be a human universal, but expecting mutual attraction to lead to the formation of long-term committed relationships is historically recent (Coontz 2005). Even in the U.S. European heritage population, the shift toward the belief that mutual attraction is the natural entry point to courtship and long term couple formation has occurred over the course of the last 250 years (Coontz 2005). Among contemporary U.S. European heritage young adults, it is common to explore the possibility of becoming a couple via courtship practices such as dating, where the potential couple engages in shared activities to assess mutual desire to form a more long term commitment (Jackson et al. 2011; Mongeau et al. 2007). In East Asian cultures, young people have historically been expected to acquiesce to their parents' choice of an appropriate spouse rather than choosing a partner based on mutual attraction (Ho 1994; Yan 2002). In Latino societies, the historical ideal has been for attraction to unfold in public spaces that can be closely supervised by parents, extended family, and members of the general community until a couple is ready to make a long term commitment that meets the approval of both sets of parents (Hirsch 2003). In the last few decades, however, the shift to love-based marriage has accelerated all over the world; the idea is popular wherever it is introduced (Coontz 2005; Hirsch 2003). Perhaps partly for this reason, the experience of falling in love appears to be similar in European, East Asian and Latino heritage groups within the U.S. (Hirsch 2003; Regan et al. 2004; Riela et al. 2010; Yan 2002) and there are also more gender similarities than differences in this domain (Riela et al. 2010).

Once couple relationships are formed, they must be maintained. Strong and thriving couple relationships are maintained through various emotion-laden processes such as shared moments of love and affection, social support for both the positive and negative events of life, and effective management of conflict. The communication of love and affection is of particular interest because it is the glue that binds couples together in love-based contexts (Coontz 2005; Hirsch 2003; Yan 2002). Although people of European, East Asian, and Latino heritage differ in their preferences for expressing emotion (as described in our Sect. 7.2), the existing literature suggests that emotion differences in subjective experience are more pronounced than emotion differences in display or physiology (e.g., Soto et al. 2005; Tsai et al. 2006). In one study of the experience and display of love, European, East Asian and Latino heritage heterosexual couples who self-reported feeling love while discussing their first date together all displayed the same set of affiliation behaviors – affirmative head nods, Duchenne smiles[2], positive gesturing with the hands, and leaning toward the partner – as they interacted in a laboratory setting

[2] Duchenne smiles are a distinctive type of smile that simultaneously engages facial muscles that raise the lips and the upper cheek below the eyes such that eyes appear to "crinkle". Duchenne smiles, also known as "felt smiles", are reliable indicators of felt positive emotion. In contrast, social smiles (or non-Duchenne smiles) are limited to mouth movements and can signal a wide variety of states.

(Gonzaga et al. 2006). Members of East Asian cultures, however, are more likely to believe that opposing feelings can co-exist (Peng and Nisbett 1999). Thus, despite similar discussion content, people of East Asian heritage are more likely to report simultaneously experiencing *both* positive and negative emotions (e.g., love and anger), while people of European heritage are likely to report experiencing either a positive *or* negative emotion (e.g., love or anger) while discussing emotion-laden topics with their partners (Shiota et al. 2010).

Social support is another important process for maintaining couple relationships. The existing research on culture and social support has seldom examined social support in the specific context of couple relationships. However, it has convincingly shown that cultures vary in the extent to which social support is openly sought and the extent to which social support seeking has negative implications for the self or the social network. For people of European heritage, receiving social support can bring unintentional harm by implying that one cannot take care of the self (e.g., Bolger and Amarel 2007). In this context, invisible social support, where one partner engages in a supportive action that the partner does not report receiving (e.g., putting gas in the car so the partner is not rushed the next morning; the receiving partner only notices that their day went smoothly) can be beneficial for the receiver's well-being. For people of East Asian heritage, openly seeking support risks disturbing or burdening the social network (Taylor et al. 2004). Kim and colleagues (2008) have shown that implicit support, where a person feels valued and cared for in interactions with members of their social network without explicitly disclosing the stressful event, is beneficial for people of East Asian heritage. For people of Latino heritage, whose version of interdependence prioritizes openly expressed positive emotion and support between family members (Sabogal et al. 1987; Keefe et al. 1979), there is some indication that women promote partner positive experience by managing social interaction in ways that reduce partner sense of threat (Herrera et al. in preparation).

Conflict is an inevitable part of life, and the ways that conflict is handled can either protect or harm couple relationships. Here again, we see that the different communication practices that are common in independent and interdependent cultures offer different routes to positive relationship outcomes. For couples of European heritage, the ability to handle conflict with humor and positivity has been shown to be associated with relationship satisfaction and stability (e.g., Gottman et al. 1998). For couples of East Asian heritage, there is some indication that negativity in the form of expressed anger and criticism is more openly expressed (Tsai et al. 2006; Williamson et al. 2012), perhaps reflecting a desire to process criticism as a route to self-improvement for the benefit of the relationship (Heine et al. 1999). This is also consistent with the greater acceptance of contradictory emotions observed in East Asian couples (Shiota et al. 2010). For couples of Latino heritage, ethnographic observations suggest that Latino couples seek to avoid and resolve conflict through indirect communication that expresses disagreement by avoiding a topic or uses subtle positivity to resolve conflict in one's favor (e.g., Hirsch 2003). These patterns, however, change with time in the U.S. Flores et al. (2004) found that more acculturated Latino husbands and wives were less likely to avoid conflict and more likely to express negativity toward each other, perhaps due to acculturation to U.S. norms of emotion expression that include acceptance of negative emotion expression in both genders.

Culturally-approved routes for handling conflict also show gender variation. For example, in "honor cultures," which include U.S. European heritage Southerners and Latinos, (a) aggressive responses to insult are socially approved and (b) the sexual behavior of women who are family or partners have implications for a man's honor and social esteem (Vandello and Cohen 2003). In a series of elegant studies, Vandello and Cohen (2003) found that men who did not respond aggressively to women partners who were discovered in infidelity were more poorly regarded than their counterparts who did respond aggressively. Further, women whose partner behaved aggressively in response to a jealousy-related honor transgression were encouraged to remain loyal to their partner (Vandello and Cohen 2003). In this case, the cultural routes for resolving conflict and preserving relationships pose challenges for both genders that are unlikely to lead to positive outcomes for women.

7.5 Cultural Exchanges in Multicultural Settings

Multicultural settings offer opportunities for acculturation to the norms of other cultures, both majority and minority. On the one hand, this may offer the benefit of a cultural "buffet" from which to pick out relationship norms that are positive personal fits. For example, immigrant Mexican women appreciate the ideals of gender equality that they perceive to be more prevalent in the U.S. than in their Mexican hometowns (e.g., Hirsch 2003). On the other hand, cultural changes are only likely to have a positive outcome when all relationship members agree to the changes. If families or partners disagree on what culture-based rules to follow, culture can become a source of distress (e.g., Cervantes et al. 1991; Hirsch 2003).

In the domain of family relationships, a great deal of research has focused on cultural gaps as a source of conflict between immigrant parents and their U.S.-born children that can harm parent-child relationships (e.g. Ahn et al. 2008). One possible cultural gap for parents and children in multicultural settings is in the arena of dating and courtship. Young adults raised in interdependent immigrant families in the U.S. have mate preferences that show consideration for parent's approval (Hynie et al. 2006) but also appreciation for the majority views of European heritage culture that regard dating and courtship as autonomous individual choices. A discrepancy in the role of family input in couple formation may thus generate conflict in immigrant East Asian and Latino families regarding appropriate courtship behavior in their children (Phinney et al. 2005). There is some indication, however, that high relationship quality can protect against the adverse effects of parent-child acculturation gaps (Schofield et al. 2008).

In the domain of couple relationships, multicultural settings are particularly interesting because of the importance of similarity between partners. Researchers initially assumed that intercultural couples (e.g., one Latino heritage partner and one European heritage partner), may be missing this vital contributor to high relationship quality (Crippen and Brew 2007). Empirical studies to date, however, have shown inconsistent results. Some studies have concluded that intercultural couples suffer from reduced relationship quality as compared to intracultural couples (e.g., Hohmann-Marriot and Amato 2008), others have shown little or no difference (e.g., Negy and Snyder 2000) and still others have shown that intercultural couples enjoy greater relationship quality as compared to intracultural couples (e.g., Troy et al. 2006). One factor that may explain the pattern of inconsistent results is the role of perceived similarity. In at least one study, intercultural couples were found to see themselves as highly similar because, like intracultural couples, they tended to focus on their shared qualities rather than their differences (Gaines et al. 2006). Another factor that may affect the relationship quality of intercultural couples is the extent to which their social network (Sprecher and Felmlee 1992) and society at large (Wilt 2011) approves of the relationship. Lack of support from parents or other valued family members, for example, may contribute to decreased couple relationship quality in interracial couples (Hohmann-Marriot and Amato 2008).

7.6 Suggestions for Future Directions

To put it plainly, the field needs more research. We need more research on positive relationship processes and we need that research to take a cultural perspective. Many key positive relationship constructs – gratitude, forgiveness, pride, and capitalization – still await multicultural investigation. We also recognize that multiculturalism encompasses a wide range of possibilities that include social class, religion, sexual orientation, and other facets that have thus far been little studied in the context of the positive psychology of relationships but also merit thoughtful investigation that will surely shed new insights on psychological processes. In particular, we see a gap in the study of intercultural couples, who are living multicultural relationships, and their biracial children. Careful studies that blend self report and observation in the laboratory and ecologically valid settings stand to shed valuable insight to relationships in multicultural contexts. We must also find ways to apply psychological knowledge to protect people from the stresses that may accompany cultural change in their family and couple relationships (Cervantes et al. 1991). For example, interventions that help families to preserve and transmit their cultural values and close-knit family ties in the face of increased acculturation may be beneficial for families and couples alike.

7.7 Conclusions

Integrating a cultural – and multicultural – perspective into the study of positive relationship processes offers an opportunity to elucidate the multiple routes to meeting the shared human need for social connectedness. For researchers, we hope our chapter provides a useful summary of current knowledge and sheds light on the knowledge gaps that need to be addressed. For clinicians and others who work on the front lines of application, we hope our chapter offers greater understanding of some of the variability in positive relationship processes observed in U.S. populations. In working with individuals in multicultural settings, we advocate a *culturally humble approach* (Hunt 2005) that is aware of multiple routes, but allows space for individuals to convey their own worldviews without another's assumptions (Kleinman 1980). In our view, the work that still needs to be done is an opportunity to generate and apply psychological knowledge in the service of enriching the lives of people across groups and circumstances.

References

Ahn, A. J., Kim, B. S. K., & Park, Y. S. (2008). Asian cultural values gap, cognitive flexibility, coping strategies, and parent-child conflicts among Korean Americans. *Cultural Diversity and Ethnic Minority Psychology, 14*, 353–363. doi:10.1037/1099-9809.14.4.353.

Bandura, A. (1976). *Social learning theory*. Englewood Cliffs: Prentice-Hall.

Bardis, P. D. (1959). A familism scale. *Marriage & Family Living, 21*, 340–341. doi:10.2307/347107.

Baumeister, R. F., & Leary, M. R. (1995). The need to belong: Desire for interpersonal attachment as a fundamental human motivation. *Psychological Bulletin, 117*, 497–529. doi:10.1037/0033-2909.117.3.497.

Berscheid, E., & Reis, H. T. (1998). Attraction and close relationships. In D. T. Gilbert, S. T. Fiske, & G. Lindzey (Eds.), *The handbook of social psychology* (4th ed., Vol. 2, pp. 193–281). New York: McGraw-Hill.

Bolger, N., & Amarel, D. (2007). Effects of social support visibility on adjustment to stress: Experimental evidence. *Journal of Personality and Social Psychology, 92*, 458–475. doi:10.1037/0022-3514.92.3.458.

Bowlby, J. (1969). *Attachment and loss: Vol. 1. Attachment*. New York: Basic Books.

Campos, J. J. (1980–1981). *Human emotions: Their new importance and their role in social referencing* (Annual Report 1–7). Research and Clinical Center for Child Development.

Campos, B., Dunkel Schetter, C., Abdou, C. M., Hobel, C., Glynn, L., & Sandman, C. (2008). Familialism, social support, and stress: Positive implications for pregnant Latinas. *Journal of Cultural Diversity and Ethnic Minority Psychology, 14*, 155–162. doi:10.1037/1099-9809.14.2.155.

Cervantes, R. C., Padilla, A. M., & Salgado de Snyder, N. (1991). The Hispanic Stress Inventory: A culturally relevant approach to psychosocial assessment. *Psychological Assessment, 3*, 438–447. doi:10.1037//1040-3590.3.3.438.

Chao, R. K., & Aque, C. (2009). Interpretations of parental control by Asian immigrant and European American youth. *Journal of Family Psychology, 23*, 342–354. doi:10.1037/a0015828.

Cheng, Y. A., & Landale, N. S. (2011). Adolescent precursors of early union formation among Asian Americans and Whites. *Journal of Family Issues, 32*, 209–236. doi:10.1177/0192513X10377066.

Coontz, S. (2005). *Marriage, a history: How love conquered marriage*. New York: Penguin.

Crippen, C., & Brew, L. (2007). Intercultural parenting and the transcultural family: A literature review. *The Family Journal, 15*, 107–115. doi:10.1177/1066480706297783.

Cross, S. E., Bacon, P. L., & Morris, M. L. (2000). The relational-interdependent self-construal and relationships. *Journal of Personality and Social Psychology, 78*, 791–808. doi:10.1037//0022-3514.78.4.191.

Desmond, M., & Lopez Turley, R. N. (2009). The role of familism in explaining the Hispanic White college application gap. *Social Problems, 56*, 311–334. doi:10.1525/sp.2009.56.2.311.

Diener, E., & Diener, C. (1996). Most people are happy. *Psychological Science, 7*, 181–185. doi:10.1111/j.1467-9280.1996.tb00354.x.

Dressler, W. W. (2004). Culture and the risk of disease. *British Medical Bulletin, 69*, 21–31. doi:10.1093/bmb/ldh020.

Dressler, W. W., Balieiro, M. C., Ribeiro, R. P., & Dos Santo, J. E. (2007). Cultural consonance and psychological distress: Examining the associations in multiple cultural domains. *Culture, Medicine and Psychiatry, 31*, 195–224. doi:10.1007/s11013-007-9046-2.

Farver, J. M., Xu, Y., Bhadha, B. R., Narang, S., & Lieber, E. (2007). Ethnic identity, acculturation, parenting beliefs, and adolescent adjustment: A comparison of Asian Indian and European American families. *Merrill-Palmer Quarterly, 53*, 184–215. doi:10.1353/mpq.2007.0010.

Flores, E., Tschann, J. M., Marin, B. V., & Pantoja, P. (2004). Marital conflict and acculturation among Mexican American husbands and wives. *Cultural Diversity and Ethnic Minority Psychology, 10*, 39–52. doi:10.1037/1099-9809.10.1.39.

Fuligni, A. J. (2007). Family obligation, college enrollment, and emerging adulthood in Asian and Latin American families. *Child Development Perspectives, 1*, 96–100. doi:10.1111/j.1750-8606.2007.00022.x.

Fuligni, A. J., Tseng, V., & Lam, M. (1999). Attitudes toward family obligations among American adolescents with Asian, Latin American, and European backgrounds. *Child Development, 70*, 1030–1044. doi:10.1111/1467-8624.00075.

Gaines, S. O., Jr., Buriel, R., Liu, J. H., & Rios, D. I. (1997). *Culture, ethnicity, and personal relationship processes*. New York: Routledge.

Gaines, S. O., Gurung, R. A. R., Lin, Y., & Pouli, N. (2006). Interethnic relationships. In J. Feeney & P. Noller (Eds.), *Close relationships: Functions, forms, and processes* (pp. 171–187). New York: Psychology Press.

Gonzaga, G. C., Turner, R. A., Keltner, D., Campos, B., & Altemus, M. (2006). Romantic love and sexual desire in close relationships. *Emotion, 6*, 163–179. doi:10.1037/1528-3542.6.2.163.

Gottman, J., Coan, J., Swanson, C., & Carrere, S. (1998). Predicting marital happiness and stability from newlywed interactions. *Journal of Marriage and the Family, 60*, 5–22. doi:10.2307/353438.

Hamilton, W. D. (1964). The genetical evolution of social behavior. Parts 1 and 2. *Journal of Theoretical Biology, 7*, 1–51. doi:10.1016/0022-5193(64)90038-4.

Heine, S. J. (2011). *Cultural psychology* (2nd ed.). New York: W. W. Norton & Company.

Heine, S. J., Lehman, D. R., Markus, H. R., & Kitayama, S. (1999). Is there a universal need for positive self-regard? *Psychological Review, 106*, 766–794. doi:10.1037//0033-295X.106.4.766.

Herrera, N., Campos, B., Keltner, D., & Gonzaga, G. C. (in preparation). Managing threat: Jealousy and relationship satisfaction in Latino couples.

Hirsch, J. S. (2003). *A courtship after marriage: Sexuality and love in Mexican transnational families*. Berkeley/Los Angeles: University of California Press.

Ho, D. Y. F. (1994). Filial piety, authoritarian moralism, and cognitive conservatism in Chinese societies. *Genetic, Social, and General Psychology Monographics, 120*(3), 347–365. Retrieved from http://hub.hku.hk/bitstream/10722/53184/1/2581.pdf?accept=1

Hohmann-Marriot, B. E., & Amato, P. (2008). Relationship quality in interethnic marriages and cohabitations. *Social Forces, 87*, 825–855. doi:10.1353/sof.0.0151.

Holloway, R. A., Waldrip, A. M., & Ickes, W. (2009). Evidence that a simpático self-schema accounts for differences in the self-concepts and social behavior of Latinos versus Whites (and Blacks). *Journal of Personality and Social Psychology, 96*, 1012–1028. doi:10.1037/a0013883.

Hrdy, S. B. (1999). *Mother nature: A history of mothers, infants, and natural selection*. New York: Pantheon.

Hunt, L. M. (2005). Beyond cultural competence: Applying humility to clinical settings. In G. E. Henderson et al. (Eds.), *The social medicine reader* (2nd ed., Vol. 2, pp. 134–136). Durham: Duke University Press.

Hynie, M., Lalonde, R. N., & Lee, N. (2006). Parent-child value transmission among Chinese immigrants to North American: The case of traditional mate preferences. *Cultural Diversity and Ethnic Minority Psychology, 12*, 230–244. doi:10.1037/1099-9809.12.2.230.

Jackson, P. B., Kleiner, S., Geist, C., & Cebulko, K. (2011). Conventions of courtship: Gender and race differences in the significance of dating rituals. *Journal of Family Issues, 32*, 629–652. doi:10.1177/0192513X10395113.

Keefe, S. E., Padilla, A. M., & Carlos, M. L. (1979). The Mexican-American extended family as an emotional support system. *Human Organization, 38*, 144–152.

Kim, H. S., Sherman, D. K., & Taylor, S. E. (2008). Culture and social support. *American Psychologist, 63*, 518–526. doi:10.1037/0003-066X.

Kleinman, A. (1980). *Patients and healers in the context of culture: An exploration of the borderland between anthropology, medicine, and psychiatry*. Berkeley/Los Angeles: University of California Press.

Magaña, S., & Smith, M. J. (2006). Health outcomes of midlife and older Latina and Black American mothers of children with developmental disabilities. *Mental Retardation, 44*, 224–234. doi:10.1352/0047-6765(2006)44[224:HOOMAO]2.0.CO;2.

Markus, H. R., & Kitayama, S. (1991). Culture and the self: Implications for cognition, emotion and motivation. *Psychological Review, 98*, 224–253. doi:10.1037/0033-295X.98.2.224.

Mason, C. A., Walker-Barnes, C. J., Tu, J., & Martinez-Arrue, R. (2004). Ethnic differences in the affective meaning of parental control behaviors. *The Journal of Primary Prevention, 25*, 59–79. doi:10.1023/B:JOPP.0000039939.83804.37.

Miller, R. S., Perlman, D., & Brehm, S. S. (2007). *Intimate relationships* (4th ed.). New York: McGraw Hill.

Mongeau, P. A., Jacobsen, J., & Donnerstein, C. (2007). Defining dates and first date goals: Generalizing from undergraduates to single adults. *Communication Research, 34*, 526–547. doi:10.1177/0093650207305235.

Montoya, R. M., Horton, R. S., & Kirchner, J. (2008). Is actual similarity necessary for attraction? A meta-analysis of actual and perceived similarity. *Journal of Social and Personal Relationships, 25*, 889–922. doi:10.1177/0265407508096700.

Morling, B., Kitayama, S., & Miyamoto, Y. (2003). American and Japanese women use different coping strategies during normal pregnancy. *Personality and Social Psychology Bulletin, 29*, 1533–1546. doi:10.1177/0146167203256878.

Negy, C., & Snyder, D. (2000). Relationship satisfaction of Mexican American and non-Hispanic White American interethnic couples: Issues of acculturation and clinical intervention. *Journal of Marital and Family Therapy, 26*, 293–304. doi:10.1111/j.1752-0606.2000.tb00299.x.

Peng, K., & Nisbett, R. E. (1999). Culture, dialectics, and reasoning about contradiction. *American Psychologist, 54*, 741–754. doi:10.1037//0003-066X.54.9.741.

Phinney, J. S., Kim-Jo, T., Osorio, S., & Vilhjalmsdottir, P. (2005). Relatedness in adolescent-parent disagreements: Ethnic and developmental factors. *Journal of Adolescent Research, 20*, 8–39. doi:10.1177/0743558404271237.

Regan, P. C., Durvasula, R., Howell, L., Ureno, O., & Rea, M. (2004). Gender, ethnicity, and the developmental timing of first sexual and romantic experiences. *Social Behavior and Personality, 32*, 667–676. doi:10.2224/sbp.2004.32.7.667.

Repetti, R. L., Taylor, S. E., & Seeman, T. E. (2002). Risky families: Family social environments and the mental and physical health of offspring. *Psychological Bulletin, 128*, 330–366. doi:10.1037/0033-2909.128.2.230.

Riela, S., Rodriguez, G., Aron, A., Xu, X., & Acevedo, B. P. (2010). Experiences of falling in love: Investigating culture, ethnicity, gender, and speed. *Journal of Social and Personal Relationships, 27*, 473–493. doi:10.1177/0265407510363508.

Ruby, M. B., Falk, C. F., Heine, S. J., Villa, C., & Silberstein, O. (2012). Not all collectivisms are equal: Opposing preferences for ideal affect between East Asians and Mexicans. *Emotion, 12*(6), 1206–1209. doi:10.1037/a0029118.

Sabogal, F., Marín, G., Otero-Sabogal, R., Marín, B. V., & Pérez-Stable, E. J. (1987). Hispanic familism and acculturation: What changes and what doesn't? *Hispanic Journal of Behavioral Sciences, 9*, 397–412. doi:10.1177/07399863870094003.

Schieffelin, B. B., & Ochs, E. (Eds.). (1986). *Language socialization across cultures*. New York: Cambridge University Press.

Schneider, M. E., & Ward, D. J. (2003). The role of ethnic identification and perceived social support in Latinos' adjustment to college. *Hispanic Journal of Behavioral Sciences, 25*, 539–554. doi:10.1177/0739986303259306.

Schofield, T. J., Parke, R. D., Kim, Y., & Coltrane, S. (2008). Bridging the acculturation gap: Parent-child relationship quality as a moderator in Mexican American families. *Developmental Psychology, 44*, 1190–1194. doi:10.1037/a0012529.

Schwartz, S. J. (2007). The applicability of familism to diverse ethnic groups: A preliminary study. *Journal of Social Psychology, 147*, 101–118. doi:10.3200/SOCP.147.2.101-118.

Shiota, M. N., Campos, B., Gonzaga, G. C., Keltner, D., & Peng, K. (2010). I love you but … : Cultural differences in complexity of emotional experience during interaction with a romantic partner. *Cognition & Emotion, 24*, 786–799. doi:10.1080/02699930902990480.

Smith, D. E. (1993). The standard North American family: SNAF as an ideological code. *Journal of Family Issues, 14*, 50–65. doi:10.1177/0192513X93014001005.

Soto, J. A., Levenson, R. W., & Ebling, R. (2005). Cultures of moderation and expression: Emotional experience, behavior, and physiology in Chinese Americans and Mexican Americans. *Emotion, 5*, 154–165. doi:10.1037/1528-3542.5.2.154.

Sprecher, S., & Felmlee, D. (1992). The influence of parents and friends on the quality and stability of romantic relationships: A three-wave longitudinal investigation. *Journal of Marriage and Family, 54*, 888–900. doi:10.2307/353170.

Taylor, S. E., Sherman, D. K., Kim, H. S., Jarcho, J., Takagi, K., & Dunagan, M. S. (2004). Culture and social support: Who seeks it and why? *Journal of Personality and Social Psychology, 87*, 354–362. doi:10.1037/0022-3514.87.3.354.

Troy, A. B., Lewis-Smith, J., & Laurenceau, J. (2006). Interracial and intraracial romantic relationships: The search for differences in satisfaction, conflict, and attachment style. *Journal of Social and Personal Relationships, 23*, 65–80. doi:10.1177/0265407506060178.

Tsai, J. L., Levenson, R. W., & McCoy, K. (2006). Cultural and temperamental variation in emotional response. *Emotion, 6*, 484–497. doi:10.1037/1528-3542.6.3.484.

Updegraff, K. A., McHale, S. M., Whiteman, S. D., Thayer, S. M., & Delgado, M. Y. (2005). Adolescent sibling relationships in Mexican American families: Exploring the role of familism. *Journal of Family Psychology, 19*, 512–522. doi:10.1037/0893-3200.19.4.512.

Vandello, J. A., & Cohen, D. (2003). Male honor and female fidelity: Implicit cultural scripts that perpetuate domestic violence. *Journal of Personality and Social Psychology, 84*, 997–1010. doi:10.1037/0022-3514.84.5.997.

Vega, W. A., Patterson, T., Sallis, J., Nader, P., Atkins, C., & Abramson, I. (1986). Cohesion and adaptability in Mexican-American and Anglo families. *Journal of Marriage and Family, 48*, 857–867. doi:10.2307/352579.

Williamson, H. C., Ju, X., Bradbury, T. N., Karney, B. R., Fang, X., & Liu, X. (2012). Communication behavior and relationship satisfaction among American and Chinese newlywed couples. *Journal of Family Psychology, 26*, 308–315. doi:10.1037/a0027752.

Wilt, J. (2011). Normal families facing unique challenges: The psychosocial functioning of multiracial couples, parents and children. *The New School Psychology Bulletin, 9*, 34–41.

Yan, Y. (2002). Courtship, love and premarital sex in a North China village. *The China Journal, 48*, 29–53. doi:10.2307/3182440.

Yeh, K.-H., & Bedford, O. (2004). Filial belief and parent-child conflict. *International Journal of Psychology, 39*, 132–144. doi:10.1080/00207590344000312.

Zambrana, R. E., Dunkel-Schetter, C., Collins, N. L., & Scrimshaw, S. C. M. (1999). Mediators of ethnic-associated differences in infant birth weight. *Journal of Urban Health, 76*, 102–116. doi:10.1007/BF02344465.

Part III
Specific Populations

Chapter 8
Positive Psychology Across the Lifespan

Jeanne Nakamura, Michael Warren, Brittany Branand, Pi-Ju Liu, Brett Wheeler, and Thomas Chan

Human development is dominated by dramatic shifts in emphasis.

Erik Erikson (1982)

Social scientists recognize that age, like gender, race, and class, constitutes a basic source of difference for individuals and societies (Settersten and Mayer 1997). This is so in two senses. First, and perhaps most familiar from a multicultural perspective, age is a component of identity. One's age group (e.g., youth) and birth cohort (e.g., "Baby Boomer") are components of one's representation of self, and how one perceives other people. Age identity is influenced by societal culture: the age-related beliefs, norms of conduct, and expectations of a society affect its members' self-experience and their attitudes and behaviors toward one another. Second, biopsychosocial functioning varies with age. Psychobiological capacities and processes vary; age differences in cognitive ability are an obvious example. Opportunities for action and patterns of interaction with the environment also vary; age-graded social contexts (e.g., school) and social roles (e.g., elder) create distinct life-worlds. Like age identity, biopsychosocial age differences are influenced by societal culture.

For these two reasons, individuals of different ages (and the same individual at different ages) to some extent occupy different cultures. The extent to which this is true varies depending on their place in the life course and the degree to which their society is age-graded. Life periods are social constructions whose borders are malleable.

The first four authors listed were respectively the lead authors on the chapter's four main sections.

J. Nakamura (✉) • M. Warren • B. Branand • P.-J. Liu • B. Wheeler • T. Chan
Division of Behavioral and Organizational Sciences, Claremont Graduate University, 1227 N. Dartmouth Ave., Claremont, CA 91711, USA
e-mail: jeanne.nakamura@cgu.edu

J. Teramoto Pedrotti and L.M. Edwards (eds.), *Perspectives on the Intersection of Multiculturalism and Positive Psychology*, Cross-Cultural Advancements in Positive Psychology 7, DOI 10.1007/978-94-017-8654-6_8,

For instance, the life course has grown more differentiated in the West. It has been argued that the idea of childhood did not emerge until the seventeenth century (Ariès 1960/1962) and the twentieth century saw the advent of both "emerging adulthood," a period characterized by extended exploration of life choices (Arnett 2004), and a sharper distinction between "young old" and "old old" (Neugarten 1974).

In addition to effects of societal culture and history, age is cross-cut by other cultural categories (e.g., class, ethnicity, gender). Age and cohort identities, and individual age periods, are valued and experienced differently in different segments of the same society. For example, college-bound teens may see themselves as no longer children but not yet adults, while teens who have left school may already identify as adults, especially if they are raising children. In childrearing, the most adaptive parenting and attachment styles vary based on cultural factors like level of environmental risk and norms about closeness and self-reliance (Thompson 1998).

Cross-culturally, awareness of age as a basis of difference emerges early. Culture affects how age is evaluated. Adolescence and old age are stigmatized in much of the West (Zebrowitz and Montepare 2000). In many cultures, *being older* is perceived as good during the first two decades of life but already by early childhood, and continuing across adulthood, *being old* is not. In a German study, young, midlife, and older adults alike reported expecting gains to decline with age and losses to increase (Heckhausen et al. 1989). Still, perceptions of life periods were differentiated: gains in some areas (wisdom, dignity) were viewed as unavailable to the young, and growth in other areas (experience, honesty) was seen as possible into old age.

This chapter is focused specifically on age-linked differences in *optimal* functioning. Increasingly, positive development is studied in positive psychology. However, positive psychology research often is silent on the question of how age or birth cohort conditions what "positive" means. Mirroring psychology more generally, researchers sometimes include age in a study but treat it purely as a nuisance variable, controlling for it but not considering what it means if age effects are found. Sometimes research on positive adulthood treats age as a variable of interest but treats the adult lifespan monolithically, leaving unclear whether differences lie between early and middle adulthood or between middle and late adulthood. Further, with noteworthy exceptions (e.g., Vaillant 2004), positive psychology has relied on cross-sectional data.

8.1 Age Differences and Positive Development Over the Lifespan

Many inquiries about the nature of age groups as distinct cultures have been *descriptive*, directed toward identifying differences with age in optimal functioning. Do strengths and other positive qualities, capacities, and processes differ across age groups or peak at different times? Are they deployed in different ways at different points in the life course or take different forms? To move beyond describing and *explain* age differences in positive functioning requires theory-guided analysis of factors in the individual, the context, and their interaction; the realm of developmental science. Development – systematic, sequential change in the person-in-context – is a major source of age differences in optimal functioning. Much of lifespan developmental theory addresses the interaction between developmental tasks and other age-related challenges on the one hand, and the person's resources for responding to these challenges on the other (McCormick et al. 2011). Psychosocial theory (Erikson 1950) pioneered developmental explanation of age-based cultures from birth to death. According to Erikson, development is propelled by the ascendance in predictable succession of eight urgent developmental issues or "crises" that require active negotiation. Relevant to positive psychology, strengths from hope to wisdom are believed to arise out of successful navigation of the successive periods of life. Later sections will highlight the crises of identity (integration of identifications), intimacy (mutuality), generativity (contribution to future generations' well-being), and ego-integrity (acceptance of one's life as lived). More recent approaches to lifespan development also provide positive perspectives on human functioning and change. Baltes and colleagues define development as a dynamic balancing of gain and loss at every age with optimal balance as the lifelong goal (Baltes and Baltes 1990; Settersten 1999). These theories are consistent with a multicultural perspective on age, avoiding the privileging of one age group and the diminishing of others as deficient forms. In particular, recent work on positive youth development and positive aging exemplify the effort to understand flourishing during every period of life (Lerner et al. 2005; Vaillant 2004). Later sections will illustrate these themes.

A science of positive psychology across the lifespan entails at least three interrelated endeavors: (a) understanding optimal functioning within the culture of different life periods on their own terms; (b) including positive pathways, and the mechanisms that account for them, alongside normative and derailed pathways; and (c) charting the developmental trajectory of each aspect of the "positive." In each case, other cultural differences (e.g., race, ethnicity, gender, etc.) may inflect the patterns found.

Illustrating the first of these tasks, the Experience Sampling Method yields rich portraits of the cultures of specific life periods. For example, Csikszentmihalyi and Larson (1984) found U.S. parents and children both spend many of their happiest moments with friends but this time occupies a large part of youths' lives versus only a small fraction of their parents'. Regarding the second task, resilience researchers are tracing the pathways through life associated with thriving despite adverse early circumstances (Masten et al. 2009). Illustrating the third task, cross-sectional data suggest that *meaning in life* increases from emerging adulthood through older adulthood while *searching* for meaning declines (Steger et al. 2009).

The following sections trace three key positive-developmental trajectories that contribute to the distinctive culture of each life period from adolescence to older adulthood: forms of well-being, romantic relationships, and the virtue of wisdom. These examples respectively highlight age differences in the affective, cognitive, and interpersonal domains (cf. Chapters 5, 6 and 7, this volume). First, changes from adolescence to older adulthood in individual well-being are discussed. Currently, the very definition of well-being is the subject of much debate. The trajectories of both eudaimonic and hedonic well-being are outlined. Second, a major contributor to well-being, romantic relationships, is discussed. Multiple lines of research have converged to suggest relationships with other people are among the main sources of well-being throughout life and across cultures. This section identifies antecedents of romantic relationships and describes how these close ties change with age. The third section describes age differences in the developmental trajectory of one virtue – the *master* virtue, some argue (Schwartz and Sharpe 2006) – wisdom. In most folk psychologies, the young are foolish and the old wise; lifespan research tells a more complex story about the wisdom attainable at different ages.

8.2 Well-Being Across the Lifespan

Eudaimonia and *hedonia* refer to two common conceptualizations of well-being. This section broadly defines eudaimonic well-being (EWB) as an individual's present well-being as indexed by the presence of "criterial goods" (e.g., positive relationships) that contribute to positive development (Ryan and Huta 2009; Ryff and Singer 1998). This view of EWB is functional in emphasizing that aspects of present well-being yield desirable future outcomes (Ryan and Huta 2009; Ryff and Singer 1998). This broad definition subsumes both traditional *indicators* of EWB (e.g., purpose in life) and what some authors argue to be *predictors* of EWB (e.g., prosocial peers). This definition facilitates a discussion of "age as culture" by allowing both psychological and contextual age-relevant constructs to fit the rubric of EWB. Just as definitions and manifestations of well-being may vary in different racial or gender groups, so too can age-relevant criterial goods suggest a shifting definition of EWB across the lifespan.

Hedonic well-being (HWB) traditionally pertains to immediate pleasure (versus pain). However, it is widely operationalized as subjective well-being: life satisfaction, positive affect, and (minimal) negative affect (Ryan and Deci 2001). Because HWB and EWB differ conceptually and empirically (Compton et al. 1996), a discussion of how both are experienced and defined in sequential portions of the lifespan is warranted. Because well-being is difficult to measure in young children, the discussion begins with adolescence.

8.2.1 Adolescence

From an EWB perspective, widespread changes during adolescence represent growth opportunities. The influential positive youth development (PYD) perspective underscores the role of both endogenous strengths (e.g., self-regulation) and contextual supports (e.g., positive adult role models) as contributors in achieving one's potential (Lerner et al. 2005). Confirmatory factor analysis offers a core PYD construct, consisting of the Five C's of Character, Confidence, Competence, Connection, and Caring (Lerner et al. 2005). Although PYD constructs may vary across cultures (Shek and Ma 2010), programs designed to foster the Five Cs have been found to protect adolescents from problem behaviors and promote healthy functioning in *both* U.S. and Hong Kong samples (Leffert et al. 1998; Sun and Shek 2012). Furthermore, the burgeoning of PYD programs for youth diverse in gender, SES, and nationality (e.g., China, El Salvador, Australia) points to a growing cross-national goal to develop these PYD goods. In sum, even U.S.-derived PYD goods may set the foundation for a flourishing adult life.

An explosion of intra-individual and contextual changes impacts adolescents' HWB. In the U.S., school schedules dictate that adolescents experience a new classroom context every hour. In addition, exposure to sex, drugs, and peer pressure increases during a time of extreme hormonal changes. It is little wonder that emotional experience is so variable during the second decade of life (Csikszentmihalyi and Larson 1984). Findings from a longitudinal study of U.S. youth suggest that general mood declines across adolescence, likely reflecting decreases in positive affect and stability in negative affect (Weinstein et al. 2007). Other factors may also interact with age-related trends as was shown in a cross-sectional study of German adolescents where girls had lower life satisfaction than boys across most ages in this group (Goldbeck et al. 2007). In sum, although providing opportunities for growth, the intense changes of adolescence are associated with overarching declines in HWB.

8.2.2 *Emerging Adulthood Through Middle Adulthood*

While many of the same criterial goods (e.g., positive relationships) of EWB remain important throughout life, their expression is tied to age-relevant issues. In U.S. adults, roughly half of one's waking hours are spent at work. Consequently, identity issues shift focus towards one's professional self-concept (Gibson 2003), and "mastery" is redefined to reflect career competencies. Interpersonally, intimacy formation is emphasized in young adulthood and generativity in middle adulthood (Erikson 1950). Importantly, normative timelines (e.g., marriage age) and value hierarchies vary by culture, uniquely shaping the interpersonal development aspect of EWB (Arnett 2004).

Based on cross-sectional data, HWB seems to decrease throughout emerging and middle adulthood, rebounding in late-middle adulthood. Mroczek and Kolarz (1998) found that positive affect decreases from age 25 through 35 in U.S. adults, and begins to increase again at 45. They also found a significant linear decrease in negative affect starting at 25. With regard to life satisfaction, cross-national data indicate that life satisfaction, like positive affect, declines throughout early and middle adulthood, then steadily increases starting at age 47 (Blanchflower and Oswald 2008). These fluctuations in life satisfaction may reflect culture- and age-normative circumstances, such as the struggles following the birth of a child in young adults in U.S. culture. This said, cultural differences in emotional complexity have been found with respect to Asian versus North American cultures. According to Spencer-Rodgers et al. (2010) Asian adults are more likely to experience a positive correlation between positive and negative affect. As only positive affect was studied by Blanchflower and Oswald (2008), more research is needed to determine whether age patterns may be more complex than these results.

8.2.3 Older Adulthood

Older adulthood is replete with changes across physical, cognitive, social, emotional, and motivational domains. EWB is redefined in terms of successful adaptation to these changes (e.g., optimizing gains while buffering losses), efficient emotion regulation, and cultivation of a sense of meaning and acceptance of one's life as a whole. With respect to adaptation, key processes that contribute to optimal aging include selection, optimization, and compensation (Baltes and Baltes 1990). For example, optimization involves focused *attention* to one's goals and *effort* to achieve them, precursors to optimal states such as flow and vital engagement (Nakamura and Csikszentmihalyi 2003). Importantly, optimization and other adaptive self-regulation processes can contribute to optimal engagement in life in the face of significant threats to well-being.

A universal salient threat in older adulthood is mortality. Socioemotional selectivity theory proposes that as awareness of mortality increases, a motivational shift occurs in which goals related to emotional meaning are prioritized above goals associated with expanding one's horizons (Samanez-Larkin and Carstensen 2011). This motivational shift leads to changes in emotion regulation strategies, such as the restructuring of one's social life in ways that fortify EWB. Specifically, older adults spend more time with close friends and family, thus increasing the likelihood of experiencing emotional meaning (Samanez-Larkin and Carstensen 2011). In addition, older adults recover faster from negative emotional states, and exhibit biases toward positive information in attention and memory (Charles et al. 2003). An example of positively-biased memory is "positive reminiscing," or recalling and reliving one's joyous experiences (Butler 1963; Charles et al. 2003). Such practices provide a context for achieving ego integrity – Erikson's final stage of psychosocial development, characterized by constructing a meaningful picture of one's life as a whole.

Interestingly, practices including positive reminiscing suggest that the culture of older adulthood is in tune with finding pleasure in present EWB processes. For example, cultivating close relationships seems to yield benefits to HWB: A cross-national meta-analysis of 286 studies (from English and German language journals) found that relationship *quality* was more strongly related to HWB than relationship *quantity* (Pinquart and Sorensen 2000). In other words, that which optimizes the present and the future may converge in later life.

A key finding with respect to HWB is that despite objective losses, older adults report similar levels of HWB as compared with younger adults – the "paradox of aging" (Kunzmann et al. 2000). A meta-analysis of 125 studies (from English and

German language journals) found that negative affect only slightly increases, and positive affect only slightly decreases, across middle and older adulthood (Pinquart 2001). Further, a study comparing U.S. participants (primarily Caucasian) and participants from China found that negative affect was lower in both older adult samples compared to their younger adult counterparts (Pethtel and Chen 2010). No main effect of age on PA was reported. However, in line with previously mentioned research, PA and NA were positively correlated in the Chinese sample. Mechanisms for this paradox of aging remain up for debate, but may be due to effective emotion regulation strategies that come online during older adulthood (as discussed above). Alternatively, HWB may be preserved due to enhanced respect from family members (e.g., in Asian cultures) or freedom from traditional child-rearing responsibilities among women of past generations. However, the maintenance processes responsible for the paradox of aging rarely keep pace with the dramatic losses experienced at the very end of life, which are associated with terminal declines in life satisfaction, at least in nationally representative samples from Germany, United Kingdom, and U.S. (Gerstorf et al. 2008). The paradox is complex, however, due to the lack of consistent findings across cultural groups; more research in non-Western and non-White populations would help to clarify this process.

In sum, development throughout life moves a person through a series of age-defined cultures with age-relevant criterial goods that define and redefine the contents of EWB. Further, the various dimensions of HWB follow age-graded patterns throughout the lifespan. Next, a consistent component of EWB and a contributor to HWB throughout life will be discussed: romantic relationships.

8.3 Romantic Relationships Across the Lifespan

Philosophy has long been engaged in studying the nature of human flourishing and thriving. In James Griffin's (1986) description of well-being, he included deep personal relationships among his top five values. Bertrand Russell (1958) defined a life well-lived as one of zest and one that is promoted by, more than anything else, being loved. In studying the significance of others, positive psychology has demonstrated that one's romantic partner, often referred to in U.S. culture as "the significant other," plays a powerful role in both HWB and EWB. The field of positive psychology extends these and other philosophical accounts of the good life and the nature of well-being as it examines the pivotal role of romantic relationships.

Research with Western populations has found the benefits of a supportive romantic relationship to be profound. Cutrona and Russell (1990) demonstrated that romantic relationships promote good health and buffer emotional stress. In a study that included three-fourths of the world's population across 55 nations, Diener (2009) found that a good relationship was the only common predictor of happiness. This said, Diener acknowledges here and in other writings (e.g., Diener and Suh 2000), that methodological issues are often a challenge in comparing culture on Western measures of well-being. In addition, what constitutes a "good relationship" varies from culture to culture.

Even within the broader U.S. culture there is evidence of racial and ethnic differences that impact the development of romantic relationships. For example, marriage for some African American women is not a protective contract promising economic benefits as often perceived by the White dominant society; rather, Burton and Tucker (2009) found that for less privileged African American women marriage held questionable benefit. Within the U.S. Latino culture, many parents place more limitations on adolescent young women than boys when it comes to romantic relationships; the traditional Latino culture and values restrict young girls from dating at an early age, while boys are allowed to date earlier (Raffaelli 2005). While these examples illuminate several cultural differences that impact romantic relationships, some studies have also demonstrated some similarities between major U.S. racial and ethnic groups (e.g., O'Sullivan et al. 2007). Bearing in mind that general findings must be taken with some caution, the following sections outline the development of romantic relationships through the different periods of the lifespan.

8.3.1 Adolescence

Although attachment during infancy sets the stage for later romantic relationships (Bretherton and Munholland 1999), romantic relationships begin during adolescence. In the culture of adolescence within the U.S., romantic relationships are normative and particularly salient (Collins and Steinberg 2006; Furman et al. 2007). For young majority culture teens, romantic relationships promote emotion regulation and help ease interpersonal communications. Although romantic interest at this time of life is characteristically short-term and lacks commitment, this affiliation with potential romantic partners precedes and prepares the teen for involvement in future committed dyadic relationships (Furman and Shomaker 2008; Shulman et al. 2011).

While teens are not searching for a deeper meaning of life in the way they will as adults, they are involved in forming their sense of identity, a necessary developmental step that will later provide the roots for that meaning. Erikson and others assert that adolescent romantic relationships assist in resolving this identity formation and preparing for mature intimacy, an essential capacity for future committed relationships (Beyers and Seiffge-Krenke 2010). In Western majority culture, the development of the ability to create and maintain romantic relationships may be one of the most important developmental tasks during adolescence.

8.3.2 Emerging Adulthood

Arnett (2011) has identified an age-based culture of emerging adulthood, and holds that the years from the late teens to the late 20s are a distinctive period of experience in U.S. social relationships. At this time, young people are involved in longer-term romantic relationships and experience stronger motivation for a lasting connection (Collins and van Dulmen 2006). In contrast to the adolescent period, romantic partners spend more time together than with others (Collins and van Dulmen 2006).

Adolescent romantic encounters are often motivated by the need to enhance status within the peer group (Brown 1999) and to fulfill one's own needs, whereas emerging adulthood relationships are marked by an increase in sensitivity to the needs of others and a balance of the needs of both partners (Shulman and Scharf 2000). Successful romantic relationships in this period provide the deeper level of commitment and interaction that fosters EWB as they begin to give color to the portrait of one's meaning and purpose in life.

8.3.3 *Middle Adulthood*

The adult romantic relationship provides positive support that builds and enhances benefits including well-being over the years (Diener and Seligman 2002; Lyubomirsky et al. 2005; Myers and Diener 1995; Vaillant 2004). Studies examining the marriage relationship have documented that in the United States, not all romantic relationships and marriages are successful as the divorce rate is in excess of 40 % for first time marriages (McCone and O'Donnell 2006). However, Gallagher and Waite (2001) report that 93 % of U.S. citizens sampled hold a happy marriage as a primary life goal. Strikingly, in the comprehensive longitudinal study of the Terman gifted men, Sears (1977) concluded that over their lifetime, these very successful men placed greater importance on achieving satisfaction in their marital relationship than in their work. It is notable, too, that denying people the right to pursue the goal of a happy marriage may have a deleterious effect on well-being. People with same-sex romantic attraction, who are denied the legal right to marry in the United States, report higher rates of minority stress and psychological distress (Rostosky et al. 2009).

Because of the profound impact of this relationship on well-being during the adult period, many researchers have sought to discover how the adult romantic relationship can be strengthened and endure. For example, Aron and Aron (1986) developed a self-expansion model that suggests that adults who continuously share novel experiences deepen their romantic partnership, expanding their sense of self and resulting well-being (Aron et al. 2004). Another, the minding theory (Omarzu et al. 2001), outlines how making the effort to pay specific attention to one's partner helps romantic relationships endure. The bulk of the literature purports that the adult romantic relationship provides the structure for long-term connectedness, the foundation for family, the pillar for building careers, and the mirror that reflects our selves.

8.3.4 *Older Adulthood*

Secure romantic relationships endure throughout the lifespan and continue to grow and provide benefits during the period of older adulthood. The culture of older adulthood allows for continuation and often a strengthening of the emotional bonds of the relationship. As one ages and perceived time on earth shortens, one reassess priorities and determines how best to spend the remaining time. Socioemotional selectivity theory (Charles et al. 2003) explains why older adults prefer to spend more time with their long-term romantic partners and less time with acquaintances or seeking new experiences. Erikson (1950) and Butler (1963) suggested that at this stage romantic relationships and well-being are strengthened by couples sharing reminiscences of their life and time together. Research has shown that shared memories strengthen romantic ties and add cohesion to one's life story, further enhancing EWB (Bazzini et al. 2007). Erikson (1982) theorized that at this life stage of ego integrity, the reflection on the development of the romantic relationship and the commitment to the romantic partner give meaning and purpose to life. Interestingly, in contrast to Erikson's thesis that older couples resolved their need for intimacy at the earlier adult stage, research has shown that older persons still maintain strivings for intimacy, suggesting that this type of striving is equally salient across the lifespan (Sheldon and Kasser 2001).

Romantic relationships throughout the lifespan are a valuable criterial good, offering the opportunity for positive development, growth, commitment, and support. While the form and function of the relationship are distinctive at each period of life, the underlying benefits to well-being are apparent throughout.

8.4 Wisdom Across the Lifespan

Throughout time and cultural traditions, the wise elder has been an archetype, indicating the old are thought to differ from the young in having greater wisdom. Nonetheless, compared with the definition of wisdom in the West, Eastern literatures have a more inclusive view that encompass the cognitive, affective, and interpersonal domains of wisdom (Takahashi 2000). In addition, not all empirical studies have supported the positive relationship between age and wisdom development (e.g., Baltes and Staudinger 2000a). Being young does not necessarily exclude people from being wise, and growing old does not automatically yield credits of wisdom (Erikson 1959). However, unlike most cognitive abilities, wisdom does not appear to decline as people age.

Since wisdom is a product of individual experiences and cultural context, the definition of wisdom varies across studies. Most paradigms recognize the cognitive component of wisdom that requires an expert knowledge system about important matters in life, which is the pragmatics of life (Baltes and Staudinger 2000b). However, Baltes and Staudinger also mentioned dealing with complex and uncertain human conditions as part of being a wise person. Ardelt (2000) referred to wisdom as overcoming self-centeredness, and developing feelings of compassion for others. Sternberg (1998) stated that wisdom involves the balance of intrapersonal, interpersonal, and extrapersonal (such as environmental or organizational) interests. Strengths of wisdom and knowledge in the Values in Action Inventory of

Strengths (VIA-IS; Peterson and Seligman 2004) include open-mindedness, perspective, and creativity as characteristics of wisdom. Lastly, Schwartz and Sharpe (2006) discussed wisdom in the Aristotelian tradition, and asserted that the moral skills and moral will to do the right thing, also called practical wisdom, is the core of all virtues. Cultural and societal groups affect the definition of wisdom as well. Among Alaska Natives, wisdom involves unspoken rules of individual contribution to the community and life experiences in each village (Lewis 2010). For Taiwanese, remaining modest and unobtrusive in social interactions is one of the factors for being wise (Yang 2001).

Culture only delineates part of the story about wisdom. As developmental tasks change across the lifespan, facets of wisdom differ among age groups, because different age groups weigh components of wisdom differently. Western research concluded that younger adults regard the cognitive component to be more central, emphasizing the learning of knowledge. Older adults are more likely to state that experience with life challenges is equally important, expressing a more complex view of wisdom (Glück and Bluck 2011). The following discussion describes the development of wisdom across the lifespan.

8.4.1 Antecedents of Wisdom

Formal knowledge taught in school does not directly lead to wisdom, but the acquisition of wisdom can be scaffolded in school and at home (e.g., Sternberg 2001). For example, moral reasoning, perspective taking, and compassion have been central developmental topics related to the acquisition of wisdom (e.g., Pasupathi and Staudinger 2001). Moral reasoning fosters the understanding of fairness and justice. Moral dilemmas involve concerns for human problems, and often require complex reasoning to provide a solution. In addition, perspective taking emerges in childhood, and recognizing others' perspective facilitates resolution of interpersonal conflicts. The development of compassion also helps overcome conflicts, since feeling compassionate connects people and leads to acknowledging others' point of view (Ardelt 2000).

Although across cultures, people do not usually relate wisdom to youth, Western studies support that adolescence and young adulthood are stages for building blocks of wisdom to develop. Pasupathi et al. (2001) argued that controlling for intelligence, wisdom-related knowledge emerges between 14 and 25. Examples of wisdom precursors include intellectual capacity and personality characteristics (Richardson and Pasupathi 2005). Cognitive capacity such as problem solving strategies increases rapidly in adolescence, and it is one of the prerequisites for higher-level thinking associated with wisdom. In addition, level of openness increases in Western adolescents, and stabilizes at around the age of 30. Since participants with the personality characteristic demonstrated a higher level of wisdom-related knowledge, wisdom can potentially be cultivated at a young age (Pasupathi et al. 2001).

8.4.2 *Wisdom in Middle and Older Adulthood*

Mastering bodies of knowledge is one of the conditions for being wise. Because acquiring an expert-level knowledge system in any field requires time for most people, it is reasonable to assume that wisdom increases as people grow old. Although the ability to operate large amounts of knowledge, which is related to fluid intelligence, declines in advanced age, crystallized intelligence, which is the knowledge of the world, does not decrease as people enter old age. As the fundamental pragmatics of life are part of the cognitive facet of wisdom, unlike most cognitive functions across the lifespan that decline, wisdom, once acquired, is a strength that does not wane.

Although relevant gains during the early years are cognitive, knowledge is only one facet of wisdom. In particular, corresponding to the affective facet of wisdom, middle-age and older adults have motivational goals to regulate emotions (e.g., Charles et al. 2003). When facing social dilemmas or interpersonal conflicts, older adults are more likely to provide wise solutions to minimize negative emotions resulting from interpersonal conflicts. A recent study supported the argument by demonstrating more advanced social reasoning skills in older adults compared to younger and middle-age adults (Grossmann et al. 2010). Similar results were presented in cross-cultural studies, but age differences in maintaining interpersonal harmony were more evident among a U.S. sample than among a sample of Japanese individuals (e.g., Grossmann et al. 2012). Additionally, studies with Western populations showed that being a wise exemplar who provides good advice benefits others' lives, and interactions with the wise foster the development of wisdom (Baltes and Smith 2008). In addition to age, non-normative events such as personal adversity and professional training can also contribute to the development of wisdom.

In sum, wisdom is certainly not a natural product of longevity. Nonetheless, if building blocks are established at a young age, wisdom is one of the virtues most likely to continue increasing during adulthood. Cognitive and physical constraints could prevent older adults from acquiring large amounts of knowledge, but when these factors are controlled for, older adults demonstrate an advantage due to greater life experience. Studies on emotional and social cognition also bolster the view that wisdom grows, such that older adults perform better when facing social conflicts.

8.5 Conclusion

Age, and relatedly birth cohort, affect each person's experience and identity. In this chapter, the cultures of different age groups were viewed from a positive lifespan-developmental perspective. Three important areas in positive psychology were highlighted: well-being, romantic relationships, and wisdom. Many directions for future research are evident, particularly with regard to studies of non-White populations within the U.S. The cultures associated with different life periods, and indeed the very definition of these periods, may differ multiculturally and evolve across historical time. Moreover, age interacts with other facets of culture discussed in this volume, including gender, ethnicity, and class. More research should address the diverse ways that age, and individual life periods, are experienced and valued in different cultures.

References

Ardelt, M. (2000). Antecedents and effects of wisdom in old age: A longitudinal perspective on aging well. *Research on Aging, 20*, 360–394.

Ariès, P. (1962). *Centuries of childhood*. New York: Vintage (Original work published 1960).

Arnett, J. J. (2004). A longer road to adulthood. In *Emerging adulthood* (pp. 3–25). New York: Oxford University Press.

Arnett, J. J. (2011). The cultural psychology of a new life stage. In L. A. Jensen (Ed.), *Bridging cultural and developmental approaches to psychology* (pp. 255–275). New York: Oxford University Press.

Aron, A., & Aron, E. N. (1986). *Love and the expansion of self: Understanding attraction and satisfaction*. New York: Hemisphere Publishing/Harper & Row.

Aron, A., Aron, E., & Norma, C. (2004). Self-expansion model of motivation and cognition in close relationships and beyond. In M. B. Brewer & M. Hewstone (Eds.), *Self and social identity* (pp. 99–123). Malden: Blackwell Publishing.

Baltes, P. B., & Baltes, M. M. (1990). Psychological perspectives on successful aging: The model of selective optimization with compensation. In P. B. Baltes & M. M. Baltes (Eds.), *Successful aging* (pp. 1–34). New York: Cambridge University Press.

Baltes, P. B., & Smith, J. (2008). The fascination of wisdom: Its nature, ontogeny, and function. *Perspectives on Psychological Science, 3*, 56–64.

Baltes, P. B., & Staudinger, U. M. (2000a). Wisdom: A metaheuristic (pragmatic) to orchestrate mind and virtue toward excellence. *American Psychologist, 55*, 122–136.

Baltes, P. B., & Staudinger, U. M. (2000b). The search for psychology of wisdom. *Current Directions in Psychological Science, 2*, 75–80.

Bazzini, D. G., Stack, E. R., Martincin, P. D., & Davis, C. P. (2007). The effect of reminiscing about laughter on relationship satisfaction. *Motivation and Emotion, 31*, 25–34.

Beyers, W., & Seiffge-Krenke, I. (2010). Does identity precede intimacy? Testing Erikson's theory on romantic development in emerging adults of the 21st century. *Journal of Adolescent Research, 25*, 387–415.

Blanchflower, D. G., & Oswald, A. J. (2008). Is well-being U-shaped over the life cycle? *Social Science & Medicine, 66*, 1733–1749. doi:10.1016/j.socscimed.2008.01.030.

Bretherton, I., & Munholland, K. A. (1999). In J. Cassidy & P. R. Shaver (Eds.), *Handbook of attachment* (pp. 89–111). New York: Guilford.

Brown, B. B. (1999). You're going out with whom? Peer group influence on adolescent romantic relationships. In W. Furman, B. B. Brown, & C. Feiring (Eds.), *Development of romantic relationships in adolescence* (pp. 291–329). New York: Cambridge University Press.

Burton, L. M., & Tucker, M. B. (2009). Romantic unions in an era of uncertainty: A post-Moynihan perspective on African American women and marriage. *The Annals of the American Academy of Political and Social Science, 621*, 132–148.

Butler, R. N. (1963). The life review. *Psychiatry, 26*, 65–76.

Charles, S. T., Mather, M., & Carstensen, L. L. (2003). Aging and emotional memory. *Journal of Experimental Psychology: General, 132*, 310–324.

Collins, W. A., & Steinberg, L. (2006). Adolescent development in interpersonal context. In N. Eisenberg, W. Damon, & R. M. Lerner (Eds.), *Handbook of child psychology* (Vol. 3, pp. 1003–1067). Hoboken: Wiley.

Collins, A., & van Dulmen, M. (2006). Friendships and romance in emerging adulthood: Assessing distinctiveness in close relationships. In J. J. Arnett & J. L. Tanner (Eds.), *Emerging adults in America* (pp. 219–234). Washington, DC: American Psychological Association.
Compton, W. C., Smith, M. L., Cornish, K. A., & Qualls, D. L. (1996). Factor structure of mental health measures. *Journal of Personality and Social Psychology, 71*, 406–413.
Csikszentmihalyi, M., & Larson, R. (1984). *Being adolescent*. New York: Basic Books.
Cutrona, C. E., & Russell, D. W. (1990). Type of social support and specific stress: Towards a theory of optimal matching. In B. R. Sarason, I. G. Sarason, & G. R. Pierce (Eds.), *Social support: An international view* (pp. 319–366). Oxford, England: Wiley.
Diener, E. (2009). *Culture and well-being: The collected works of Ed Diener*. New York: Springer.
Diener, E., & Seligman, M. E. P. (2002). Very happy people. *Psychological Science, 13*, 81–84.
Diener, E., & Suh, E. M. (2000). *Culture and subjective well-being*. Cambridge, MA: MIT Press.
Erikson, E. H. (1950). *Childhood and society*. New York: Norton.
Erikson, E. H. (1959). *Identity and the life cycle*. New York: International Universities Press.
Erikson, E. H. (1982). *The life cycle completed: A review*. New York: Norton.
Furman, W., & Shomaker, L. B. (2008). Patterns of interaction in adolescent romantic relationships. *Journal of Adolescence, 31*, 771–788.
Furman, W., Ho, M. J., & Low, S. M. (2007). The rocky road of adolescent romantic experience: Dating and adjustment. In R. Engels, M. Kerr, & H. Stattin (Eds.), *Friends, lovers, and groups: Key relationships in adolescence* (pp. 61–80). New York: Wiley.
Gallagher, M., & Waite, L. (2001). *The case for marriage*. New York: Doubleday.
Gerstorf, D., Ram, N., Rocke, C., Lindenberger, U., & Smith, J. (2008). Decline in life satisfaction in old age. *Psychology and Aging, 23*, 154–168.
Gibson, D. E. (2003). Developing the professional self-concept: Role model construals in early, middle, and late career stages. *Organization Science, 14*, 591–610.
Glück, J., & Bluck, S. (2011). Laypeople's conceptions of wisdom and its development: cognitive and integrative views. *Journal of Gerontology, 66B*, 321–324.
Goldbeck, L., Schmitz, T. G., Besier, T., Herschbach, P., & Henrich, G. (2007). Life satisfaction decreases during adolescence. *Quality of Life Research, 16*, 969–979.
Griffin, J. (1986). *Well-being*. Oxford, England: Clarendon.
Grossmann, I., Na, J., Varnum, M. E. W., Park, D. C., Kitayama, S., & Nisbett, R. E. (2010). Reasoning about social conflicts improves into old age. *PNAS, 107*, 7246–7250.
Grossmann, I., Karasawa, M., Izumi, S., Na, J., Varnum, M. E. W., Kitayama, S., & Nisbett, R. E. (2012). Aging and wisdom: Culture matters. *Psychological Science, 23*, 1059–1066.
Heckhausen, J., Dixon, R. A., & Baltes, P. B. (1989). Gains and losses in development throughout adulthood as perceived by different adult age groups. *Developmental Psychology, 25*, 109–121.
Kunzmann, U., Little, T. D., & Smith, J. (2000). Is age-related stability of subjective well-being a paradox? Cross-sectional and longitudinal evidence from the Berlin Aging Study. *Psychology and Aging, 15*, 511–526.
Leffert, N., Benson, P. L., Scales, P. C., Sharma, A. R., Drake, D. R., & Blyth, D. A. (1998). Developmental assets: Measurement and prediction of risk behaviors among adolescents. *Applied Developmental Science, 2*, 209–230.
Lerner, R. M., Lerner, J. V., Almerigi, J. B., Theokas, C., Phelps, E., Gestsdottir, S., et al. (2005). Positive youth development, participation in community youth development programs, and community contributions of fifth-grade adolescents. *Journal of Early Adolescence, 25*, 17–71.
Lewis, J. P. (2010). Successful aging through the eyes of Alaska Natives: Exploring generational differences among Alaska Natives. *Journal of Cross-Cultural Gerontology, 25*, 385–396.
Lyubomirsky, S., King, L., & Diener, E. (2005). The benefits of frequent positive affect: Does happiness lead to success? *Psychological Bulletin, 131*, 803–855.
Masten, A. S., Cutuli, J. J., Herbers, J. E., & Reed, M.-G. J. (2009). Resilience in development. In S. J. Lopez & C. R. Snyder (Eds.), *Handbook of positive psychology* (2nd ed., pp. 117–131). New York: Oxford University Press.
McCone, D., & O'Donnell, K. (2006). Marriage and divorce trends for graduates of the U.S. Air Force Academy. *Military Psychology, 18*, 61–75.

McCormick, C. M., Kuo, S. I., & Masten, A. S. (2011). Developmental tasks across the life span. In K. L. Fingerman, C. A. Berg, J. Smith, & T. C. Antonucci (Eds.), *Handbook of life-span development* (pp. 117–139). New York: Springer.

Mroczek, D. K., & Kolarz, C. M. (1998). The effect of age on positive and negative affect: A developmental perspective on happiness. *Journal of Personality and Social Psychology, 75*(5), 1333–1349. doi:10.1037/0022-3514.75.5.1333.

Myers, D. G., & Diener, E. (1995). Who is happy? *Psychological Science, 6*, 10–19.

Nakamura, J., & Csikszentmihalyi, M. (2003). The construction of meaning through vital engagement. In C. L. M. Keyes & J. Haidt (Eds.), *Flourishing* (pp. 83–104). Washington, DC: American Psychological Association.

Neugarten, B. L. (1974). Age groups in American society and the rise of the young-old. *Annals of the American Academy of Political and Social Science, 415*, 187–198.

Omarzu, J., Whalen, J., & Harvey, J. H. (2001). How well do you mind your relationship? A preliminary scale to test the minding theory of relating. In J. Harvey & A. Wenzel (Eds.), *Close romantic relationships* (pp. 345–356). Mahwah: Lawrence Erlbaum Associates.

O'Sullivan, L. F., Cheng, M. M., Harris, K. M., & Brooks-Gunn, J. (2007). I wanna hold your hand: The progression of social, romantic and sexual events in adolescent relationships. *Perspectives on Sexual and Reproductive Health, 39*, 100–107.

Pasupathi, M., & Staudinger, U. M. (2001). Do advanced moral reasoners also show wisdom? *International Journal of Behavioral Development, 25*, 401–415.

Pasupathi, M., Staudinger, U. M., & Baltes, P. B. (2001). Seeds of wisdom: Adolescents' knowledge and judgment about difficult life problems. *Developmental Psychology, 37*, 351–361.

Peterson, C., & Seligman, M. (2004). *Character strengths and virtues*. New York: Oxford University Press.

Pethtel, O., & Chen, Y. (2010). Cross-cultural aging in cognitive and affective components of subjective well-being. *Psychology and Aging, 25*, 725–729. doi:10.1037/a0018511.

Pinquart, M. (2001). Age differences in perceived positive affect, negative affect, and affect balance in middle and old age. *Journal of Happiness Studies, 2*, 375–405.

Pinquart, M., & Sorensen, S. (2000). Influences of socioeconomic status, social network, and competence on subjective well-being in later life: A meta-analysis. *Psychology and Aging, 15*, 187–224.

Raffaelli, M. (2005). Adolescent dating experiences described by Latino college students. *Journal of Adolescence, 28*, 559–572.

Richardson, M. J., & Pasupathi, M. (2005). Young and growing wiser. In R. J. Stenberg & J. Jordan (Eds.), *A handbook of wisdom: Psychological perspectives* (pp. 139–159). Cambridge, England: Cambridge University Press.

Rostosky, S. S., Riggle, E. D. B., Horne, S. G., & Miller, A. D. (2009). Marriage amendments and psychological distress in lesbian, gay, and bisexual (LGB) adults. *Journal of Counseling Psychology, 56*, 56–66.

Russell, B. (1958). *The conquest of happiness*. New York: Liveright (Original work published 1930).

Ryan, R. M., & Deci, E. L. (2001). On happiness and human potentials: A review of research on hedonic and eudaimonic well-being. *Annual Review of Psychology, 52*, 141–166.

Ryan, R. M., & Huta, V. (2009). Wellness as healthy functioning or wellness as happiness: The importance of eudaimonic thinking. *Journal of Positive Psychology, 4*, 202–204.

Ryff, C. D., & Singer, B. (1998). The contours of positive human health. *Psychological Inquiry, 9*, 1–28.

Samanez-Larkin, G. R., & Carstensen, L. L. (2011). Socioemotional functioning and the aging brain. In J. Decety & J. T. Cacioppo (Eds.), *The handbook of social neuroscience* (pp. 507–521). New York: Oxford University Press.

Schwartz, B., & Sharpe, K. E. (2006). Practical wisdom: Aristotle meets positive psychology. *Journal of Happiness Studies, 7*, 377–395.

Sears, R. R. (1977). Sources of life satisfactions of the Terman gifted men. *American Psychologist, 32*, 119–128.

Settersten, R. A. (1999). *Lives in time and place*. Amityville: Baywood.
Settersten, R. A., & Mayer, K. U. (1997). The measurement of age, age structuring, and the life course. *Annual Review of Sociology, 23*, 233–261.
Shek, D. L., & Ma, C. S. (2010). Dimensionality of the Chinese Positive Youth Development Scale: Confirmatory factor analyses. *Social Indicators Research, 98*, 41–59.
Sheldon, K. M., & Kasser, T. (2001). Getting older, getting better? Personal strivings and psychological maturity across the life span. *Developmental Psychology, 37*, 491–501.
Shulman, S., & Scharf, M. (2000). Adolescent romantic behaviors and perceptions. *Journal of Research on Adolescence, 10*, 99–118.
Shulman, S., Davila, J., & Shachar-Shapira, L. (2011). Assessing romantic competence among adolescents. *Journal of Adolescence, 34*, 397–406.
Spencer-Rodgers, J., Peng, K., & Wang, L. (2010). Dialecticism and the co-occurrence of positive and negative emotions across cultures. *Journal of Cross-Cultural Psychology, 41*, 109–115.
Steger, M. F., Oishi, S., & Kashdan, T. B. (2009). Meaning in life across the life span. *Journal of Positive Psychology, 4*, 43–52.
Sternberg, R. J. (1998). A balance theory of wisdom. *Review of General Psychology, 2*, 347–365.
Sternberg, R. J. (2001). Why schools should teach for wisdom: The balance theory of wisdom in educational settings. *Educational Psychologist, 36*, 227–245.
Sun, R. F., & Shek, D. L. (2012). Positive youth development, life satisfaction and problem behaviour among Chinese adolescents in Hong Kong: A replication. *Social Indicators Research, 105*, 541–559. doi:10.1007/s11205-011-9786-9.
Takahashi, M. (2000). Toward a culturally inclusive understanding of wisdom: Historical roots in the east and west. *International Journal of Aging & Human Development, 51*, 217–230.
Thompson, R. (1998). Early sociopersonality development. In N. Eisenberg (Ed.), *Handbook of child psychology* (Vol. 3, pp. 25–104). New York: Wiley.
Vaillant, G. E. (2004). Positive aging. In P. A. Linley & S. Joseph (Eds.), *Positive psychology in practice* (pp. 561–578). New York: Wiley.
Weinstein, S. M., Mermelstein, R. J., Hankin, B. L., Hedeker, D., & Flay, B. R. (2007). Longitudinal patterns of daily affect and global mood during adolescence. *Journal of Research on Adolescence, 17*, 587–600.
Yang, S.-Y. (2001). Conceptions of wisdom among Taiwanese Chinese. *Journal of Cross-Cultural Psychology, 32*, 662–680.
Zebrowitz, L. A., & Montepare, J. M. (2000). Too young, too old: Stigmatizing adolescents and elders. In T. F. Heatherton, R. E. Kleck, M. R. Hebl, & J. G. Hull (Eds.), *The social psychology of stigma* (pp. 334–373). New York: Guilford Press.

Chapter 9
Positive Psychology and Gender

Matt Englar-Carlson and Rebekah Smart

The promise of positive psychology in many ways should appeal to those interested in the psychology of gender. After all, a psychology focused on the conditions and processes that promote optimal functioning in people and institutions (Gable and Haidt 2005) serves as a significant counter to pathology-based psychology, and thus could advance a more meaningful understanding of all genders. Most psychological scholars of gender, like those in multicultural psychology, take a sociopolitical view of psychology, mental health, and social change, and this is not often seen in positive psychology. Heavily influenced by feminist psychology (both psychology of women and men; Brown 2010), a focused analysis of gender by means of examining power and privilege in any given society would need to be incorporated into a positive psychology perspective in order to be relevant. Whereas the end goal of the elevation of strengths and optimal health for all genders in pursuit of happiness and the "good life" is a goal shared by many, how the scholarly field of positive psychology has conceptualized, accounted for, and addressed gender is still a cause for discussion.

This chapter will review the different discussions and debate about the utility of positive psychology for work within the psychology of gender. For us, a deeper examination raises a series of questions about how positive psychology and gendered concerns intersect, and impact people of all genders. Further, the very nature of the historical relationship of power, privilege, and gender creates vastly different conditions for the connection of positive psychology to ideas around masculinity and femininity. This chapter will survey the existing research and critiques of positive psychology and gender with a goal of identifying future areas of scholarly

---

M. Englar-Carlson, Ph.D. (✉) • R. Smart
Department of Counseling, California State University, Fullerton,
Fullerton, CA 92834-6868, USA
e-mail: mattec@fullerton.edu; rsmart@fullerton.edu

J. Teramoto Pedrotti and L.M. Edwards (eds.), *Perspectives on the Intersection of Multiculturalism and Positive Psychology*, Cross-Cultural Advancements in Positive Psychology 7, DOI 10.1007/978-94-017-8654-6_9,

inquiry and investigation. In line with Levant and Silverstein's (2005) observation, it is critical to note that it is problematic to only discuss one aspect of diversity (e.g., gender) without full consideration of the impact of other identities (e.g., race, ethnicity, sexual orientation, etc.). We wanted to acknowledge this upfront, as we do not want to repeat oversights previously contained in the feminist and multicultural literature (Reid 2002).

9.1 An Initial Examination of Positive Psychology and Gender

One of the greatest shifts in psychology has been the increased sensitivity and awareness given to cultural diversity issues, including the influence of gender roles (American Psychological Association 2003). Among other identity factors, sex and gender are recognized as powerful organizing variables in peoples' lives and experiences (Brown 2010). From a social constructivist view, notions of femininity and masculinity, and thus the lived lives of any individual are defined by cultural, historical, socioeconomic, and institutional forces (Smiler 2004). Based on the sociopolitical reality of privilege and power, men, women, and transgender individuals have different experiences. Whereas understanding the positive and healthy aspects of these cultural influences and identity has promise, positive psychology risks overlooking and dismissing real societal, structural and lived reality when it does not incorporate a contextual view (McNulty and Fincham 2012). In addition, Gable and Haidt (2005) note that for some in positive psychology, "the aim is to build up what we know about *human* resilience, strength, and growth to integrate and complement the existing knowledge base" (p. 107). This statement indicates that for some researchers, the emphasis in positive psychology has been on universal, or "human" findings that are by definition devoid of cultured multiple identities that include gender. This is problematic as gender, as well as other cultural facets, are seemingly taken out of the equation and not considered complex and influential determinants in people's lives (Eagly and Diekman 2003). A key principle of feminist therapy is that people's experiences are honored for what they are with an emphasis on gender-based phenomenon (Brown 2010); therefore, the lack of specific attention to gendered/cultured experiences is concerning.

Another concern about focusing on "positive" gendered traits (either "feminine" or "masculine") is that it essentializes those traits as belonging exclusively to a gender and reinforces stereotypes. For example, scholarly work on "positive masculinity" has been criticized as promoting essentialism in that it inhibits the deconstruction of gender roles and limits social change (Addis et al. 2010). Further, it is erroneous to assume that there is only one perspective of a "positive trait" for different genders, as different cultures have varying ideas of what is "positive" for each respective gender (Pedrotti 2011). Traits are not universally positive across the globe, as a multitude of contextual cultural factors influence how traits are perceived and performed (Pedrotti et al. 2009). Transgender individuals may also be able to incorporate aspects of masculinity and femininity into their identity in ways that are positive for them (Riggle et al. 2011).

However, there are differing perspectives on the role of culture in evaluating and examining strengths. Pedrotti (2011) described the emergence of two camps within positive psychology: the "culture-free" camp and the more recent "culturally embedded" camp. Seligman and Csikszentmihalyi (2000) exemplify the culture-free perspective, which holds that universal strengths exist, and that empirical science is objective enough to determine universal strengths. This view of positive psychology has been criticized as ethnocentric, overly individualistic, and prescriptive in its values (Becker and Marecek 2008). The culturally-embedded approach to positive psychology instead incorporates culture and context (including facets such as gender) into positive psychology and takes the position that one must consider culture when interpreting any type of behavior (Pedrotti and Edwards 2009). Findings from positive psychology can be used to encourage people to adopt behavior, attitudes, and beliefs that are helpful to them (Gable and Haidt 2005), but cultural context must play a role in determining which traits are "most helpful."

As the social change of institutions and the redefinition of gender roles is a core focus in the psychology of gender (Brown 2010; Levant and Pollack 1995), the historical absence of an activist or contextual focus positions positive psychology as a more traditional approach to psychology. In that sense, for many feminist thinkers positive psychology as presented thus far has not been able to address many fundamental concerns. Further, an understanding of the psychology of gender suggests that what is good for people is reducing sexism, discrimination, and other institutionalized forms of oppression that restrict people's lives. Thus positive psychology research could look at successful ways to examine the impact the pursuit of social change has on happiness and well-being.

9.2 Women, "Femininity," and Positive Psychology

A brief review of some of the feminist history is worth noting before examining positive psychology and women's gender, as feminist theories and therapies have utilized the concepts of *empowerment* and *strength-based approaches* for some time.

9.2.1 Feminist Therapy's History of Strength-Based Work and Empowerment

Prior to the 1970s, the field of psychology paid little attention to the social and gendered contexts of women's lives. The Women's Movement in the U.S. and consciousness-raising groups that examined rape and domestic violence in the context of women's oppression were essential to the critique of psychology and the subsequent changes in the field (Evans et al. 2005). Among the criticisms of mainstream psychology were bias in diagnosis, the pathologizing of traits that women had been socialized to adopt (e.g., nurturing seen as overly dependent); viewing so-called "healthy" women as dependent, passive, and highly emotional (from the famous study by Broverman et al. 1970); pathologizing women who defied traditional female traits; and failing to consider the impact of women's social context (e.g., gender, poverty, inequality) on their mental health (Worell and Johnson 2001). An overarching theme in the feminist critique was countering the dominant narrative that male (White male) was the "norm" and those who did not conform to a White male worldview were deviant. However, as groundbreaking as this critique was, it was still linked almost entirely to a White, middle-class, heterosexual perspective; the experiences of women of color, women living in poverty, and women who were not exclusively heterosexual were largely ignored until much later (Evans et al. 2005).

One of the hallmarks of emerging feminist therapies was a revaluing of so-called feminine traits. Worell and Johnson's (2001) integrative model of feminist practice includes the principle *Female Perspectives Are Valued*: "Goals reflecting this principle include helping the client to identify her personal strengths, trusting her own experience, translating perceived weakness into strengths, and bonding with other women" (p. 323). As the authors pointed out, this principle is grounded in cultural feminism, a branch of feminism that re-values previously disparaged traits associated with women. An influential example of this kind of revaluing was Gilligan's work in the 1980s on moral development, in which she challenged prevailing theory with research that suggested that girls and women were not less moral than boys or men but that they had an equally important but different kind of morality, one based on *care* rather than on *justice* (Sherblom 2008). In the context of the times, the notion that women's morality was equally valuable to men's and possibly superior, was inspiring for many. The problem with this approach, as many have noted, is that it essentializes "women's nature," insinuating that a trait common to some women in some circumstances is inherent to all women in all circumstances; this in turn is enormously problematic, both theoretically and practically (Grant 1993). Grant contended that the "revalorization of the feminine" (p. 10) should be understood as an important strategy for its time but that suggesting that the newly valued traits are inherent to all people of one gender is untenable.

Further, as important as the work of Gilligan was, she was criticized by many for grounding her research and theory in the experience of small samples of presumably middle class White girls, and so not only did many interpret her work as "the truth" about women, but they failed to consider that "women" in this context meant only one subset of women. Indeed, what are considered traditionally feminine traits (e.g., nice, non-dominant, nurturing, and fragile) derive from stereotypes across many cultures (Goodwin and Fiske 2001), but not all. For example, "women" should not show anger or pride from this viewpoint; however, given the historical context of work outside the home, this gender norm is less common in African American culture (Durik et al. 2006). Because the dominant culture's views prevail, African American women have been pathologized as "less feminine" as compared to White women throughout history (Collins 1997), even perhaps with regard to distinctions drawn from times of slavery.

Many feminist therapists resist essentializing so-called feminine traits, but do seek to validate all women's experiences and empower them. For example, Lenore Walker, the early leading advocate of women in battering relationships shifted the focus from "victim" to "survivor," explored women's strengths, and worked on empowering them (Choate 2008). The focus on strengths has been used in many areas of work with girls and women and in 1997 the feminist national conference identified strength-based approaches as key to feminist therapy (Johnson 2003).

Brown (2010) asserted that analysis of external contributors to distress and analysis of privilege and patriarchy (power) are essential to feminist therapy; any therapy that does not do that simply serves the status quo. Indeed, one of the central historical feminist criticisms was that established therapies could passively reinforce gendered power differentials (Worell and Johnson 2001); for example, by being "neutral" and not attending to power dynamics between partners in a heterosexual relationship or by being "colorblind" and not attending to cultural influences in the potentially different power dynamics of a Latino couple versus a White couple.

9.2.2 Positive Psychology and the Psychology of Women

There is little explicit consideration of women's gender (in a sociocultural or sociopolitical context) in the positive psychology literature. However, there are aspects of overlap and compatibility between psychology of women/feminist psychology and positive psychology. In a comprehensive text on women by feminist editors, O'Leary and Bhaju (2006) wrote about *resilience* and *empowerment*, stating: "Paralleling the positive psychology movement, but not well integrated into it, have been theories advanced by feminist psychologists who actively rejected many of the traditional assumptions of the male dominated medical model of psychology with its emphasis on pathology" (pp. 157–158). However, they make little other reference to positive psychology. Similarly, Choate (2008) and Johnson (2003) indicated a benign compatibility between positive psychology and feminist therapy, but with little detail about positive psychology. Both authors only noted that the two perspectives share a focus on empowerment and using strengths, and a reduced focus on pathology.

Numerous works (Burns 2010; Elston and Boniwell 2011) using the umbrella of positive psychology have focused on utilizing strengths in women clients but with no real reference to gender per se, and no examination of their sociocultural or sociopolitical contexts. Becker and Marecek (2008) expressed concern that when Seligman and Csikszentmihalyi (2000) wrote their foundational article on positive psychology at the start of Seligman's presidency of the American Psychological Association (APA), they did not include any kind of social analysis—no "interrogation of power, privilege, and social hierarchy" (p. 596). The culturally embedded camp of positive psychology, as described earlier, attempts to broaden the focus of Seligman and others on universal strengths to a viewpoint that asserts that while strengths are rightly acknowledged and valued, the contexts in which these qualities emerge influence their utility and consequences (Pedrotti 2011). There appears to be room for social analysis in this perspective, although it is not emphasized.

Building on the culturally embedded perspective and adding emphases from feminist theory and the APA's 2007 psychological guidelines, we suggest that a positive psychology approach to working with girls and women from all backgrounds should include the following: (a) exploring previously disparaged traits or identities in new ways and helping clients, when appropriate, to identify positive aspects within them; (b) helping clients to draw more positive conclusions about themselves by viewing their behaviors within their sociocultural-political contexts; (c) understanding symptoms as a means of coping rather than as inherent pathology; (d) exploring personal qualities through the client's worldview and intersecting identities; (e) exploring gender role conflict within a client's culture and subcultures; and (f) recognizing the positive and innovative ways in which girls and women navigate multiple and conflicting gendered demands within societies that are often rapidly changing.

A few authors have illustrated some or all of these points. Using the example of working with biracial girls and women, Edwards and Pedrotti (2004) acknowledged the very real experiences of stereotype threat, prejudice specifically directed at biracial women (rather than men), and identity struggles that can happen; however, they also suggested that historically disparaged traits associated with being biracial, such as being hopelessly "marginalized" and stuck between cultures, should be reconsidered to include potentially positive aspects, such as having the ability to navigate two cultures, being able to draw from a rich heritage, and developing coping skills. Johnson (2003) wrote a case study of a teenage girl who was acting out at home and at school. Utilizing positive psychology, feminist therapy, and strengths-based interventions, she worked with both daughter and parents on identifying their own strengths (through specifically developed questionnaires as well as in therapy) as a way of building rapport and setting the stage for positive action. She also helped the parents to recognize how their own cultural and gender biases had prevented them from recognizing their daughter's strengths. In the end, the parents were better able to accept what they perceived as more typically masculine qualities (seeking independence) in their daughter, and in this case, Johnson helped the daughter and parents come to terms with gender non-conforming behavior.

Tzou et al. (2012) used "Positive Feminist Therapy" (PFT) to work with Chinese women going through divorce. They integrated empowerment feminist therapy, positive psychology's emphasis on strengths and resilience, and systems theory. In the case example of a woman who struggled greatly with the decision to leave her marriage, the therapist worked to acknowledge both internal and external strengths, such as loyalty to family, various positive relationships, and education. Tzou et al. (2012) maintained that the following techniques were critical to the therapy: *power-, gender role-, and social location analysis*, as well as *reframing* and *active problem-solving skills*. Although the authors stressed that work with every client must be individualized and cultural norms respected, clearly this approach holds the possibility for encouraging clients to analyze oppressive forces (familial, institutional, cultural) in their lives. The therapist never pushes for particular action, but may help clients weigh risks and benefits of acting on their insight, given the cultural backdrop.

Aspects of positive psychology are consistent with the long-held feminist strategies of empowerment and strength-based approaches, but without the inclusion of a social and power analysis positive psychology has potential to harm women by maintaining the status quo and reinforcing essentialist notions. Taking a culturally embedded approach within positive psychology might be able to make it more relevant for women in all their diversity. However, we emphasize that without using the lens of power and privilege, even culturally embedded positive psychology runs the risk of sanctioning or promoting traits simply because they are valued within a cultural context. This presents complex and difficult issues with regard to perceptions of "women's traits," particularly those traits that were forged, at least in part, within the context of oppression. For example, Rudman and Glick (2001) described how the idea of women's "communal" nature and "niceness" developed within the context of subordination to men. Niceness and communality can be viewed as desirable traits and normative for many women, but if researchers and therapists are not aware of the historical context and the price paid by women, they may support these traits without question and inadvertently support a troubling status quo. More pointedly, Lamb (2005) questioned the emphasis used by some in positive psychology for cultivating the trait of "forgiveness." Her concern is that forgiveness therapy often revolves around women's issues (victims of violence, infidelity, abandonment), and that women have historically had to develop traits like forgiveness in order to survive even though it was not always optimal for their well-being. Qualities that tend to be highly valued in the abstract and from a particular vantage point (i.e., people in power) may harm people (in this case, women) who have less privilege and power. Finally, the willingness to view psychological traits not as innately positive or negative (McNulty and Fincham 2012), but rather as dependent on the context in which they emerge, could spur future research to focus on the complexities of gender with other intersecting identities, such as culture, socioeconomic status, sexual orientation, and physical and mental ability/disability.

9.3 Men, Masculinity, and Positive Psychology

The past 30 years have seen a flurry of scholarly activity focused on understanding the psychology of men and masculinity (see Brooks and Good 2005; Englar-Carlson 2006; O'Neil 2012). One shift was recognizing the wide variation within male cultures when multiple identities are considered (Smiler 2004). It is common to use the term "masculinities" rather than "masculinity" to acknowledge the various conceptions of male gender roles associated with an intersection of multiple identities (e.g., rural, working class adult White masculinities may take a different form than urban teenage Mexican American masculinities; Kimmel and Messner 2012). There is also the understanding that certain forms of masculinities are more socially central and associated with authority, social power, and influence (Connell and Messerschmidt 2005). In Western society, the dominant ideal of masculinity has moved from an upper-class aristocratic image to a more rugged and self-sufficient ideal (Kimmel 2011). Thus traditional masculinity can be viewed as the dominant (referred to as "hegemonic" masculinity) form of masculinity and thus highly influential of what members of a culture take to be normative.

Drawing on the Feminist Movement in larger society and the psychology of women, the psychology of men brought attention to the gendered identity of men and questions of how sexist norms within Western contexts have impacted men (O'Neil 2012). Though men had developed much of psychology, it had not focused on men as gendered individuals. A new framework titled the new psychology of men questioned "traditional [Western] norms for the male role, such as the emphases on competition, status, toughness, and emotional stoicism," (Levant and Pollack 1995, p. 1) and framed many of the problems associated with men (aggression and violence, homophobia, misogyny, detached fathering, and neglect of health) as resulting from the male socialization process in which rigid forms of masculinity are emphasized. A driving factor behind this model was the compiling of male-specific data and examining the underlying causes of the ever-growing physical and mental health disparities across every racial group between men and women (see Courtenay 2011; O'Neil 2012).

In a substantial literature review on the psychology of men, O'Neil (2012) noted the collected data on the lives of boys and men are sobering. In the United States, despite having greater socioeconomic advantages than women, in every ethnic group the age-adjusted death rate has been found to at least 50 % higher for men than women (Department of Health and Human Services as cited in Courtenay et al. 2011). Courtenay et al. noted the health disparities that exist between men of various ethnic and racial backgrounds (e.g., African American men die 6 years younger than European American men) and how that is associated with distinctions between the leading causes of death (e.g., the death rate of HIV is among the five leading causes highest for African America and Latinos but not among the leading causes for any other group of men) and specific health risk behaviors (Asian American men report riskier habits than other groups of men for behavior related to preventative health). An observation of the existing research on the psychology of men led Brooks and Silverstein (1995) to the conclusion that there was a "dark" or "toxic" side to traditional conceptualizations of masculinity, and that a masculinity crisis exists with men of all racial groups (Levant 1997). Isacco et al. (2012) noted that based on the entirety of this research it is easy to take an essentialist perspective and conclude that traditional masculinity, or masculinity as a whole is always negative. However, they added the critical distinction that traditional masculinity *per se* is not associated with negative outcomes, but rather the rigid, restrictive, sexist enactment of one idea of "traditional" male roles. Similar to positive psychology's assertion that the field of psychology had neglected examining strengths, assets, and well-being (Seligman and Csikszentmihalyi 2000), there is a growing awareness that the psychology of men and masculinity has primarily explored the "toxic" side of men's lives with little examination of healthy masculinity and how that is enacted for men of different racial, ethnic, and cultural backgrounds.

9.3.1 Positive Masculinity

Before examining the application of positive psychology, it is important to note the shift toward the positive, health, or strengths of men entered the scholarly discourse with a fair amount of critique and feedback (Addis et al. 2010; Levant 2008). With feminist roots, and many scholars identifying as feminist or profeminist (Szymanski et al. 2002), the field is aligned with a strong activist stance of reducing patriarchal power, male dominance, male sexism, and the restructuring of masculinity itself (Baird et al. 2007; Levant 1997). Further, much of the scholarly work in the new psychology of men focuses on the myriad problems associated with men or acted out by men on women and society (interpersonal violence, anger, aggression, etc.); and men themselves were rarely conceptualized as a marginalized group. The whole idea of empowering men or identifying "strengths" would seem foreign, or downright antithetical to someone working to reduce male power and sexism.

One question is why there might be a shift now toward looking at strengths and positive aspects of men. O'Neil (2012) noted the study of men and masculinity has a short history in psychology, and that only in the past 30 years have men's psychological processes been studied. There is now a firm understanding in Western societies how restricted gender roles affect men and women to the point where the damaging effects of patriarchal sexism on men is slowly emerging as a social justice issue (Englar-Carlson 2009; Kiselica and Woodford 2007). Overall, the field has identified what is not working with men, yet it seems to struggle with advancing a model of how to make life better or even what better might *be* for men. O'Neil (2012) summarized this, stating the psychology of men needs to emphasize more healthy criteria for being male.

Clearly, the new psychology of men provided a much needed gender-sensitive lens through which to view boys and men, however, the model largely emphasized deficit models of male development and a remedial helping approach designed to help men recover from the damaging effects of constricted masculinity on themselves and others (Kiselica 2011; Kiselica and Englar-Carlson 2010; Kiselica et al. 2008; O'Neil and Lujan 2009). Some in the field of psychology of men and masculinity have questioned if something else about men was missing in the scholarly literature, namely that not all men experience gender role conflict or maintain rigid masculine roles, but these men were seldom studied or referenced. Further, some questioned if everything about traditional masculinity was necessarily bad, and if there were contextualized settings where aspects of traditional masculinity could be adaptive and prosocial. When the existing research in the field was rigidly applied to men in clinical settings without an assessment of one's gender role and cultural context, it was easy to overlook the actual experiences of male clients and the man himself (Stevens and Englar-Carlson 2010). If the majority of scholarly work seemed to focus on the dark, or negative masculinity, it is not surprising that "positive masculinity" was the term used to refer to qualities of traditional masculine roles that are more positive, strength-based, and potentially used to better the lives of men and those around them (Isacco et al. 2012). For the most part, a focus on male strengths, empowerment, and even social justice are largely absent in the psychology of men literature (O'Neil 2012). The past few years have seen the emergence of more comprehensive research that explores how men of various cultural identities navigate their own traditional masculinity in adaptive ways.

Drawing upon theoretical traditions in psychotherapy that have elevated the role of client strengths and available resources as a focal point of intervention (see Duncan et al. 2004), Kiselica and Englar-Carlson (2010) proposed the Positive Psychology/Positive Masculinity (PPPM) model as a strength-based complement to the existing new psychology of men. A goal of this framework is to help boys and men distinguish and embrace healthy and constructive aspects of masculinity, noting that aspects of traditional male norms such as self-reliance, risk-taking behaviors, and a male relational style can also be viewed from a positive and adaptive lens. These male strengths are reported as social constructions, noting they are neither male-specific (e.g., women show courage, are heroic, and use humor) nor based on biologically-determined sex differences between men and women, and therefore can be considered *universal* strengths across genders from a Western perspective (Kiselica et al. 2008). However, within one's cultural context, boys and men are often socialized to develop and demonstrate these positive qualities and behaviors, which are then modeled for others and passed down in male-particular ways (Pleban and Diez 2007). This positive male socialization process is rarely discussed in the psychological literature on boys, men, and masculinity, with the possible exception of the work on generative fatherhood, which accentuates how fathers and grandfathers from a broad range of cultural backgrounds often care for the next generation (Hawkins and Dollahite 1996). Further, Kiselica and Englar-Carlson (2010) cautioned how cultural and contextual factors may influence the definition, development, and expression of male strengths. For example, a man raised in Caucasian American culture may view male self-reliance and autonomy as a strength, whereas a man raised in a more collectivist environment may see self-reliance as undermining of the community, and therefore place more value in fulfilling family or community obligations. In addition, Kiselica et al. (2008) cautioned that these strengths are not universally positive; rather they are adaptive in some settings and maladaptive in others. It is the ability to be flexible in the enactment of these norms and the knowledge to know when it is adaptive that is critical.

It is important to note that work in positive masculinity is primarily theoretical, with the exception of one known research article by Hammer and Good (2010). That study examined the relationship between traditional Western conceptualizations of masculine norms, positive psychology strengths and psychological well-being. They found endorsement of some masculine norms (risk-taking, dominance, primacy of work, and pursuit of status) to be associated with positive psychology constructs of personal courage, autonomy, endurance, and resilience. Other Western masculine norms such as winning, emotional control, self-reliance, and pursuit of status were associated with lower levels of positive psychology constructs. This study provided empirical evidence of the existence of strengths associated with traditional ways of enacting masculinity in the Western context. The authors suggested future research could examine these relations within specific groups of men (e.g., men of color, gay and bisexual men, working class men), and explore the attributes that each context views as being strengths for men. Positive masculinity is clearly in the beginning stages of development, and further empirical investigation is needed.

9.3.2 Clinical Applications

Davies et al. (2010) worked with similar ideas in a clinical setting and coined the term "possible masculinities," as a way for men of varying backgrounds to examine a positive view of attitudes, norms, and behaviors. Many clinicians adopt a deficit model with men, asking "What brought you here? and What can you do differently?" Possible masculinity focuses more on an aspiration approach, asking "What kind of man do you want to be in the future? and What's stopping you from being that man?" Possible masculinity incorporates the range of masculinities as the goal of a man's aspirational self is driven individually by each man and connected to his cultural context (Isacco et al. 2012).

Many in the field of the psychology of men have focused specifically on emotional expression. Males tend to be capable of recognizing and expressing a wide range of emotions, yet observed differences in emotional expression for males tend to be influenced by social contexts and the willingness to express emotions, not ability (Wong and Rochlen 2005). In a chapter in *Positive Psychology: Exploring the Best in People,* Wong and Rochlen (2008) examined three perspectives on men's emotional lives: essentialism, gender role socialization, and social constructionism. They stated that social constructionism is a more complex and nuanced approach to understanding masculinities as it is more of a positive, strengths-based way of seeing the emotional lives of men. They use the example of solution-focused therapy's use of "exceptions" to explore men's difficulty with expressing emotion to "construct a more affirming picture of men's emotional life" (p. 159). Wong and Rochlen's (2008) approach focuses on looking for ways in which men *are* expressive and in which context so that a more comprehensive and hopeful view is taken, thus an individual man is not reduced to a non-emotional male stereotype.

9.3.3 Additional Areas of Inquiry

There are many other areas where positive psychology and the psychology of men may overlap in meaningful ways. Certainly, scholars and health practitioners are merging different areas of scholarship by recognizing the negative outcomes associated with the restrictive and rigid enactment of masculinity and acknowledging how many men live their lives in an adaptive, pro-social manner. This often necessitates a broader, deeper contextual understanding of men and their cultural context. For example, many men in the United States are choosing to be "stay-at-home dads" at an increasing rate and finding satisfaction with this historically non-traditional role in their families (Rochlen et al. 2008). The assumption is that many men may improve their health and the health of their families and communities if they adhere less rigidly to traditional masculinity norms and are free to assume non-traditional roles and identities.

Another example is examining fathers of Latino origin. *Machismo* is a popular cultural stereotype of Latino men thought to have only negative connotations of aggression and chauvinistic behavior (Arciniega et al. 2008). Thus Latino fathers are portrayed as dominant, withdrawn, and harsh disciplinarians. However, there is little data to support this image (Saracho and Spodek 2008). Recent research has stressed *caballerismo* (the positive side of machismo; Glass and Owen 2010), which includes dignity, honor, respect, familial responsibility, and a father's role as a provider (Arciniega et al. 2008; Falicov 2010). This conceptualization draws together changing gender role expectations for fathers and men of Latino heritage (Gutmann 2007). Research by Cruz et al. (2011) found that fathers of Mexican origin who endorse positive machismo are more like to be involved and have positive relationships with their children. This is one of many recent studies that emphasizes both quantity and quality as the dimensions that capture positive father involvement (Pleck 2010).

Further, there is a growing collection of work capturing the experiences of men who are not succumbing to traditional male stereotypes. In a qualitative study, Hernandez (2002) chronicled the efforts of inner-city, Chicano, adolescent fathers who were model sons, brothers, and fathers in the face of grinding poverty, crime, and limited life options. These stories highlighted the resilience of these young men as they embraced responsibility and parenthood. Exploring the narratives of 20 African American men from a wide range of family backgrounds, ages, geographical locations, sexualities, and occupations, White (2008) focused on the creative agency to redefine the assumptions and practices of manhood, create social change, and establish egalitarian relationships with women, children, and other men. Riggle et al. (2008) studied the many positive aspects of being a gay man. All of this research is notable for providing a broader understanding of men and masculinities that is tied to societal and cultural context.

It appears in many ways that research on positive psychology and men and masculinity parallels the evolution in positive psychology from the "culture-free" perspective to culturally "embedded" (Pedrotti and Edwards 2009). For many years the psychology of men generated important, however, often unidirectional research that highlighted the hazards of being male. Though primarily theoretical, initial efforts (Davies et al. 2010; Kiselica et al. 2008; Kiselica and Englar-Carlson 2010) helped establish that a "positive psychology of men" existed and had value. Future research can examine how men from the full range of masculinities lead healthy lives and how so-called positive and negative traits are contextualized.

9.4 Transgender Individuals and Positive Psychology

Although enormous gender variancy has existed throughout human history, the binary gender system of only male and female continues to dominate as normative (Goldner 2011). The binary system and homophobia also serve to promote and enforce the notions that masculinity belongs to men and femininity belongs to women; those who do not conform (e.g., "effeminate" men, masculine women) are pathologized (Goldner 2011). Kitzinger (2001) pointed out that transsexuals (original authors' wording) could be seen as maintaining the binary system when they are conceptualized within it, as in "women in men's bodies (or vice verse)" (p. 283), but transsexuality has increasingly come to mean gender variation outside the binary system. For example, someone may choose to keep a penis *and* have breast implants; others may reject both male and female labels; and some construct their trans, queer, or other identities with no surgery at all (Kitzinger 2001).

In spite of the long human history of gender variance, people who do not conform to conventional identities have rarely been free to express themselves. Singh et al. (2011) outline the persecution and oppression of transgender people. Even as much of U.S. society becomes more tolerant of non-heterosexual sexual orientation, it is not tolerant of people who seem to violate the "rules" of gender. There is scant literature within positive psychology that has addressed transgender issues; however, there is potential within the field using the culturally embedded framework, to make important contributions. Singh et al. (2011) used a phenomenological qualitative approach to examining resilience strategies in 21 transgender people, identifying significant strengths in a group that endures considerable adversity. Newfield et al. (2006) examined health-related quality of life in female-to-male (FTM) transgender individuals. Though finding this population reported significant mental health needs, those receiving hormones treatment had a significantly higher quality of life. Riggle et al. (2011) examined the self-reported positive aspects of a transgender identity and identified eight positive identity themes that could be used to develop strength-based therapeutic approaches.

This is an area with which positive psychology is familiar and can do more work: drawing out the positive. Like the work of cultural feminists, this is an important step in changing the overly negative and pathologizing dialogues, not only in the broader society but within the helping professions as well (e.g., the diagnostic system). However, as has been discussed, to stop there runs the risk of essentializing traits in a very diverse group of people, not to mention the problematic issue of valorizing traits forged under oppression.

Perhaps one of the greatest gifts of the tremendous variability and fluidity in gender identities is that the binary system and the linkage between men and masculinity and women and femininity can be truly challenged if people are free to express who they are. All people, not just transgender people, would benefit from this. Positive psychologists could approach every individual with the awareness that given their biological sex, sexual orientation, levels of perceived masculinity and femininity, and current gender identity, there is a host of qualities and experiences, many of them positive. For example, working with the person's unique expressions of masculinity and femininity, cultural contexts, and sexual orientation, the positives and negatives of having both male and female biology can be explored.

9.5 Conclusion

This chapter has focused on developing an understanding about the connections and disconnections between positive psychology and the psychology of gender. One commonality between positive psychology and the psychology of men and women and transgender people is that they are all relatively new areas of inquiry and focus, thus they are dynamic fields that are rapidly growing in complexity. These four areas share the aspirational goal of the betterment of society, yet the psychology of gender reminds positive psychology that gender and other salient cultural identities have sociopolitical consequences for individuals and societies that should not be ignored. We recommend a continued exploration of and focus on viewing traits as neither innately positive nor negative, but rather as dependent on context, and viewing positive and negative as potentially interrelated. In addition, we believe that positive psychology would do well to articulate its relationship to feminist and multicultural theory, and that it has the potential to be a leader in gender freedom.

References

Addis, M., Mansfield, A., & Syzdek, M. (2010). Is "masculinity" a problem?: Framing the effects of gendered social learning in men. *Psychology of Men & Masculinity, 11*, 77–90.

American Psychological Association. (2003). Guidelines on multicultural education, training, research, practice and organizational change for psychologists. *American Psychologist, 58*, 377–402.

American Psychological Association. (2007). Guidelines for psychological practice with girls and women. *American Psychologist, 62*, 949–979.

Arciniega, G. M., Anderson, T. C., Tovar-Blank, Z. G., & Tracey, T. J. G. (2008). Toward a fuller conception of machismo: Development of a traditional machismo and caballerismo scale. *Journal of Counseling Psychology, 55*, 19–33.

Baird, M., Szymanski, D., & Ruebelt, S. (2007). Feminist identity development and practice among male therapists. *Psychology of Men & Masculinity, 8*, 67–78.

Becker, D., & Marecek, J. (2008). Positive psychology: History in the remaking? *Theory and Psychology, 18*, 591–604.

Brooks, G. R., & Good, G. E. (Eds.). (2005). *The new handbook of psychotherapy & counseling with men: A comprehensive guide to settings, problems, & treatment approaches* (Rev. ed.). San Francisco: Jossey-Bass.

Brooks, G. R., & Silverstein, L. B. (1995). Understanding the dark side of masculinity: An interactive systems model. In R. F. Levant & W. S. Pollack (Eds.), *A new psychology of men* (pp. 280–336). New York: Basic Books.

Broverman, I. K., Broverman, D. M., Clarkson, F. E., Rosenkrantz, P. S., & Vogel, S. R. (1970). Sex-role stereotypes and clinical judgments of mental health. *Journal of Consulting and Clinical Psychology, 34*, 1–7.

Brown, L. S. (2010). Feminist therapy. In J. Carlson & M. Englar-Carlson (Eds.), *Theories of psychotherapy series*. Washington, DC: American Psychological Association.

Burns, G. W. (Ed.). (2010). *Happiness, healing, enhancement: Your casebook collection for applying positive psychology in therapy*. Hoboken: Wiley.

Choate, L. H. (2008). *Girls' and women's wellness: Contemporary counseling issues and interventions*. Alexandria: American Counseling Association.

Collins, P. H. (1997). The meaning of motherhood in black culture and black mother/daughter relationships. In M. M. Gergen & S. N. Davis (Eds.), *Toward a new psychology of gender: A reader* (pp. 325–340). New York: Routledge.

Connell, R. W., & Messerschmidt, J. W. (2005). Hegemonic masculinity: Rethinking the concept. *Gender and Society, 19*, 829–885.

Courtenay, W. H. (2011). *Dying to be men*. New York: Routledge.

Courtenay, W. H., McCreary, D. R., & Merighi, J. R. (2011). Gender and ethnic differences in health beliefs and behaviors. In W. H. Courtenay (Ed.), *Dying to be men* (pp. 241–250). New York: Routledge.

Cruz, R., King, K., Widaman, K., Leu, J., Cauce, A., & Conger, R. (2011). Cultural influences on positive father involvement in two-parent Mexican-origin families. *Journal of Family Psychology, 25*, 731–740.

Davies, J., Shen-Miller, D., & Isacco, A. (2010). The men's center approach to addressing the health crisis of college men. *Professional Psychology: Research and Practice, 41*, 347–354.

Duncan, B. L., Miller, S. D., & Sparks, J. A. (2004). *The heroic client: A revolutionary way to improve effectiveness through client-directed, outcome-informed therapy*. San Francisco: Jossey Bass.

Durik, A. M., Hyde, S. J., Marks, A. C., Roy, A. L., Anaya, D., & Schultz, G. (2006). Ethnicity and gender stereotypes of emotion. *Sex Roles, 54*, 429–445.

Eagly, A. H., & Diekman, A. B. (2003). The malleability of sex differences in response to changing social roles. In L. G. Aspinwall & U. M. Staudinger (Eds.), *A psychology of human strengths: Fundamental questions and future directions for a positive psychology* (pp. 103–115). Washington, DC: American Psychological Association.

Edwards, L., & Pedrotti, J. (2004). Utilizing the strengths of our cultures: Therapy with biracial women and girls. *Women & Therapy, 27*(1/2), 33–43.

Elston, F., & Boniwell, I. (2011). A grounded theory study of the value derived by women in financial services through a coaching intervention to help them identify their strengths and practice using them in the workplace. *International Coaching Psychological Review, 6*, 16–32.

Englar-Carlson, M. (2006). Masculine norms and the therapy process. In M. Englar-Carlson & M. A. Stevens (Eds.), *In the room with men: A casebook of therapeutic change* (pp. 13–48). Washington, DC: American Psychological Association.

Englar-Carlson, M. (2009). Men and masculinity: Cultural, contextual, and clinical considerations. In C. Ellis & J. Carlson (Eds.), *Cross cultural awareness and social justice in counseling* (pp. 89–120). New York: Routledge.

Evans, K. M., Kincade, E. A., Marbley, A. F., & Seem, S. R. (2005). Feminism and feminist therapy: Lessons from the past and hopes for the future. *Journal of Counseling and Development, 83*, 269–277.

Falicov, C. J. (2010). Changing constructions of machismo for Latino men in therapy: "The devil never sleeps". *Family Process, 49*, 309–329.

Gable, S. L., & Haidt, J. (2005). What (and why) is positive psychology. *Review of General Psychology, 9*, 103–110.

Glass, J., & Owen, J. (2010). Latino fathers: The relationship among machismo, acculturation, ethnic identity, and paternal involvement. *Psychology of Men & Masculinity, 11*, 251–261.

Goldner, V. (2011). Trans: Gender in free fall. *Psychoanalytic Dialogues, 21*, 159–171.

Goodwin, S. A., & Fiske, S. T. (2001). Power and gender: The double-edged sword of ambivalence. In R. K. Unger (Ed.), *Handbook of the psychology of women and gender* (pp. 358–366). New York: Wiley.

Grant, J. (1993). *Fundamental feminism: Contesting the core concepts of feminist theory*. New York: Routledge.

Gutmann, M. C. (2007). *The meanings of macho: Being a man in Mexico City*. Berkley: University of California Press.
Hammer, J., & Good, G. (2010). Positive psychology: An empirical examination of beneficial aspects of endorsement of masculine norms. *Psychology of Men & Masculinity, 11*, 303–318.
Hawkins, A. J., & Dollahite, D. C. (Eds.). (1996). *Generative fathering: Beyond deficit perspectives*. Thousand Oaks: Sage.
Hernandez, R. (2002). *Fatherwork in the crossfire: Chicano teen fathers struggling to take care of business* (Report No. JSRI-WP-58). East Lansing: Michigan State University, Julian Samora Research Institute (ERIC Document Reproduction Services No. ED 471 926).
Isacco, A., Talovic, E., Chromik, L., & Yallum, N. (2012). Addressing men's mental health through a strength-based approach. In J. M. Rippe (Ed.), *Lifestyle medicine* (2nd ed., pp. 369–381). Boca Raton: CRC Press.
Johnson, N. G. (2003). On treating adolescent girls: Focus on strengths and resiliency in psychotherapy. *Journal of Clinical Psychology/In Session, 59*, 1193–1203.
Kimmel, M. (2011). *Manhood in America: A cultural history* (3rd ed.). New York: Oxford University Press.
Kimmel, M., & Messner, M. (Eds.). (2012). *Men's lives* (9th ed.). New York: Prentice Hall.
Kiselica, M. S. (2011). Promoting positive masculinity while addressing gender role conflicts: A balanced theoretical approach to clinical work with boys and men. In C. Blazina & D. Shen-Miller (Eds.), *An international psychology of men: Theoretical advances, case studies, and clinical innovations* (pp. 127–156). New York: Routledge.
Kiselica, M. S., & Englar-Carlson, M. (2010). Identifying, affirming, and building upon male strengths: The positive psychology/positive masculinity model of psychotherapy with boys and men. *Psychotherapy: Theory, Research, Practice, Training, 47*, 276–287.
Kiselica, M. S., & Woodford, M. S. (2007). Promoting healthy male development: A social justice perspective. In C. Lee (Ed.), *Counseling for social justice* (pp. 111–135). Alexandria: American Counseling Association.
Kiselica, M. S., Englar-Carlson, M., Horne, A., & Fisher, M. (2008). A positive psychology perspective on helping boys. In M. S. Kiselica, M. Englar-Carlson, & A. Horne (Eds.), *Counseling troubled boys: A guidebook for professionals* (pp. 31–48). New York: Routledge.
Kitzinger, C. (2001). Sexualities. In R. K. Unger (Ed.), *Handbook of the psychology of women and gender* (pp. 272–285). New York: Wiley.
Lamb, S. (2005). Forgiveness therapy: The context and conflict. *Journal of Theoretical and Philosophical Psychology, 25*, 61–80.
Levant, R. F. (1997). The masculinity crises. *The Journal of Men's Studies, 5*, 221–231.
Levant, R. F. (2008). How do we understand masculinity? An editorial. *Psychology of Men & Masculinity, 9*, 1–4.
Levant, R. F., & Pollack, W. S. (Eds.). (1995). *The new psychology of men*. New York: Basic Books.
Levant, R. F., & Silverstein, L. S. (2005). Gender is neglected in both evidence based practices and "treatment as usual". In J. C. Norcross, L. E. Beutler, & R. F. Levant (Eds.), *Evidence-based practice in mental health: Debate and dialogue on the fundamental questions* (pp. 338–345). Washington, DC: American Psychological Association.
McNulty, J. K., & Fincham, F. D. (2012). Beyond positive psychology? Toward a contextual view of psychological process and well-being. *American Psychologist, 67*, 101–110.
Newfield, E., Hart, S., Dibble, S., & Kohler, L. (2006). Female-to-male transgender quality of life. *Quality of Life Research, 15*, 1447–1457.
O'Leary, V. E., & Bhaju, J. (2006). Resilience and empowerment. In J. Worell & C. D. Goodheart (Eds.), *Handbook of girls' and women's psychological health* (pp. 157–165). New York: Oxford University Press.
O'Neil, J. M. (2012). The psychology of men and boys in the year 2010: Theory, research, clinical knowledge, and future directions. In E. Altmaier & J. Hansen (Eds.), *The Oxford handbook of counseling psychology* (pp. 375–408). New York: Oxford University Press.
O'Neil, J. M., & Lujan, M. L. (2009). Preventing boy's problems in schools through psychoeducational programming: A call to action. *Psychology in the Schools, 46*, 257–266.

Pedrotti, J. (2011). Broadening perspectives: Strategies to infuse multiculturalism into a positive psychology course. *Journal of Positive Psychology, 6*, 506–513.

Pedrotti, J. T., & Edwards, L. M. (2009). The intersection of positive psychology and multiculturalism in counseling. In J. G. Ponterotto, J. M. Casas, L. A. Suzuki, & C. M. Alexander (Eds.), *Handbook of multicultural counseling* (3rd ed., pp. 165–174). Thousand Oaks: Sage.

Pedrotti, J., Edwards, L., & Lopez, S. (2009). Positive psychology within a cultural context. In S. Lopez & C. Snyder (Eds.), *The Oxford handbook of positive psychology* (2nd ed., pp. 49–57). New York: Oxford University Press.

Pleban, F. T., & Diez, K. S. (2007). Fathers as mentors: Bridging the gap between generations. In S. E. Brotherson & J. M. White (Eds.), *Why fathers count: The importance of fathers and their involvement with children* (pp. 307–318). Harriman: Men's Studies Press.

Pleck, J. H. (2010). Paternal involvement: A revised conceptualization and theoretical linkages with child outcomes. In M. E. Lamb (Ed.), *The role of the father in child development* (5th ed., pp. 58–93). Hoboken: Wiley.

Reid, P. T. (2002). Multicultural psychology: Bringing together gender and ethnicity. *Cultural Diversity and Ethnic Minority Psychology, 8*, 103–114.

Riggle, E., Whitman, J., Olson, A., Rostosky, S., & Strong, S. (2008). The positive aspects of being a lesbian or gay man. *Professional Psychology: Research and Practice, 39*, 210–217.

Riggle, E., Rostosky, S., McCants, L., & Pascule-Hague, D. (2011). The positive aspects of a transgendered self-identification. *Psychology & Sexuality, 2*, 147–158.

Rochlen, A., Suizzo, M., McKelley, R., & Scaringi, V. (2008). "I'm just providing for my family": A qualitative study of stay-at-home fathers. *Psychology of Men & Masculinity, 9*, 193–206.

Rudman, L. A., & Glick, P. (2001). Prescriptive gender stereotypes and backlash toward agentic women. *Journal of Social Issues, 57*, 743–762.

Saracho, O. N., & Spodek, B. (2008). Demythologizing the Mexican American father. *Journal of Hispanic Higher Education, 7*, 79–96.

Seligman, M., & Csikszentmihalyi, M. (2000). Positive psychology: An introduction. *American Psychologist, 55*, 5–14.

Sherblom, S. (2008). The legacy of the 'care challenge': Re-envisioning the outcome of the justice-care debate. *Journal of Moral Education, 37*, 81–89.

Singh, A. A., Hayes, D. G., & Watson, L. S. (2011). Strength in the face of adversity: Resilience strategies of transgender individuals. *Journal of Counseling and Development, 89*, 20–27.

Smiler, A. P. (2004). Thirty years after the discovery of gender: Psychological concepts and measures of masculinity. *Sex Roles, 50*, 15–26.

Stevens, M. A., & Englar-Carlson, M. (2010). Counseling men. In J. A. Erickson-Cornish, B. A. Schreier, L. I. Nadkarni, L. H. Metzger, & E. R. Rodolfa (Eds.), *Handbook of multicultural counseling competencies* (pp. 195–230). New York: Wiley.

Szymanski, D. M., Baird, M. K., & Kornman, C. (2002). The feminist male therapist: Attitudes and practices for the 21st century. *Psychology of Men & Masculinity, 3*, 22–27.

Tzou, J. Y., Kim, E., & Waldheim, K. (2012). Theory and practice of positive feminist therapy: A culturally responsive approach to divorce therapy with Chinese women. *International Journal for the Advancement of Counselling, 34*, 143–158.

White, A. (2008). *Ain't I a feminist, too? African American men speak out fatherhood, friendship, forgiveness, and freedom.* New York: State University of New York Press.

Wong, Y. J., & Rochlen, A. (2005). Demystifying men's emotional behavior: New directions and implications for counseling and research. *Psychology of Men & Masculinity, 6*, 62–72.

Wong, Y. J., & Rochlen, A. (2008). Re-envisioning men's emotional lives: Stereotypes, struggles, and strengths. In S. J. Lopez (Ed.), *Positive psychology: Exploring the best in people* (pp. 149–165). Westport: Greenwood Publishing Company.

Worell, J., & Johnson, D. (2001). Therapy with women: Feminist frameworks. In R. K. Unger (Ed.), *Handbook of the psychology of women and gender* (pp. 317–329). New York: Wiley.

Chapter 10
Religion, Spirituality, and Positive Psychology: Strengthening Well-Being

Melissa D. Falb and Kenneth I. Pargament

10.1 Introduction

Views toward religion have long been highly polarized, particularly within the field of psychology, where psychologists themselves show generally lower rates of religious belief and affiliation than the general public (Gross and Simmons 2009). In particular, both within and outside of psychology, many individuals view religion as a destructive force, ignoring its many positive implications and benefits. On the other hand, others view religion as essential to health and well-being, ignoring its potentially negative repercussions, such as those that arise for individuals who utilize negative coping strategies and experience spiritual struggles.

Over the last several decades, increasing attention has been given to the role of spirituality and religion in both mental and physical health. For example, from 1965 to 2000, there was a 727 % rise in the average number of health-related research articles published per year dealing with spirituality (Weaver et al. 2006). Contemporary psychologists and other health care providers and scientists are also increasing their attempts to integrate religion and spirituality into their research and clinical practice. This interest takes a variety of forms and includes topic areas such as coping, prayer, meditation, spiritual modeling, religious attachment, spiritual transformation, sanctification, and the integration of spirituality within various forms of psychotherapy. In addition, the advent of the field of positive psychology has opened up certain topics that have particular religious and spiritual relevance, such as hope (Berg et al. 2008), forgiveness (Wade and Worthington 2005), gratitude (Emmons and McCullough 2003), humility (Krause 2010), resilience (Bonanno 2004), and compassion (Gilbert 2005) to increased psychological investigation.

M.D. Falb, M.A. (✉) • K.I. Pargament, Ph.D.
Psychology Department, Bowling Green State University, Bowling Green, OH 43403, USA
e-mail: mdfalb@gmail.com

J. Teramoto Pedrotti and L.M. Edwards (eds.), *Perspectives on the Intersection of Multiculturalism and Positive Psychology*, Cross-Cultural Advancements in Positive Psychology 7, DOI 10.1007/978-94-017-8654-6_10,

These trends have been accompanied by a more balanced and nuanced approach to the role that religion and spirituality can play in people's overall well-being and functioning (Pargament et al. 2013). Currently, there is ample empirical support for the position that religion and spirituality can serve as both a positive and negative force in people's lives (See Ano and Vasconcelles 2005 for a review).

In this chapter, we assert that whether religion is primarily a constructive or destructive force depends largely on the kind of religion we are considering and the ways in which the individual interacts with and expresses that religion. As a prelude to this discussion, it is critical to provide a definition of religion, and of its partner construct, spirituality.

10.2 Defining Religion and Spirituality

Historically, religion has been, and continues to be, defined in a variety of ways (see Zinnbauer and Pargament 2005). Classically, religion was a broad-based construct involving beliefs, practices, relationships, and emotions that served a variety of purposes (James 1902). More recently, religion has been defined more narrowly as an institutionally-based set of beliefs and practices and increasingly, religion has been contrasted with spirituality. In this comparison, religion has often been viewed as institutional, restrictive, ritualized, and negative in character in contrast to spirituality which has been viewed as personal, freeing, spontaneous, and positive in character (Koenig et al. 2012). However, this polarization has been critiqued and found to be inadequate (Zinnbauer and Pargament 2005). In particular, this polarization is needlessly constrictive, limits investigation within the field, and oversimplifies the complex, multi-dimensional, and overlapping nature of these concepts.

For simplification, in this chapter we will focus on the common ground involving religion and spirituality, rather than their differences. Specifically, we focus on religion and spirituality as they are involved in individuals' attempts to discover, sustain, and transform objects of significance in the individual's life (see Pargament 2007). Generally, religion occurs within the context of institutions, beliefs, and traditions whose goal is the facilitation of this search, and, most importantly, the search for higher, spiritual ends. Spirituality refers specifically to the individual's search for a relationship with the sacred, which may or may not occur in an institutional context (Pargament 2007). Significance refers to any object of value, for example loving relationships, purpose in life, virtues, material success, and self-development. The sacred refers to any aspect of life that has been sanctified or deemed worthy of veneration, for example religious figures, leaders, or symbols, noble truths, and vocations. Both significance and the sacred may manifest themselves in a variety of dimensions of life, including the social, psychological, physical, material, and divine. Using this broad definition helps underscore the diversity of forms and functions of religious and spiritual experience and expression, and to avoid the polarized debate often encountered in this field. In this way, we hope to maintain a focus on the conversation at hand: religion/spirituality at its best, at its worst, and how religion/spirituality can be utilized to enhance well-being among diverse populations.

10.3 Religion/Spirituality at Its Best

In times of stress, people often draw on religion and spirituality as vital resources for coping (Pargament 1997). In religion and spirituality, people find a variety of ways of understanding and dealing with challenging life situations. These coping methods include benevolent religious reframing of negative situations, religious support, rites of passage, meditation and prayer, purification rituals, and conversion. Empirical studies have shown that these methods of religious coping are generally helpful to people and, moreover, appear to predict outcomes above and beyond the effects of secular coping methods (Pargament 1997, 2011). Religious resources serve a number of key psychological, social, and spiritual functions.

10.3.1 Community and Social Connection

Among the positive effects of religion is the sense of community, connectedness, and identity it provides participants. Nearly a century ago, Emile Durkheim (1912/1954), emphasized the social function of religion, stressing the communal activities and bonds religious participation offers. In his *Elementary Forms of Religious Life*, he described religion as an "eminently collective thing" and gave special emphasis to the moral community religion creates (Durkheim 1912/1954, p. 47). In addition to subjective reports of the benefits of religion's social functions, several research studies provide empirical evidence supporting this view.

For example, church attendance appears to be beneficial on a number of levels. In a meta-analysis of 44 studies of healthy and 13 studies of unhealthy samples, Chida et al. (2009) found that religiosity and spirituality, measured primarily by involvement with a religious community were correlated with decreased mortality rates among healthy samples, even after controlling for potentially confounding behaviors. In particular, religious attendance (at least once a week) had a greater protective effect on mortality than organizational activity generally. Similarly, religious service attendance has been found to be associated with lower risk of developing major depression (Maselko et al. 2009) and to be a protective factor against suicide attempts (Rasic et al. 2011).

Additionally, several studies suggest that church-based support offers health benefits above and beyond those provided by secular support. In one study, Krause (2006) found that church-based emotional support reduced the health effects of financial strain, but secular support from family and friends did not, suggesting there is something unique about church-based social support. These stress-buffering effects were found among African Americans, but not among Whites. Similar results were found among Mexican Americans (Krause and Bastida 2010), where church-based support was linked with an increased sense of personal control and better health. These studies, and others, suggest that the sense of community from spiritual support may be especially beneficial to racial and ethnic minority populations. This may be due in part to the importance of community versus individual identity among many non-White groups, as well as to the central social role the Church often plays among minority groups who have experienced a long-standing history of prejudice and discrimination.

10.3.2 *Self-Regulation and Self-Control*

A second benefit of religion is its ability to help individuals learn self-regulation and self-control. Clearly, morality forms a central component of religions across cultures, as evidenced by moral codes such as Judaism and Christianity's Ten Commandments and Buddhism's five precepts, as well as the moral elements inherent in many religious concepts, including, notably, Heaven and Hell. An important function of religion, then, is to help individuals develop the skills and ability to adhere to appropriate standards of moral conduct. Such self-regulation not only enhances individual well-being, but has important benefits for interpersonal relationships and society as a whole.

Religion facilitates self-control in a variety of ways. These methods of improving self-regulation include offering clear instructions regarding right and wrong (e.g. commandments, precepts); providing motivation to engage in moral behavior (e.g. salvation, reincarnation, enlightenment); assisting in self-monitoring (e.g. prayer, meditation, confession); helping to manage temptation and inappropriate desires (e.g. gender segregation, celibacy); assisting in emotion regulation (e.g. encouraging faith in God's benevolence/wisdom); enforcing beliefs about successful self-regulation (e.g. personal responsibility); and reinforcing guilt to teach lessons, prevent amoral behavior, and enhance prosocial actions (Geyer and Baumeister 2005).

Empirical studies support the regulatory function of religion as well. McCullough and Willoughby (2009) reviewed evidence from diverse religions and cultures that religion promotes self-control, self-monitoring, and self-regulation, that religion influences the selection, pursuit, and organization of goals, and that some of the positive health outcomes of religion are likely due to self-regulatory functions. In addition, a meta-analysis of 71 studies of personality correlates of religiousness across 19 countries (Saroglou 2010) showed a relationship between religion and several personality variables, including conscientiousness, a trait related to self-control and self-discipline. This relationship of conscientiousness with religion held across religiosity, spirituality, and fundamentalism, suggesting that self-control may be important across many aspects of the religious experience. These findings were consistent across age, gender, country, and religion.

10.3.3 *Meaning and Meaning-Making*

Another positive aspect of religion is its function as a source of meaning (for reviews, see Park 2005, 2007). While meaning is certainly important in other fields, including psychology (e.g. Wong and Fry 1998), religion is distinctively concerned with ultimate values and sacred matters. Indeed, for millennia, it has been primarily religion to which individuals turn in their efforts to seek and create meaning in their lives. Some have suggested that religion's ability to provide meaning at least partly accounts for its powerful and positive influence on health and well-being (George et al. 2002). A range of research has demonstrated an association between the meaning-making function of religion and well-being.

For example, several studies show an association of the meaning and peace aspect of spiritual well-being with quality of life. In a study of two samples of patients with colorectal cancer, Salsman et al. (2011) found meaning and peace to be a more potent predictor of health-related quality of life than faith. While both facets were positively associated with all aspects of health quality (physical, social and emotional), faith was not a significant predictor of health quality when controlling for meaning/peace. Similar findings have been identified in other populations, including older adults (Homan and Boyatzis 2010) and cancer patients (Yanez et al. 2009). These findings suggest that religion and spirituality may produce their effects, in part, through the sense of meaning and peace they offer people.

In addition, other studies have shown significant relationships between the meaning making function of religion/spirituality and positive outcomes. Mahoney et al. (2005) found that religion and spirituality assist individuals in the pursuit of meaningful goals. In particular, spiritual strivings were related to increased joy and happiness in a community sample of adults. In a study of the neural correlates of religious and secular meaning, Inzlicht et al. (2009) found a link between religious belief and activity in the anterior cingulate cortex, a brain system related to anxiety and self-regulation. Based on these findings, they suggest that religion helps prevent anxiety by providing meaning systems which inform behavior as well as predictions about oneself and the world.

The meaning making function of religion is also salient to Terror Management Theory (TMT; Solomon et al. 1991). TMT asserts that religion provides individuals with a particularly well-suited method for making sense of fears of mortality and of death. This is due to religious beliefs' often comprehensive nature, their promise of immortality, and the difficulty of disconfirming basic religious tenets (Vail et al. 2010). In particular, individuals with more intrinsic religiousness – who strive for meaning and value via religious belief rather than using religion for more utilitarian purposes (extrinsic religiousness) – show lower levels of fear of death (Jonas and Fischer 2006). This increased intrinsic religiousness appears to serve a terror management function, particularly in the face of uncontrollable adverse events, including illness, death, and terrorism, and to mitigate the tendency for individuals to react negatively toward those with differing worldviews. The meaning-making function of religion thus has positive benefits in both the physical and psychological realms.

10.3.4 Comfort and Anxiety Reduction

Another function of religion and spirituality illustrated by terror management theory is that of emotional comfort and anxiety reduction. The meanings created by religion in particular can serve the additional function of buffering anxiety in the face of one's own mortality and death. Indeed many religious beliefs provide an alternate point of view that gives life purpose, value, and existence beyond the death of the body. This anxiety-reducing function of religion, especially as related to fear of death, is supported by a wealth of empirical studies (see Soenke et al. 2013).

In another particularly interesting qualitative study, Pevey et al. (2008) directly asked dying patients with a range of medical conditions if and how religion brought them comfort. Many respondents directly acknowledged feeling comforted by their religious beliefs when facing death. In particular, they noted the importance of several specific aspects of their religion, including cosmic order (the belief that God is in control), divine relations (having a personal relationship with God), and belief in an afterlife.

The idea of a comforting function of religion is not new. The relief from anxiety provided by religious belief was noted by early and eminent psychologists, including Freud, one of the first and most emphatic to stress the role of religion in alleviating anxiety (Freud 1927/1961). In addition, contemporary psychological approaches such as attachment theory suggest that, like attachment to parents, attachment to God-figures can provide security and reduce distress (Kirkpatrick 2005). This comforting and anxiety-reducing function is an especially salient and long-standing example of the positive functions that religion and spirituality can serve.

10.3.5 Sense of Transcendence

Finally, the transcendent function of religion and spirituality provides an additional potential source of positive physical and psychological outcomes. Spiritual transcendence can be defined as "the capacity of individuals to stand outside of their immediate sense of time and place and to view life from a larger, more objective perspective … in which a person sees a fundamental unity underlying the diverse strivings of nature" (Piedmont 1999, p. 988). This capacity for transcendence can contribute to enhanced well-being, above and beyond that predicted by personality factors. For example, Piedmont's Spiritual Transcendence Scale (STS; 1999) has been shown to uniquely predict a range of psychological outcomes, including perceived social support, interpersonal orientation, vulnerability to stress, self-actualization, purpose in life, and pro-social behavior (Piedmont 1999, 2001).

The STS is particularly relevant to a cross-cultural discussion of religion/spirituality. In an attempt to identify aspects of spirituality common to diverse traditions, the scale was developed with input from theological experts in many faiths, including Buddhism, Hinduism, Lutheranism, Catholicism, Quakerism, and Judaism. As might be expected then, Piedmont's findings appear to hold cross-culturally. In a study with Hindus, Christians, and Muslims, Piedmont and Leach (2002) found support for the STS with individuals from multiple faiths in an international context. The scale appeared internally consistent overall and was predictive of psychological outcomes, such as positive affect, negative affect, and purpose in life, providing evidence of the universal nature of the transcendent aspect of spirituality.

A related line of research looks at the imbuing of significant objects with transcendent or sacred qualities. Numerous studies suggest that such "sanctification" produces positive benefits. For example, sanctification of strivings (Mahoney et al. 2005), marriage (Mahoney et al. 1999), nature (Tarakeshwar et al. 2001), and sexual intercourse (Murray-Swank et al. 2005) have been shown to lead to positive outcomes, including greater meaning, commitment, and satisfaction, increased collaboration, and more investment of energy and resources. Findings from this body of research suggest that imbuing objects with transcendent or sacred qualities has benefits that go beyond simple perceptions of objects as important (see Pargament et al. 2005a) and beyond the benefits of general religiousness (DeMaris et al. 2010).

Similarly, research on meditation has found a range of beneficial effects for participants learning a spiritual versus a secular form of meditation. In a study comparing migraine sufferers who learned a spiritual meditation technique to those who learned a non-spiritual meditation technique Wachholtz and Pargament (2008) found that spiritual meditators showed greater decreases headache frequency, anxiety, and negative mood, and greater increases in pain tolerance, self-efficacy, spiritual experiences, and existential well-being compared to secular meditators. Thus, the transcendent component when added to meditation appears to provide positive benefits compared to meditation techniques that lack this element.

10.4 Religion/Spirituality at Its Worst

Despite the many positive effects of religion and spirituality, it would be short-sighted to neglect the negative consequences of some forms of religious and spiritual expression. Due to this chapter's focus on positive psychology and well-being, however, this side of the discussion will be deliberately short and the reader is referred to other sources for a more in-depth approach to the negative side of religion and spirituality. Three topics are noteworthy in this area and will be covered briefly These include hatred toward out groups, religion as a source of struggle and despair, and rigidity, authoritarianism, and prejudice.

10.4.1 Hatred Toward Out Groups

One harmful effect of religion is its role as a source of hatred toward those outside of a particular religious tradition. Although it is important to note that this can apply outside of religious contexts, out group hatred is unfortunately no stranger to religious groups. Despite clear evidence of this phenomenon across gender, age, national, racial, ethnic, and political lines, out group hatred can be particularly insidious when it arises within a distorted or disintegrated religious context, in which religious tenets and beliefs are used in hurtful, rigid, discriminatory, or even aggressive ways.

This can take many forms, including terrorism (Jones 2006), genocide (Waller 2013), and reactions to what one considers a sacred violation or desecration (Pargament et al. 2007; Raiya et al. 2008). The vilification of those outside one's own religious group can yield a range of aggressive and insidious effects, varying from the bias and hostility seen in desecration to the murder and genocide found during times of war.

10.4.2 Religion as a Source of Struggle and Despair

An additional source of problematic outcomes arising from religion relates to spiritual struggles (for an overview, see Exline and Rose 2005). Spiritual struggles can be defined as questions, uncertainty or conflict about sacred matters relating to God, spiritual relationships, or within oneself (Pargament et al. 2005b). Such struggles often grow out of various life problems, including accidents, illnesses, abuse, crime, natural disasters, and other traumas. Specific spiritual struggles can include anger toward God, struggles with personal sin, perceived spiritual attacks (e.g. harm or possession by evil forces), and social problems within religious institutions (e.g. sexual abuse by clergy, misogyny or homophobia within the Church; Pargament et al. 2005b). Such spiritual struggles have consistently been shown to be associated with a range of negative psychological effects, including depression, anxiety, distress, paranoid ideation, obsessive–compulsiveness, and somatization (Ano and Vasconcelles 2005; McConnell et al. 2006). The effects of spiritual struggles on mental health appear to be far-reaching in both the short and long term (Pirutinsky et al. 2011).

10.4.3 Rigidity, Authoritarianism, and Prejudice

Finally, certain forms of religious belief and religious expression appear to be linked to rigidity, authoritarianism, and prejudice. Specifically, fundamentalism (the belief in one fundamental, correct, inerrant set of religious teachings which must be followed in order to have a special relationship with God and to oppose forces of evil) is closely linked to authoritarian beliefs, including prejudice against outsiders, submission to authority, and aggressive punishment of lawbreakers (Altemeyer and Hunsberger 1992). Similarly, extrinsic religiosity and religious fundamentalism have been shown to be associated with higher levels of racism, particularly when stemming from authoritarian attitudes (submission/aggression), rather than from fundamentalist values (conformity/tradition) (Laythe et al. 2001). It is important to note that authoritarian attitudes can be found not only in "fundamentalist" religions, but to some degree in all denominations. While certain religious styles and denominations appear to foster prejudice more than others, any religion can be used in a way that discriminates against those who are different.

10.5 Applications and Implications

Moving beyond an exploration of the positive and negative effects of religion and spirituality, it is important to think about ways in which the spiritual and religious side of existence can be integrated more fully into human growth and development. How can religion and spirituality be more consistently utilized in constructive, life-enhancing ways? How can the negative repercussions of religion and spirituality be minimized or even transformed? Can partnerships and collaboration between secular and religious/spiritual groups lead to further enrichment of human life, relationships, and health? These are some of the vital questions the final section of this paper will address.

One important strategy in utilizing psychological interventions and programs to enhance human growth and development is to foster the constructive aspects of religiousness and spirituality. This approach builds on the inherent strengths and benefits which accrue to those who draw on religious and spiritual resources, both individually and in community. Helping people cope in ways that lead to positive outcomes is essential. Many religious and spiritual communities and practices emphasize such resources, including forgiveness, collaboration, support, reappraisal, and connection (Pargament 1997). In addition, interventions can draw on religious and spiritual resources among individuals and communities to enhance physical health. Such programs have targeted numerous health outcomes, such as smoking cessation (Samuel-Hodge et al. 2009), weight loss (Kennedy et al. 2005), and fruit and vegetable consumption (Resnicow et al. 2004). These and other promising programs have focused on African American churches (Allicock et al. 2013).

Reducing the destructive aspects of religion and spirituality is another strategy for enhancing quality of life and well-being. For example, given the negative repercussions of spiritual struggles, strategies which reduce such struggles can be a beneficial step toward reducing distress. In one such intervention, Gear et al. (2008) developed and evaluated a 9 week spiritually integrated group treatment for college students experiencing spiritual struggles. The program was not only successful at reducing spiritual struggles, but also decreased psychological distress and increased emotion regulation skills, coping ability, and alignment between personal behaviors and stated spiritual values. Similar interventions have shown success in reducing negative religious coping and negative God images (Oman et al. 2007) and reducing depression and spiritual struggles among HIV patients (Tarakeshwar et al. 2005). The effectiveness of these programs suggests that spiritual struggles, though perhaps inevitable for many, do not inevitably lead to problems; rather, they can be addressed through interventions which facilitate a process of positive growth and transformation.

Rather than focus on treating problems that grow out of religion and spirituality, it is possible and reasonable to prevent such problems before they occur. One example of such a proactive approach is the spiritual fitness component of the Army's recent initiative, the Comprehensive Soldier Fitness program (Cornum et al. 2011). The spiritual fitness module of the program (Pargament and Sweeney 2011) is intended to help soldiers anticipate and deal with spiritual struggles before they occur. Based on the awareness that spirituality can serve significant motivating and developmental purposes, the program is intended to facilitate the human search for truth, self-understanding, meaning, and purpose rather than waiting for problems to arise. Although the program has yet to be evaluated, its premise of preventative intervention appears promising, especially given the positive effects of similar (treatment-based) approaches cited above.

A third consideration for taking advantage of the life-enhancing aspects of religion and spirituality is through the use of creative partnerships and collaborative relationships between religious individuals and communities. Because most Americans report that religion and/or spirituality are important to them (Pew 2008), implementing programs through this channel can have far-reaching effects. Religious and spiritual communities are widely available, and offer numerous resources and influence. Indeed, some research supports the idea that interventions implemented through religious communities are more effective and reliable than those implemented through secular channels (Wuthnow et al. 2004). Religiously and spiritually oriented community interventions may or may not incorporate religious language, content, and practices and may start inside or outside of religious and spiritual contexts. Such interventions often use community psychology methods – such as prevention, empowerment, self/program evaluation, and needs assessment – to enhance individual and community growth and development. They target wide-ranging social and personal problems, including poverty, racism, crime, incarceration, hunger, housing and homelessness, immigration, and a range of physical and mental health conditions (Maton 2013).

Finally, a further approach is to consider the potential for negative aspects of religion to have positive effects. For example, spiritual struggles, despite many negative repercussions, have the potential for contributing to positive change and growth. Important historical religious exemplars (e.g. Jesus, Buddha) faced significant struggles on their paths toward spiritual maturity; such struggles may in fact have been essential. More recent examples include Mahatma Gandhi and Martin Luther King, Jr., who faced significant spiritual dilemmas in their non-violent oppositions to gross injustice. They used experiences of humiliation which might have become catalysts for violence to instead fuel a process of deep transformation (Jones 2006). Research supports this notion that religious/spiritual struggle (as measured by negative religious coping) can sometimes lead to positive outcomes such as post-traumatic growth. For example, Pargament et al. (1998) found that despite links between negative religious coping and poorer physical and mental health, negative coping was also associated with stress-related growth across three samples. Other studies have supported these findings across diverse religious groups, including Jewish and Christian clergy (Proffitt et al. 2007) and U.S. Muslims experiencing negative interpersonal desecrations after the 9/11 attacks (Abu Raiya et al. 2011). These findings suggest that negative religious coping, despite harmful effects in some circumstances and for some people, can be a source of growth among diverse populations. Further research in this area can lead to a better understanding of how the negative aspects of religion can be not just minimized, but addressed in ways that lead to positive, long-lasting transformation.

In summary, religion and spirituality are not in and of themselves inherently beneficial or problematic. Rather, whether they serve primarily as positive or negative forces in people's lives depends on characteristics of the belief system, as well as how individuals interact with and express their religion and spirituality. Although there are relevant and stark examples of the ways religion and spirituality can be detrimental to human health and relationships, there is also abundant evidence of the ways this aspect of life can be used as a force for good, can improve physical and mental well-being, and can lead to positive growth and transformation.

References

Abu Raiya, H., Pargament, K. I., & Mahoney, A. (2011). Examining coping methods with stressful interpersonal events experienced by Muslims living in the United States following the 9/11 attacks. *Psychology of Religion and Spirituality, 3*, 1–14. doi:10.1037/a0020034.

Allicock, M., Resnicow, K., Hooten, E. G., & Campbell, M. K. (2013). Faith and health behavior: The role of the African American church in health promotion and disease prevention. In K. Pargament (Ed.-in-Chief), J. Exline, & J. Jones (Assoc. Eds.), *APA handbooks in psychology: APA handbook of psychology, religion, and spirituality: Vol. 1*. Washington, DC: American Psychological Association.

Altemeyer, B., & Hunsberger, B. (1992). Authoritarianism, religious fundamentalism, quest, and prejudice. *The International Journal for the Psychology of Religion, 2*, 113–133. doi:10.1207/s15327582ijpr0202_5.

Ano, G. G., & Vasconcelles, E. B. (2005). Religious coping and psychological adjustment to stress: A meta-analysis. *Journal of Clinical Psychology, 61*, 461–480. doi:10.1002/jclp.20049.

Berg, C. J., Snyder, C. R., & Hamilton, N. (2008). The effectiveness of a hope intervention in coping with cold pressor pain. *Journal of Health Psychology, 13*, 804–809. doi:10.1177/1359105308093864.

Bonanno, G. A. (2004). Loss, trauma, and human resilience: Have we underestimated the human capacity to thrive after extremely aversive events? *American Psychologist, 59*, 20–28. doi:10.1037/0003-066X.59.1.20.

Chida, Y., Steptoe, A., & Powell, L. H. (2009). Religiosity/spirituality and morality: A systematic quantitative review. *Psychotherapy and Psychosomatics, 78*, 81–90. doi:10.1159/000190791.

Cornum, R., Matthews, M. D., & Seligman, M. E. P. (2011). Comprehensive soldier fitness: Building resilience in a challenging institutional context. *American Psychologist, 66*, 4–9. doi:10.1037/a0021420.

DeMaris, A., Mahoney, A., & Pargament, K. I. (2010). Sanctification of marriage and general religiousness as buffers of the effects of marital inequity. *Journal of Family Issues, 31*, 1255–1278. doi:10.1177/0192513X10363888.

Durkheim, E. (1912/1954). *The elementary forms of religious life* (J. Swain, Trans.). New York: The Free Press.

Emmons, R. A., & McCullough, M. E. (2003). Counting blessings versus burdens: An experimental investigation of gratitude and subjective well-being in daily life. *Journal of Personality and Social Psychology, 84*, 377–389. doi:10.1037/0022-3514.84.2.377.

Exline, J. J., & Rose, E. (2005). Religious and spiritual struggles. In R. F. Paloutzian & C. L. Park (Eds.), *Handbook of the psychology of religion and spirituality* (pp. 315–330). New York: Guilford Press.

Freud, S. (1927/1961). *The future of an illusion*. New York: W.W. Norton and Company.

Gear, M. R., Faigin, C. A., Gibbel, M. R., Krumrei, E., Oemig, C., McCarthy, S. K., & Pargament, K. I. (2008). The winding road: A promising approach to addressing the spiritual struggles of college students. *Spirituality in Higher Education Newsletter, 4*, 1–8.

George, L. K., Ellison, C. G., & Larson, D. B. (2002). Explaining the relationships between religious involvement and health. *Psychological Inquiry, 13*, 190–200.

Geyer, A. L., & Baumeister, R. F. (2005). Religion, morality and self-control: Values, virtues, and vices. In R. F. Paloutzian & C. L. Park (Eds.), *Handbook of the psychology of religion and spirituality* (pp. 412–432). New York: Guilford Press.

Gilbert, P. (Ed.). (2005). *Compassion: Conceptualizations, research and use in psychotherapy*. New York: Routledge.

Gross, N., & Simmons, S. (2009). The religiosity of American college and university professors. *Sociology of Religion, 70*, 101–129. doi:10.1093/socrel/srp026.

Homan, K. J., & Boyatzis, C. J. (2010). Religiosity, sense of meaning, and health behavior in older adults. *The International Journal for the Psychology of Religion, 20*(3), 173–186. doi:10.1080/10508619.2010.481225.

Inzlicht, M., McGregor, I., Hirsh, J. B., & Nash, K. (2009). Neural markers of religious conviction. *Psychological Science, 20*, 385–392. doi:10.1111/j.1467-9280.2009.02305.x.

James, W. (1902). *The varieties of religious experience: A study in human nature*. New York: Longmans, Green and Co.

Jonas, E., & Fischer, P. (2006). Terror management and religion: Evidence that intrinsic religiousness mitigates worldview defense following mortality salience. *Journal of Personality and Social Psychology, 9*, 553–567. doi:10.1037/0022-3514.91.3.553.

Jones, J. W. (2006). Why does religion turn violent? A psychoanalytic exploration of religious terrorism. *Psychoanalytic Review, 93*(2), 167–190.

Kennedy, B. M., Paeratakul, S., Champagne, C. M., Ryan, D. H., Harsha, D. W., McGee, B., Johnson, G., Deyhim, F., Forsythe, W., & Bogle, M. L. (2005). A pilot church-based weight loss program for African-American adults using church members as health educators: A comparison of individual and group intervention. *Ethnicity & Disease, 15*, 373–378.

Kirkpatrick, L. A. (2005). *Attachment, evolution, and the psychology of religion*. New York: Guilford Press.

Koenig, H. G., King, D., & Carson, V. (2012). *Handbook of religion and health* (2nd ed.). New York: Oxford University Press.

Krause, N. (2006). Exploring the stress-buffering effects of church-based and secular social support on self-rated health in late life. *Journal of Gerontology B: Social Sciences, 61B*, S35–S43.

Krause, N. (2010). Religious involvement, humility, and self-rated health. *Social Indicators Research, 98*, 23–39. doi:10.1007/s11205-009-9514-x.

Krause, N., & Bastida, E. (2010). Church-based social relationships, belonging, and health among older Mexican Americans. *Journal for the Scientific Study of Religion, 50*, 397–409. doi:10.1111/j.1468-5906.2011.01575.x.

Laythe, B., Finkel, D., & Kirkpatrick, L. A. (2001). Predicting prejudice from religious fundamentalism and right-wing authoritarianism: A multiple-regression approach. *Journal for the Scientific Study of Religion, 40*, 1–10. doi:10.1111/0021-8294.00033.

Mahoney, A., Pargament, K. I., Jewell, T., Swank, A., Scott, E., Emery, E., & Rye, M. (1999). Marriage and the spiritual realm: The role of proximal and distal religious constructs in marital functioning. *Journal of Family Psychology, 13*, 321–338. doi:10.1037/0893-3200.13.3.321.

Mahoney, A., Pargament, K. I., Cole, B., Jewell, T., Magyar, G. M., Tarakeshwar, N., Murray-Swank, N., & Phillips, R. (2005). A higher purpose: The sanctification of strivings in a community sample. *The International Journal for the Psychology of Religion, 15*, 239–262. doi:10.1207/s15327582ijpr1503_4.

Maselko, J., Gilman, S. E., & Buka, S. (2009). Religious service attendance and spiritual well-being are differentially associated with risk of major depression. *Psychological Medicine, 39*, 1009–1017. doi:10.1017/S0033291708004418.

Maton, K. I. (2013). Addressing religion and psychology in communities: The congregation as intervention site, community resource, and community influence. In K. Pargament (Ed.-in-Chief), J. Exline, & J. Jones (Assoc. Eds.), *APA handbooks in psychology: APA handbook of psychology, religion, and spirituality: Vol. 1*. Washington, DC: American Psychological Association.

McConnell, K. M., Pargament, K. I., Ellison, C. G., & Flannelly, K. J. (2006). Examining the links between spiritual struggles and symptoms of psychopathology in a national sample. *Journal of Clinical Psychology, 62*, 1469–1484. doi:10.1002/jclp.20325.

McCullough, M. E., & Willoughby, B. L. B. (2009). Religion, self-regulation, and self-control: Associations, explanations, and implications. *Psychological Bulletin, 135*, 69–93. doi:10.1037/a0014213.

Murray-Swank, N. A., Pargament, K. I., & Mahoney, A. (2005). At the crossroads of sexuality and spirituality: The sanctification of sex by college students. *The International Journal for the Psychology of Religion, 15*, 199–219. doi:10.1207/s15327582ijpr1503_2.

Oman, D., Shapiro, S. L., Thoresen, C. E., Flinders, T., Driskill, J. D., & Plante, T. G. (2007). Learning from spiritual models and meditation: A randomized evaluation of a college course. *Pastoral Psychology, 55*, 473–493. doi:10.1007/s11089-006-0062-x.

Pargament, K. I. (1997). *The psychology of religion and coping: Theory, research, practice*. New York: Guilford Press.

Pargament, K. I. (2007). *Spiritually integrated psychotherapy: Understanding and addressing the sacred*. New York: Guilford Press.

Pargament, K. I. (2011). Religion and coping: The current state of knowledge. In S. Folkman (Ed.), *Oxford handbook of stress, health, and coping* (pp. 269–288). New York: Oxford University Press.

Pargament, K. I., & Sweeney, P. J. (2011). Building spiritual fitness in the Army: An innovative approach to a vital aspect of human development. *American Psychologist, 66*, 58–64. doi:10.1037/a0021657.

Pargament, K. I., Smith, B. W., Koenig, H. G., & Perez, L. (1998). Patterns of positive and negative religious coping with major life stressors. *Journal for the Scientific Study of Religion, 37*, 710–724.

Pargament, K. I., Magyar-Russell, G. M., & Murray-Swank, N. A. (2005a). The sacred and the search for significance: Religion as a unique process. *Journal of Social Issues, 61*, 665–687. doi:10.1111/j.1540-4560.2005.00426.x.

Pargament, K. I., Murray-Swank, N., Magyar, G. M., & Ano, G. (2005b). Spiritual struggle: A phenomenon of interest to psychology and religion. In W. R. Miller & H. D. Delaney (Eds.), *Judeo-Christian perspectives on psychology: Human nature, motivation, and change* (pp. 245–268). Washington, DC: American Psychological Association.

Pargament, K. I., Trevino, K., Mahoney, A., & Silberman, I. (2007). They killed our Lord: The perception of Jews as desecrators of Christianity as a predictor of anti-Semitism. *Journal of the Scientific Study of Religion, 46*, 143–158. doi:10.1111/j.1468-5906.2007.00347.x.

Pargament, K. (Ed.-in-Chief), Exline, J., Jones, J., Mahoney, A., & Shafranske, E. (Assoc. Eds.). (2013). *APA handbooks in psychology: APA handbook of psychology, religion, and spirituality*. Washington, DC: American Psychological Association.

Park, C. L. (2005). Religion and meaning. In R. F. Paloutzian & C. L. Park (Eds.), *Handbook of the psychology of religion and spirituality* (pp. 295–314). New York: Guilford Press.

Park, C. L. (2007). Religiousness/spirituality and health: A meaning systems perspective. *Journal of Behavioral Medicine, 30*, 319–328. doi:10.1007/s10865-007-9111-x.

Pevey, C. F., Jones, T. J., & Yarber, A. (2008). How religion comforts the dying: A qualitative inquiry. *Omega – Journal of Death and Dying, 58*, 41–59. doi:10.2190/OM.58.1.c.

Pew Forum on Religion & Public Life. (2008). *U.S. religious landscape survey*. Retrieved June 9, 2012 from religions.pewforum.org/pdf/report-religious-landscape-study-full.pdf

Piedmont, R. L. (1999). Does spirituality represent the sixth factor of personality? Spiritual transcendence and the five-factor model. *Journal of Personality, 67*, 985–1013. doi:10.1111/1467-6494.00080.

Piedmont, R. L. (2001). Spiritual transcendence and the scientific study of spirituality. *Journal of Rehabilitation, 67*, 4–14.

Piedmont, R. L., & Leach, M. M. (2002). Cross-cultural generalizability of the spiritual transcendence scale in India: Spirituality as a universal aspect of human experience. *American Behavioral Scientist, 45*, 1888–1901. doi:10.1177/0002764202045012011.

Pirutinsky, S., Rosmarin, D. H., Pargament, K. I., & Midlarsky, E. (2011). Does negative religious coping accompany, precede, or follow depression among Orthodox Jews? *Journal of Affective Disorders, 132*, 401–405. doi:10.1016/j.jad.2011.03.015.

Proffitt, D., Cann, A., Calhoun, L. G., & Tedeschi, R. G. (2007). Judeo-Christian clergy and personal crisis: Religion, posttraumatic growth and well being. *Journal of Religion and Health, 46*, 219–231. doi:10.1007/s10943-006-9074-1.

Raiya, H. A., Pargament, K. I., Mahoney, A., & Trevino, K. (2008). When Muslims are perceived as a religious threat: Examining the connection between desecration, religious coping, and anti-Muslim attitudes. *Basic and Applied Social Psychology, 30*, 311–325. doi:10.1080/01973530802502234.

Rasic, D., Robinson, J. A., Bolton, J., Bienvenu, O. J., & Sareen, J. (2011). Longitudinal relationships of worship attendance and spirituality with major depression, anxiety disorders, and suicidal ideation and attempts: Findings from the Baltimore epidemiologic catchment area study. *Journal of Psychiatric Research, 45*, 848–854. doi:10.1016/j.jpsychires.2010.11.014.

Resnicow, K., Campbell, M. K., Carr, C., McCarty, F., Wang, T., Periasamy, S., Rahotep, S., Doyle, C., Williams, A., & Stables, G. (2004). Body and soul: A dietary intervention conducted through African-American churches. *American Journal of Preventative Medicine, 27*, 97–105. doi:10.1016/j.amepre.2004.04.009.

Salsman, J. M., Yost, K. J., West, D. W., & Cella, D. (2011). Spiritual well-being and health-related quality of life in colorectal cancer: A multi-site examination of the role of personal meaning. *Supportive Care in Cancer, 19*, 757–764. doi:10.1007/s00520-010-0871-4.

Samuel-Hodge, C. D., Keyserling, T. C., Park, S., Johnston, L. F., Gizlice, Z., & Bangdiwala, S. I. (2009). A randomized trial of a church-based diabetes self-management program for African-Americans with type 2 diabetes. *Diabetes Education, 35*, 439–454. doi:10.1177/0145721709333270.

Saroglou, A. (2010). Religiousness as a cultural adaptation of basic traits: A five-factor model perspective. *Personality and Social Psychology Review, 14*, 108–125. doi:10.1177/1088868309352322.

Soenke, M., Landua, M. J., & Greenberg, J. (2013). Sacred armor: Religion's role as a buffer against the anxieties of life and the fear of death. In K. Pargament (Ed.-in-Chief), J. Exline, & J. Jones (Assoc. Eds.), *APA handbooks in psychology: APA handbook of psychology, religion, and spirituality: Vol. 1*. Washington, DC: American Psychological Association.

Solomon, S., Greenberg, J., & Psyzczynski, T. (1991). A terror management theory of social behavior: The psychological functions of self-esteem and cultural worldviews. *Advances in Experimental Social Psychology, 24*, 93–159. doi:10.1016/S0065-2601(08)60328-7.

Tarakeshwar, N., Swank, A. B., Pargament, K. I., & Mahoney, A. (2001). Theological conservatism and the sanctification of nature: A study of opposing religious correlates of environmentalism. *Journal for the Scientific Study of Religion, 42*, 387–404. doi:10.2307/3512131.

Tarakeshwar, N., Pearce, M. J., & Sikkema, K. J. (2005). Development and implementation of a spiritual coping group intervention for adults living with HIV/AIDS: A pilot study. *Mental Health, Religion & Culture, 8*, 179–190. doi:10.1080/13694670500138908.

Vail, K. E., III, Rothschild, Z. K., Weise, D. R., Solomon, S., Pyszczynski, T., & Greenberg, J. (2010). A terror management analysis of the psychological functions of religion. *Personality and Social Psychology Review, 14*, 84–94. doi:10.1177/1088868309351165.

Wachholtz, A. B., & Pargament, K. I. (2008). Migraines and meditation: Does spirituality matter? *Journal of Behavioral Medicine, 31*, 351–366. doi:10.1007/s10865-008-9159-2.

Wade, N. G., & Worthington, E. L., Jr. (2005). In search of a common core: Content analysis of interventions to promote forgiveness. *Psychotherapy: Theory, Research, Practice, Training, 4*, 160–177. doi:10.1037/0033-3204.42.2.160.

Waller, J. E. (2013). Religion and evil in the context of genocide. In K. Pargament (Ed.-in-Chief), J. Exline, & J. Jones (Assoc. Eds.), *APA handbooks in psychology: APA handbook of psychology, religion, and spirituality: Vol. 1*. Washington, DC: American Psychological Association.

Weaver, A. J., Pargament, K. I., Flannelly, K. J., & Oppenheimer, J. E. (2006). Trends in the scientific study of religion, spirituality, and health: 1965–2000. *Journal of Religion and Health, 45*, 208–214. doi:10.1007/s10943-006-9011-3.

Wong, P. T. P., & Fry, P. S. (Eds.). (1998). *The human quest for meaning: A handbook on psychological research and clinical applications*. Mahwah: Erlbaum.

Wuthnow, R., Hackett, C., & Hsu, B. Y. (2004). The effectiveness and trustworthiness of faith-based and other service organizations: A study of recipient's perceptions. *Journal for the Scientific Study of Religion, 43*, 1–17.

Yanez, B., Edmondson, D., Stanton, A. L., Park, C. L., Kwan, L., Ganz, P. A., & Blank, T. O. (2009). Facets of spirituality as predictors of adjustment to cancer: relative contributions of having faith and finding meaning. *Journal of Consulting and Clinical Psychology, 77*, 730–741. doi:10.1037/a0015820.

Zinnbauer, B. J., & Pargament, K. I. (2005). Religiousness and spirituality. In R. F. Paloutzian & C. L. Park (Eds.), *Handbook of the psychology of religion and spirituality* (pp. 21–42). New York: Guilford Press.

Chapter 11
Social Class Mobility and Positive Psychology

William Ming Liu and Allison Allmon

11.1 Positive Psychology and Social Class

Positive psychology provides a way to understand the unique challenges and strengths that are present among individuals in the lower social classes. The purpose of this chapter is to highlight the strengths of the lower social class and how these may be used to aid in meeting unique challenges, since there is much bias towards this status (Liu 2011). In order to explore positive psychology's contributions to our understanding of the lower social class the following definitions will be reviewed: social class, social mobility, upward mobility bias, and habitus. A brief introduction to social class mobility and positive psychology will follow this review. Finally, the authors present the Mobility Typology (Liu 2011) as a framework for understanding how people in lower social classes navigate social transitions. For brevity, only the two quadrants of the Mobility Typology which focus on individuals in the lower social class, *entitled* and *distressed*, are explored.

11.1.1 Definitions

Throughout this chapter, the authors choose to use the term *social class* rather than *socioeconomic status* (SES). As Liu (2011) has suggested in his review of extant social class and SES literature, there is confusion and conflation among researchers as to the definition of both social class and SES. Social class and SES have been used by various researchers to represent an aggregate of variables that

W.M. Liu, Ph.D. (✉) • A. Allmon
N328 Lindquist Center, Psychological and Quantitative Foundations,
The University of Iowa, Iowa City, IA 52242, USA
e-mail: william-liu@uiowa.edu

J. Teramoto Pedrotti and L.M. Edwards (eds.), *Perspectives on the Intersection of Multiculturalism and Positive Psychology*, Cross-Cultural Advancements in Positive Psychology 7, DOI 10.1007/978-94-017-8654-6_11,

revolve around income, education, occupation, resources, wealth, power, affluence, and poverty to name a few. Because of this interchangeability in psychological literature and the conflation of terms, Liu and his colleagues (Liu and Ali 2005; Liu et al. 2004) chose the term social class because of its nominal ease in connecting it to classism. Classism, with respect to social class, is a co-construct that must operate in tandem much like race and racism – one cannot happen without the other.

Liu and colleagues (2006) elaborated further on the important intersections of social class with race and racism and extrapolated these affects to other identities such as gender and age. Historically, Whiteness was codified and legitimized as a racial group that had political power (i.e., the right to vote) as well as economic power (i.e., land ownership). The roots of poverty, classism, and racism are linked to the socio-political (e.g., the unequal distribution of power), socio-historical (e.g., biased and inaccurate histories of peoples), and socio-structural (e.g., legal, education, and economic systems) forces that marginalize and oppress (Liu and Ali 2005). Poverty, classism, and economic/resource inequality are not merely unfortunate consequences of American capitalism, but integral to the "healthy" functioning of the American economy. Zinn (1991) suggests, for instance, that the founders and authors of the Constitution were fully cognizant of the divide between the poor and rich, Black and White. Their motivation was to retain privilege and wealth for those who had it (i.e., land-owning wealthy White men), and suppress dissent and protest related to poverty and debt. The founders believed God ordained those with riches due to providence and hard work and sought to codify power and privilege among a certain group of men. Built into this assumption, of course, was the belief that wealth and poverty were "natural" aspects of human society, without regard and acknowledgement for family wealth and privilege passed through multiple generations (Zinn 1991). As generations of the privileged sought and gained access to power and resources (e.g., government subsidies, tax waivers, special access) due merely to their status, the division between rich and poor grew. In effect, the rich gained momentum while the poor stagnated. The poor and others who faced the brunt of economic inequality were often racial minority groups, women, and Whites who were not deemed part of the privileged classes. And although the focus of this chapter is the understanding of social class from a positive psychology lens, the authors acknowledge the importance of looking at the intersectionality of identities including social class, gender, and race. Specifically, individuals are multifaceted and cannot be examined solely within the vacuum of their social class identities.

For mental health providers and researchers, the extension of this historical ideology is the Upward Mobility Bias (Liu 2011). This is the perception that all individuals have an innate need and "should" be moving upward through the social classes; that upward mobility is always healthy and normal; and that failing to either move upward or to maintain one's higher social class is the fault of the individual in transition. In contrast to this bias, the authors present the Mobility Typology as a means to understand social class transitions within a positive psychology context through the exploration of strengths that a client brings to therapy.

11.1.1.1 Social Class Transitions

Social class transition refers to the individual's experience of traversing upward (i.e., moving to a higher social class), downward (i.e., moving to a lower social class), and laterally (i.e., moving between equal social classes), from one's current social class group. Related to this idea is the concept of social class resources, such as intrapersonal (e.g., ability to withstand frustration), interpersonal (i.e., social networks, support, and friends), or material capital (i.e., money, home), that may be used and transformed given any situation. These resources are apparent and readily used and accessible for the individual.

As an example, the affluent have access to quantitatively more resources than those in lower social classes. They are able to transform raw resources such as money into social class relevant apparati like expensive clothing, large homes, educational attainment, and social networking. The use of resources in these social class specific ways allows the affluent individual to remain congruent with the expectations of others in his/her social class and to continue to solidify his/her position vis-à-vis their resource allocations.

As an example of how individuals in secure and resource abundant contexts are able to feel in control of their environment and be effective in their lives, affluent individuals are easy exemplars of the intersection of social class and positive psychology. In this chapter, however, the authors challenge the perception by some psychologists that those in lower social-class contexts lack agency or are constantly struggling. The authors use this literature to understand how people in lower social classes may navigate social class transitions, thus demonstrating important strengths and resilience.

11.1.1.2 Habitus

Bourdieu (1977) described an individual's habitus, or worldview, as being shaped by their environment. Positive psychology holds that individuals' perception of strengths and challenges, and therefore their habitus, are culturally defined and normed (Snyder et al. 2011). Thus, positive psychology provides a way for individuals to be understood within their own habitus. One factor that impacts an individual's habitus is their social class. Middle social class habitus includes a position of equality and expectation, where teachers and coaches are partners and questioning and debate are encouraged (Lareau 2003). This is starkly discrepant from the habitus of lower social class individuals, which consists of respect for adults as authority figures, and accomplishment through "natural growth" (Lareau 2003, p. 1). The perceived norms of society are built on middle social class habitus; individuals of the lower social class may not know how to operate on middle social class habitus (Abelev 2009). Abelev conducted a qualitative study of successful (defined as now members of the middle social class) adults who were members of the lower social class as a child and found that the primary reason for success was access to middle social class habitus. This included access through mentorships to high-performing schools, scholarships, and customized education plans. Additional studies of individuals who have succeeded in transitioning from the lower social class to the middle social class have provided reasons in the following three areas: intervening conditions (mentors, school), external factors (e.g., motivational support from family, community, peer groups, school- highly valued promote adjustment, expectations), and internal factors (e.g., perseverance, self-esteem, coping strategies, relationships, goal-orientation) (Ellis 2011). These transition reasons are dependent upon access to resources and knowledge about interacting within the middle class milieu (Abelev 2009).

11.1.2 Social Class Mobility and Positive Psychology

Among the many topics related to social class such as classism and stratification, one of the most difficult to understand is social mobility. Is social mobility only upward through social classes or is social mobility downward as well? Moreover, what makes someone successful when he/she moves into a new social class whereas for other individuals, being in a new social class creates distress? Although most psychological and sociological theories related to social class focus on stratifying individuals into discrete social class groups (i.e., middle-class) (Liu 2011), there is relatively little psychology and counseling research into social mobility (Nelson et al. 2006). Yet psychology, especially positive psychology, has much to contribute to the understanding of social mobility. From individuals who choose to downshift (Schor 2000, 2004) from hectic financial lives to agrarian existences, to those who continue to work and save and strive for upward mobility, positive psychology offers a glimpse into the ways in which people construct and make meaning from their choices and contexts. Positive psychology asserts that strengths and challenges are identified and developed as a function of cultural norms and environment (Lopez and Snyder 2009). That is, what may be considered a strength in one culture may not be in another (e.g., deference to authority). Positive psychology provides a way for psychologists to conceptualize the strengths individuals bring to understand and thrive within their economic world. From a subjective approach to understanding social class, this means that a positive psychological perspective allows clinicians and researchers to see people within a similar social class situation (i.e., lower-income) as having different self and situational perceptions about social mobility. Not everyone within a lower-income environment has the same social class worldview.

Having provided definitions of terms associated with social class, the authors now review the literature on the strengths of those in lower social classes. Next, the Mobility Typology will be described. While the typology certainly may cover the experiences of social class mobility and transition from affluent social classes to lower social classes, for illustration and brevity, the authors choose to focus on people who transition from lower to higher social classes. The authors describe the typology and elaborate on the personal experiences specifically among those who might be considered entitled and distressed types. As part of the description the authors provide a case example and discuss counseling and research implications.

11.2 Strengths and Challenges of the Lower Class

There is extensive empirical literature identifying the risk factors associated with members of the lower social class or poor. However, there is a dearth of literature examining the strengths among this social class (Israel and Jozefowicz-Simbeni 2009; Shumba 2010). The scant literature may be a result of the current operational definition and measurement of strengths and the negative perceptions associated with members of the lower social class present in research. The economic assumptions that upward mobility constitutes psychological strength are violated when researchers try to explore interpersonal and intrapsychic strengths among those in lower social classes. Related to this problem is the potential minimization of contextual and social problems (i.e., poverty) if intrapsychic strengths are found (Liu et al. 2009; Nguyen et al. 2012; Sanchez et al. 2011). Clearly, exploring strengths in the lower social class requires that researchers examine, identify, and disband any biases that they may have about this population (Clauss-Ehlers 2008).

There is immense within-group heterogeneity among the social classes (Liu et al. 2004; Masten and Sesma 1999; Obradovic et al. 2009). Socio-economic status does not necessarily correlate with risk and may depend on the personal environment of the individual (Masten et al. 2009). Individuals are multidimensional with many multicultural and personal factors, other than social class, that may add to their strengths (e.g., spirituality, family support). In the following section, the challenges and risk factors associated with lower social class will be discussed, as well as the resilience factors and strengths.

11.2.1 Lower Social Class and Risk Factors

There is extensive literature on the risk factors associated with lower social class or poor individuals (e.g., Bradley and Corwyn 2002; Slavin 1998). Individuals who are born into the lower social class or poverty may begin life at a disadvantage, due to substandard pre-natal and post-natal care and day care (Slavin 1998). Lower social class and poverty has been demonstrated to negatively impact physical health (Adler et al. 2000; Barger et al. 2009; Iwasaki 2006; Link and Phelan 1995; Ostrove et al. 2000; Starfield et al. 2002), mental health (Masten et al. 1993), school and academic achievement (e.g., Obradovic et al. 2009; Powers 1996), child development (e.g., Bradley and Corwyn 2002; Powers 1996), behavioral characteristics (McLloyd 1998), and social-emotional functioning (Kamper 2008; Mossakowski 2008).

Additionally, there may be a lasting impact of childhood lower socioeconomic class. For example, Mossakowski (2008) found increased reports of depression among individuals who were among the lower social class as a child. Furthermore, while the assertion that poverty increases creativity has received literary and theoretical support (e.g., Simonton 2009) it has not been empirically supported (e.g., Roley 2009). Instead, researchers have found less creativity among individuals of the lower social class when compared to middle social class (e.g., Strauss 1968; Roley 2009; Zhang and Postiglione 2001). Of course one problem related to findings in studies such as this is the privilege given by researchers to what is considered "creative." In environments where autonomy is valued and nurtured, creativity may reflect independence, while in other social class groups which may value adherence to social norms, creativity may reflect congruence to group norms and expectations.

Individuals in the lower social class are labeled 'at-risk' due to the risk factors (e.g., negative association between lower social class and physical health, mental health, child development, academic achievement) gleaned from the aforementioned research. However, this may be related to the focus of the research itself or the perceptions of the researcher (e.g., look for middle social class strengths, creativity; Strauss 1968). The concepts often explored and operationalized as strengths may be conceptually biased, such as the liberties taken by researchers to define 'creativity' in the aforementioned research. When conceptual inequality is present in studies it may minimize the strengths of the lower social class due to opportunity and exposure to middle or upper class resources. The use of traditional measures of strength (or what is believed to be a strength) may not be applicable across social class. For example, lack of exposure to resources for traditional creative outlets (e.g., the arts) likely impacts the use of those outlets among the lower class. It is for reasons such as this that it is imperative that researchers and practitioners remain vigilant in dispelling personal biases and developing an understanding of these variables through the lens of each social class.

11.2.2 Lower Social Class Strengths and Resilience

Despite the risk factors associated with the lower social class and the societal norm of middle social class habitus, members of the lower social class continue to persevere through their circumstances. Their resiliency or withstanding adverse circumstances (Masten 2011; Ong et al. 2009) inherently includes strengths. Banerjee (1998) asserted that, "strength typically evokes images of power, vigor, energy, wealth, and assets; people who have strengths are aspiring, capable, talented, and courageous" (p. 45); however strengths will need to be redefined in order for positive psychologists to seek out the strengths of the lower social class. Rapp's (1993) strength's model may provide one conceptual framework for identifying strengths among individuals of the lower social class. Rapp's model includes both personal (wants, desires, skills, abilities, confidence) and environmental (opportunities, resources, supports) strengths. Banerjee's (1998) study used Rapp's (1993) model to examine the personal and community strengths of 40 economically poor individuals in Calcutta, India. Banerjee (1998) found that although these individuals were economically poor, they had both individual and community strengths. These strengths, although not adequately explored (Israel and Jozefowicz-Simbeni 2009; Shumba 2010), include positive personal and behavioral characteristics (e.g., personality, intelligence), a sense of control and self-efficacy, and prosocial behaviors.

Israel and Jozefowicz-Simbeni (2009) study provided a rare opportunity for members of the lower social class to self-identify strengths. This study of homeless families explored mother-perceived strengths of their children. The mothers identified multiple child strengths including positive personality and behavioral characteristics, intelligence and academic achievement, and positive physical attributes, suggesting not only the presence, but also awareness for self-identification of Rapp's (1993) personal and environmental strengths among the lower social class.

Self-concept can impact academic motivation, engagement, and achievement (Aldridge et al. 1999; Pierce 1994). Lachman and Weaver (1998) found that poor individuals who had a sense of control (vs. poor individuals who did not) felt efficacy in their environment and that other people did not constrain them. Lachman and Weaver operationalized sense of control with two dimensions: (1) personal mastery (i.e., one's sense of efficacy or effectiveness in carrying out goals) and (2) perceived constraints (i.e., to what extent one believes there are obstacles or factors beyond one's control that interfere with reaching goals). This sense of control, or belief in one's capabilities, may be a protective factor among poor individuals. Contrarily, other research has demonstrated that individuals from a lower social class may be less likely to develop a positive self-concept (Gwirayi and Shumba 2007). Individuals in the lower social class may feel control and subsequent self-efficacy through means that are different from those in the middle or upper class. Due to their habitus, individuals in the middle social class may have the opportunity to rely on their school system or neighborhood to provide them with a sense of security, while those of the lower social class may not (Abelev 2009). Therefore, individuals in the lower social class may rely on habitus consistent ways of gaining a sense of control. Research is needed in order to explore these ways.

When individuals of the lower social class advance to middle social class they are labeled 'resilient' (Mendez et al. 2002). Resilience can be defined as "the capacity of a dynamic system to withstand or recover from significant challenges that threaten its stability, viability, or development" (Masten 2011, p. 494). The labels prescribed to individuals of the lower social class are not consistent with this definition of resiliency because resilience does not inherently imply improvement, but rather withstanding. Ong et al.'s (2009) review of the literature on resilience asserts that resilience may be more appropriately defined for individuals of the lower social class as a positive adaptation in the context of risk. Additionally, "resilience is a dynamic developmental process" (Luthar et al. 2000, p. 546). Therefore lower social class strengths may be more appropriately explored as meaningful short-term adaptation to daily stress, rather than stable traits. The review concludes that there is a need to know more than which assets and social resources are associated with positive adaptation; rather there is a need to consider how factors contribute to resilience in face of the daily challenges of being a member of the lower social class.

The introduction of a resource (e.g., financial, food, safety) may have a greater impact for the lower social class than other social classes (Diener and Biswas-Diener 2009; Diener and Oishi 2000). Gaining resources helped to increase a sense of well-being among poor individuals (defined as those who did not have their basic needs such as shelter, food, and safety met) (Diener and Biswas-Diener 2009; Diener and Oishi 2000). Additionally, Diener and Biswas-Diener found that the relationship between income and happiness tends to be much stronger in poor nations. However, it is important to note that although changes among the income of lower social class individuals had a strong impact on well-being, overall levels of well-being continue to be higher among middle social class or wealthy individuals (Diener and Biswas-Diener 2009).

Across four studies Piff and colleagues (2010) found that when compared to their upper class counterparts, individuals in the lower class acted in a more prosocial fashion. These studies provided evidence that individuals in the lower class exhibited more generosity, more support for charity, more trust behavior toward a stranger, and more helping behavior toward a person in distress even when doing so was costly to themselves. These studies suggest that the reasons for acting in a more prosocial fashion were greater commitment to egalitarian values and feelings of compassion and may be consistent with values found in the lower class habitus.

Rather than a wholly negative worldview among those in lower social classes, therefore, some of the literature identified here suggests points of strength and resiliency. In part, those studies that point to strengths among the lower social classes tend to show how individuals are able to identify necessary resources (intrapersonal, interpersonal, material, social) for them to survive and even thrive (e.g., Banerjee 1998; Lachman and Weaver 1998; Piff et al. 2010). Building on the framework of resource use here and in Liu (2011), the authors present a typology that describes the experiences of people who have experienced social class transition and their resource use as a means of adaption to their new context.

11.3 Mobility Typology

The Mobility Typology (Liu 2011) focuses on the personal experiences of individuals as they experience social class transitions (see Fig. 11.1). Using this typology within a positive psychology perspective helps to provide an understanding of the strengths that individuals in each cell possess and how these individuals may construct meaning from their contexts. This typology may apply to a diverse group of individuals experiencing social class transitions. From homeless veterans to college students to business owners, each experiences his/her own form of transition and a unique cognitive appraisal of his/her experience. In describing each experience, two factors were apparent and these form the axis of the typology. First, the individual

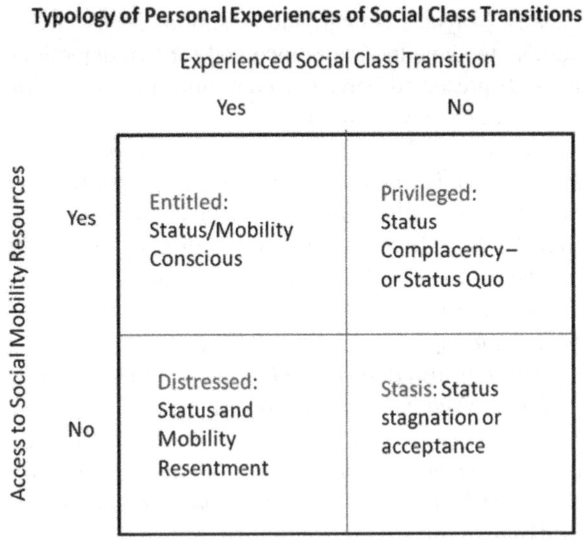

Fig. 11.1 Mobility Typology

experienced what he/she regarded as a social class transition. This transition may be upward and a form of social class ascending from working-class to middle-class, for instance. These experiences may have been in the form of increasing income, property, or educational level. Transition was also downward such as moving from owning one's own business to working as a clerk in another person's business. Downward transition also implicates the loss of resources, property, or status. The second axis was the person's access to resources. Simply stated, did or does the individual have access to resources as part of their social class transition? As the individual moved upward, for example, were there adequate resources (personal, interpersonal, social, material) that facilitated or eased the transition? These resources may be intrapersonal (e.g., ability to withstand frustration), interpersonal (i.e., social networks, support, and friends), material (i.e., money, home), to name a few. These resources are apparent and readily used and accessible for the individual.

To both of these questions, the Mobility Typology provides two discrete answers, yes and no (See Fig. 11.1). If the answer were yes to the questions of experiencing transition and having access to resources, then the first quadrant is titled "Entitled" wherein the individual is status and mobility conscious. If the individual experienced transition but did not have access to resources, the then the individual may fall into the quadrant of "Distressed" wherein the individual may have status and mobility resentment. If the individual did not experience transition and still had access to resources, then the individual may fall into the quadrant of "Privileged" wherein the individual is status accepting. Finally, if the person did not experience transition and did not have access to resources, the person may be in the quadrant of "Stasis" wherein he or she is either in stagnation or status acceptance.

Because the focus of this chapter is on individuals who are in lower social classes, only two cells will be delineated (Entitled and Distressed). In this case, for ease of illustration, the authors chose a case study, Wayne, who is moving upward in social classes. Wayne's background is similar for both illustrations and allows for the authors to show the issues involved for two depictions of Wayne (entitled and distressed) presented here. For continuity in explanation the authors adapt Wayne's case to fit each type presented.

Wayne is a 52-year old White male. He is homeless and resides at a medium sized homeless shelter in a rural city in the Midwest. Wayne has had periods of homelessness throughout his adult life, and recently was homeless as a result of a divorce from his wife. He has a history of substance use, most significantly alcohol abuse, and he has been cycling in and out of treatment centers for 10 years. He also has an inconsistent work history and he has held manual labor work (e.g., dishwashing, house painting) throughout his adult life.

Wayne is also a talented photographer. His photographs have been shown in art galleries around the country and he has been publically recognized for his talent. Each time he becomes sober and works on his photography, and each time he becomes recognized for his talent, Wayne slips back into his alcoholism. When he is drunk, he blames the recognition and attention he is receiving as the cause of his drinking.

11.3.1 Entitled

The entitled individual experienced a social class transition either upward or downward and may be the result of a decision may have not been in the control of the individual (i.e., a layoff) or it may have been a deliberate life choice (i.e., education, promotion, down-shifting). In this type, what buffered the transition is access to resources. Because the individual experienced a social class transition, one strength a client may have is that he/she is aware of social class differences, understands the difficulty of negotiating a new lifestyle within a different social class context, and as a result, the individual possesses a consciousness about status and mobility. In this first example, Wayne's background is used to illustrate the Entitled cell.

11.3.1.1 Wayne as an Entitled Individual

Wayne's entitlement attitudes are most apparent during his psychological treatment. As part of his treatment, the psychologist recommends he take a course on photography at a nearby community college. Although he has never been formally trained in photography, Wayne is excited to discuss portraitures and photography with knowledgeable and like-minded others. He recognized the course as an important resource that would allow him to focus on an important interest and talent, and through his photographs, he hopes to salvage his sobriety.

At first, Wayne is a good student in class. He engages with the instructor and other students, presents his photographs for critique, and supports his classmates. The instructor recognizes Wayne's talent and recommends he submit his photographs to a national magazine. Overtime, Wayne continually seeks individual attention from the instructor as well as additional support for gallery and other public showings. As the course continues, rather than asking for this special attention outside of class, Wayne openly demands it in class, and begins to disregard his relationships with his classmates.

11.3.1.2 Strengths and Challenges

One of the most apparent strengths for Wayne, or other entitled individuals, is an ability and capacity to adapt to new social class situations and environments. The individual perceives and uses available resources. In some cases the individual may be faced with fewer resources (e.g., being laid off), but the individual is willing and able to adapt and restructure resources to the new situational demands; in essence, the individual feels entitled to use available and seek out new resources. The most meaningful challenge for this individual is the perception from others may be that the person has become "selfish" or "egocentric" in his/her use of resources. So the challenge for the individual is not to deplete his/her resources quickly since, for some in lower social classes, replenishing social and material resources is difficult (Gallo et al. 2005).

11.3.2 Distressed

For the distressed individual, he/she experienced a social class transition either upward or downward, but without any readily accessible or available resources. Resources may be present, but the individual may not have been able to recognize the appropriate resource in a new context. Take for instance the first-generation college student who comes from a working-class background and finds him or herself in an affluent and privileged environment like a university or college. The university or college may provide transition services (a form of resource) for the first-generation student, but because "social activities," for example, are not seen by the first-generation college student as directly pertinent to his/her academic success; the student may limit or not participate in any social support activities. What arises from this context may be an appraisal of resentment for being in a new social class context. In this second example, Wayne's background is used to illustrate the Distressed cell.

11.3.2.1 Wayne as a Distressed Individual

As Wayne's photography talents become recognized, he is continually requested by private and community organizations to come and speak about his experiences as a "homeless man." Many times he is paid a nominal fee but most frequently he finds himself at galas, luncheons, and dinners populated by wealthy and affluent philanthropists and community leaders. He finds himself abruptly transitioning between two worlds: the homeless shelter where he shares a dormitory room with 40 other men and the private ballrooms of hotels.

He recognizes his rising distress and anxiety related to these social class transitions. When he goes to these philanthropic events, he goes alone; he is often ill- or under-dressed for the event. He tells people he does not like these events anymore and would rather avoid them. The shelter staff and other residents often reply with assurances that "things will get better" and "he deserves the attention for his talent." Wayne starts to resent his success and public attention. He is unsure how to navigate these new situations and he does not have anyone available to assist him.

11.3.2.2 Strengths and Challenges

Emotional distress resulting from social class transitions (upward or downward) is an important psychological signal to which the individual must be aware. Distress, in the long-term, certainly is detrimental for the individual's psychological and physical health, but in the short-term, it is the organism's alerting the person to "take care of itself" as seen in Wayne's case. For psychologists, an expression of distress by the client may be an important early warning from the body and mind that the person must find a means to adapt or suffer damage. Of course the most significant challenge for the individual is to change his/her perceptions to seek out resources. Without recognizing the connection of psychological distress to social class transitions, the distress may be attributed by the client and psychologist to other sources (e.g., relationships). Chronic distress is linked to physical health problems (Sapolsky 2005) and psychologically, the experience of social class transition without adequate or necessary resources may result in feelings and attitudes of resentment.

11.4 Implications and Conclusion

The Mobility Typology (Liu 2011), focuses on the personal experiences, including the strengths and challenges, of individuals as they experience social class transitions. As demonstrated in the aforementioned case illustrations, positive psychology provides an understanding of the strengths that individuals in each cell possess and how these individuals may construct meaning from their contexts. Those utilizing a positive psychological framework, both within research and practice, could work with individuals to identify available forms of resources that are helpful and assistive of their social class transition. These resources may be social support networks such as their family of origin. Practitioners may work with clients to bridge social support networks between their social class or origin and their new social class context and then overtime, help the client to integrate these networks. Changing the dialogue may help the client move from identifying only stressors and "problems" in their transitions and social class contexts to identifying personal and external strengths that will help them "withstand" the stressors and demands of a new environment. This suggestion is valid for those moving upward as it is for those who have experienced downward transitions too. Identifying personal strengths (e.g., resiliency and adaptability), and helping the individual feel a sense of control (Sapolsky 2005) will have long and far reaching positive outcomes. As research in positive psychology and social class begins to grow it is imperative that researchers remain vigilant about dispelling personal biases and developing an understanding of variables through the lens of each social class.

References

Abelev, M. S. (2009). Advancing out of poverty: Social class worldview and its relation to resilience. *Journal of Adolescent Research, 24*, 114–141. doi:10.1177/0743558408328441.

Adler, N. E., Epel, E. S., Castellazzo, G., & Ickovics, J. R. (2000). Relationship of subjective and objective social status with psychological and physiological functioning: Preliminary data in health white women. *Health Psychology, 19*, 586–592. doi:10.1037/0278-6133.19.6.586.

Aldridge, J. M., Huang, T., & Fraser, B. J. (1999). Investigating classroom environment in Taiwan and Australia with multiple research methods. *Journal of Educational Research, 93*, 48–61. doi:10.1080/00220679909597628.

Banerjee, M. M. (1998). Strengths in a slum: A paradox? *Journal of Applied Social Sciences, 22*(1), 45–58.

Barger, S. D., Donoho, C. J., & Wayment, H. A. (2009). The relative contributions of race/ethnicity, socioeconomic status, health, and social relationships to life satisfaction in the United States. *Quality of Life Research: An International Journal of Quality of Life Aspects of Treatment, Care, & Rehabilitation, 18*, 179–189. doi:10.1007/s11136-008-9426-2.

Bourdieu, P. (1977). *Outline of a theory of practice*. New York: Cambridge University Press.

Bradley, R. H., & Corwyn, R. F. (2002). Socio-economic status and child development. *Annual Review of Psychology, 53*, 371–399. doi:10.1146/annurev.psych.53.100901.135233.

Clauss-Ehlers, C. S. (2008). Sociocultural factors, resilience, and coping: Support or a culturally sensitive measure of resilience. *Journal of Applied Developmental Psychology, 29*, 197–212. doi:10.1016/j.appdev. 2008.02.004.

Diener, E., & Biswas-Diener, R. (2009). Will money increase subjective well-being?: A literature review and guide to needed research. In E. Diener (Ed.), *The science of well-being: The collected works of Ed Diener* (pp. 119–154). New York: Springer.

Diener, E., & Oishi, S. (2000). Money and happiness: Income and subjective well-being across nations. In E. Diener & E. M. Suh (Eds.), *Subjective well-being across cultures* (pp. 185–218). Cambridge, MA: MIT Press.

Ellis, W. T. (2011). Against the odds; Academic resilience among high-ability African American adolescents living in rural poverty. *Dissertation Abstracts International Section A: Humanities and Social Sciences*, 3218.

Gallo, L. C., Bogart, L. M., Vranceanu, A. M., & Matthews, K. M. (2005). Socioeconomic status, resources, psychosocial experiences, and emotional responses: A test of the reserve capacity model. *Journal of Personality and Social Psychology, 88*, 386–399. doi:10.1037/0022-3514.88.2.386.

Gwirayi, P., & Shumba, A. (2007). A preliminary study of the relationship between students' self-concept and academic achievement in Zimbabwe. *Journal of Psychology in Africa, 17*, 119–122.

Israel, N., & Jozefowicz-Simbeni, D. M. H. (2009). Perceived strengths of urban girls and boys experiencing homelessness. *Journal of Community & Applied Social Psychology, 19*, 156–164. doi:10.1002/casp.987.

Iwasaki, Y. (2006). Counteracting stress through leisure coping: A prospective health study. *Psychology, Health & Medicine, 11*, 209–220. doi:10.1080/13548500500155941.
Kamper, G. (2008). A profile of effective leadership in some South African high-poverty schools. *South African Journal of Education, 28*, 1–18.
Lachman, M. E., & Weaver, S. L. (1998). Sociodemographic variations in the sense of control by domain: Findings from the MacArthur studies of midlife. *Psychology and Aging, 13*, 553–562. doi:10.1037/0882-7974.13.4.553.
Lareau, A. (2003). *Unequal childhoods: Class, race, and family life*. Berkeley: University of California Press.
Link, B. G., & Phelan, J. (1995). Social conditions as fundamental causes of disease. *Journal of Health and Social Behavior, 35*, 80–94, Extra Issue: Forty Years of Medical Sociology: The State of the Art and Directions for the Future. Article Stable URL: http://www.jstor.org/stable/2626958.
Liu, W. M. (2011). *Social class and classism in the helping professions: Research, theory, and practice*. Thousand Oaks: Sage.
Liu, W. M., & Ali, S. R. (2005). Addressing social class and classism in vocational theory and practice: Extending the emancipatory communitarian approach. *The Counseling Psychologist, 33*, 189–196. doi:10.1177/0011000004272269.
Liu, W. M., Ali, S. R., Soleck, G., Hopps, J., Dunston, K., & Picket, T. (2004). Using social class in counseling psychology research. *Journal of Counseling Psychology, 51*, 3–18. doi:10.1037/0022-0167.51.1.3.
Liu, W. M., Hernandez, J., Mahmood, A., & Stinson, R. (2006). The link between poverty, classism, and racism in mental health. In D. W. Sue & M. G. Constantine (Eds.), *Racism as a barrier to cultural competence in mental health and educational settings* (pp. 65–86). New York: Wiley.
Liu, W. M., Stinson, R., Hernandez, J., Shepard, S., & Haag, S. (2009). A qualitative examination of masculinity, homelessness, and social class among men in a transitional shelter. *Psychology of Men and Masculinity, 10*, 131–148. doi:10.1037/a0014999.
Lopez, S. J., & Snyder, C. R. (Eds.). (2009). *Oxford handbook of positive psychology* (2nd ed.). New York: Oxford University Press.
Luthar, S. S., Cicchetti, D., & Becker, B. (2000). The construct of resilience: A critical evaluation and guidelines for future work. *Child Development, 71*, 543–562. doi:10.1017/S0954579400004156.
Masten, A. S. (2011). Resilience in children threatened by extreme adversity: Frameworks for research, practice, and translational synergy. *Development and Psychopathology, 23*, 493–506. doi:10.1017/S0954579411000198.
Masten, A. S., & Sesma, A. (1999). Risk and resilience among children homeless in Minneapolis. *CURA Reporter, 29*, 1–6. Retrieved from http://www.cura.umn.edu/sites/cura.advantagelabs.com/files/publications/29-1-Masten-Sesma.pdf
Masten, S., Miliotis, D., Graham- Bermann, S. A., Ramirez, M., & Neemann, J. (1993). Children in homeless families: Risks to mental health and development. *Journal of Consulting and Clinical Psychology, 61*, 335–343. doi:10.1037/0022-006X.61.2.335.
Masten, A. S., Cutuli, J. J., Herbers, J. E., & Reed, M. J. (2009). Resilience in development. In S. J. Lopez & C. R. Snyder (Eds.), *The Oxford handbook of positive psychology* (pp. 117–131). New York: Oxford University Press.
McLoyd, V. C. (1998). Socioeconomic disadvantage and child development. *American Psychologist, 53*, 185–204.
Mendez, J. L., Fantuzzo, J., & Cicchetti, D. (2002). Profiles of social competence among Low income African American preschool children. *Child Development, 73*, 1085–1100.
Mossakowski, K. N. (2008). Dissecting the influence of race, ethnicity, and socioeconomic status on mentalhealthinyoungadulthood. *ResearchonAging, 30*,649–671.doi:10.1177/0164027508322693.
Nelson, M. L., Englar-Carlson, M., Tierney, S., & Hau, J. (2006). Class jumping into academia: Multiple identities for counseling academics. *Journal of Counseling Psychology, 53*, 1–14. doi:10.1037/0022-0167.53.1.1.

Nguyen, C. M., Liu, W. M., Hernandez, J. O., & Stinson, R. (2012). Problem-solving appraisal, gender role conflict, help-seeking behavior and psychological distress among men who are homeless. *Psychology of Men and Masculinity, 13*, 270–282. doi:10.1037/a0025523.

Obradovic, J., Long, J. D., Cutuli, J. J., Chan, C. K., Hinz, E., Heistad, D., et al. (2009). Academic achievement of homeless and highly mobile children in an urban school district: Longitudinal evidence of risk, growth, and resilience. *Development and Psychopathology, 21*, 493–518. doi:10.1017/S0954579409000273.

Ong, A. D., Bergeman, C. S., & Boker, S. M. (2009). Resilience comes of age: Defining features in later adulthood. *Journal of Personality, 77*, 1777–1804. doi:10.1160011/j.1467-6494.2009.x.

Ostrove, J. M., Adler, N. E., Kupperman, M., & Washington, A. E. (2000). Objective and subjective assessments of socioeconomic status and the relationship to self-rated health in an ethnically diverse sample of pregnant women. *Health Psychology, 19*, 613–618. doi:10.1037/0278-6133.19.6.613.

Pierce, I. J. (1994). Importance of classroom climate for at-risk learners. *Journal of Educational Research, 88*, 37–43. doi:10.1080/00220671. 1994.9944832.

Piff, P. K., Kraus, M. W., Côté, S., Cheng, B. H., & Keltner, D. (2010). Having less, giving more: The influence of social class on prosocial behavior. *Journal of Personality and Social Psychology, 99*, 771–784. doi:10.1037/a0020092.

Powers, D. A. (1996). Social background and social context effects on young men's idleness transitions. *Social Science Research, 25*, 50–72. doi:10.1006/ssre. 1996.0003.

Rapp, C. A. (1993). Theory, principles, and methods of the strengths model of case management. In M. Harris & H. C. Bergman (Eds.), *Case management for mentally ill patients: Theory and practice* (pp. 143–164). Langhorne: Harwood Academic Publishers.

Roley, S. E. (2009). Creativity, cultural proficiency and self-efficacy in rural school principals: The relationship to reducing the achievement gap for low-income students. *Dissertation Abstracts International Section A: Humanities and Social Sciences*, 430.

Sanchez, F. J., Liu, W. M., Leathers, L., Goins, J., & Vilain, E. (2011). The subjective experience of social class and upward mobility among African American men in graduate school. *Psychology of Men and Masculinity, 12*, 368–382. doi:10.1037/a0024057.

Sapolsky, R. (2005). Sick of poverty. *Scientific American, 293*, 92–99.

Schor, J. B. (2000). *Do Americans shop too much?* Boston: Beacon.

Schor, J. B. (2004). *Born to buy: The commercialized child and the new consumer culture*. New York: Scribner.

Shumba, A. (2010). Resilience in children of poverty. *Journal of Psychology in Africa, 20*, 211–214.

Simonton, D. K. (2009). Creativity. In S. J. Lopez (Ed.), *The Oxford handbook of positive psychology* (pp. 261–269). New York: Oxford University Press.

Slavin, R. E. (1998). *Show me the evidence: Proven and promising programs for America's schools*. New York: Corwin.

Snyder, C. R., Lopez, S. J., & Pedrotti, J. T. (2011). *Positive psychology: The scientific and practical exploration of human strengths*. Thousand Oaks: Sage.

Starfield, B., Riley, A. W., Witt, W. P., & Robertson, J. (2002). Social class gradients in health during adolescence. *Journal of Epidemiology and Community Health, 56*, 354–361. doi:10.1136/jech.56.5.354.

Strauss, M. A. (1968). Communication, creativity, and problem-solving ability of middle-and working-class families in three societies. *The American Journal of Sociology, 73*, 417–430.

Zhang, L. F., & Postiglione, G. A. (2001). Thinking styles, self-esteem, and socio-economic status. *Personality and Individual Differences, 31*, 1333–1346. doi:10.1016/S0191-8869(00)00227-0.

Zinn, H. (1991). *Declarations of independence: Cross-examining American ideology*. New York: Harper Collins.

Chapter 12
Disability and Positive Psychology

Michael L. Wehmeyer and Karrie A. Shogren

Positive psychology refers the pursuit of understanding optimal human functioning and well-being. Disability is, alternatively, typically understood to refer to deficient human functioning. As such, disability and positive psychology would seem to be incompatible constructs; optimal human functioning versus deficient human functioning. In this chapter, we frame disability in a modern paradigm within typical human functioning that obviates the apparent incompatibility of disability and positive psychology and discuss the emerging body of literature on positive psychology and disability.

12.1 Disability

Historically, *disability* was understood as an extension of a medical model that conceived health as an *interiorized state* of functioning and health problems as an individual pathology; as a problem *within* the person (Wehmeyer et al. 2008). Within such a context, disability was understood to be medical in nature and a characteristic of a person. By the late 1970s, it became evident that individual pathology models offered a far too narrow perspective for describing, understanding, and addressing the lives of people affected by a chronic or pervasive health condition, including disability. In 1980, the World Health Organization (WHO) introduced a multidimensional model of human functioning, called the *International Classification of Impairments, Disabilities, and Handicaps (ICIDH)*, that proposed different

---

M.L. Wehmeyer, Ph.D. (✉) • K.A. Shogren
Kansas University Center on Developmental Disabilities, University of Kansas,
1200 Sunnyside Avenue, Room 3136, Lawrence, KS 66045, USA
e-mail: wehmeyer@ku.edu; shogren@ku.edu

J. Teramoto Pedrotti and L.M. Edwards (eds.), *Perspectives on the Intersection of Multiculturalism and Positive Psychology*, Cross-Cultural Advancements in Positive Psychology 7, DOI 10.1007/978-94-017-8654-6_12,

perspectives for looking at human functioning and for describing the consequences of diseases. The ICIDH perspective for describing the impact of a health condition or pathology on human functioning were: (a) the *exteriorization of a pathology* in body anatomy and functions; (b) *objectified pathology* as expressed in the person's activities (e.g. adaptive behavior skills), and (c) the *social consequences of pathology* (e.g. participation in social life domains; WHO 1980).

Subsequent versions of the WHO systems, most recently the *International Classification of Functioning, Disability, and Health* (*ICF*; WHO 2001), emphasized the impact of contextual and environmental factors on health status. They recognized that limitations in human functioning are not necessarily linear or causal consequences of pathology, but that human functioning should be conceived as multiple interactive processes where each factor can influence each dimension of functioning and each other factor either directly or indirectly.

Within the ICF (WHO 2001), disability is understood in the context of typical human functioning. Human functioning is an umbrella term encompassing all body functions, activities, and participation. *Body functions* refer to the physiological functions of body systems, including psychological functions. *Body structures* refer to anatomical parts of the body, such as organs, limbs, and their components. *Activities* refer to the execution of a task or action by an individual. *Participation* is involvement in life situations (WHO 2001). Disability, within the ICF (WHO 2001) system, serves as an umbrella term for limitations in human functioning involving impairments, activity limitations, or participation restrictions. *Impairments* are problems in body function or body structure, such as significant deviation or loss. *Activity limitations* are difficulties an individual may have in executing activities. *Participation restrictions* are problems an individual may experience in involvement in life situations (WHO 2001).

The importance of this shift in understanding disability from an interiorized state in which the disability resides within or is a characteristic of the person, to an exteriorized state (conceptualized as limitations in typical activities and participation impacted by contextual factors), is significant. The WHO (2001) ICF model and other similar models of disability are referred to as "functional" models. This is both because of their grounding in typical human functioning, and because they draw from social-ecological models that look at human behavior as a function of the fit or interaction between the person and his or her capacities and the demands of the environment or context (Wehmeyer et al. 2008).

The benefits of conceptualizing disability within a person-environment fit/interaction model are manifold, the first being that the locus of the intervention within this approach is distributed between enhancing the capacity of the person and changing the expectations or characteristics of the environment or context. Further, such models are strengths-based, emphasizing a person's capacities and abilities, as opposed to the historic emphasis on incapacity and defect. The ICF (WHO 2001) classification is one in which disability is manifested as a state of functioning that exists only within the fit between the person's capacities and the context in which the person functions. Finally, these person-environment engagement models emphasize the development of individualized supports to both increase personal capacity and provide accommodations for or modifications to the environment or context, and move away from creating static "programs" for service delivery that are based primarily on levels or types of disabilities (Schalock et al. 2010).

It is within this relatively new way of conceptualizing disability that nascent efforts to examine issues of positive psychology and disability have emerged. Because disability is understood in the context of typical human functioning within such conceptualizations, positive psychology's intent to understand optimal human functioning becomes increasingly relevant to understanding how to enable people with disabilities to enhance their functioning and quality of life. It is important to note, as well, that this is still an emerging area within disability research. Shogren et al. (2007) analyzed 30 years (1975–2004) of peer-reviewed articles from journals in the field of intellectual disability to identify the degree to which research focused on the capacities and strengths of people with intellectual disability. In the earliest decade, only 20 % of published articles had a strengths focus, climbing to just over 30 % during the second decade, and peaking at 50 % during the 10 years between 1995 and 2004. Thus half of the published research articles in the most recent decade surveyed were still deficits-focused, suggesting that research in positive psychology and disability is still emerging.

12.2 Disability and Diversity

The experience of a disability is a source of diversity in the lives of people in and of itself. Like other areas of diversity, the experience of having a disability co-occurs with other factors, such as gender, race, or ethnicity. We know little about the impact of these co-occurring experiences, other than to suggest that the presence of a disability often exacerbates issues of prejudice and discrimination experienced by such other factors (Rousso and Wehmeyer 2001). There is, as Rousso and Wehmeyer argued, a double jeopardy associated with the co-occurrence of disability and gender, race, or ethnicity that uniquely impacts someone experiencing both.

In the area, for example, of gender and disability issues, research shows that girls and young women with disability achieve less positive adult-related outcomes than do their male peers with disability (Rousso and Wehmeyer 2001). This is most evident in the area of employment. Doren and Benz (2001) reviewed the literature pertaining to gender and employment outcomes, finding that:

- Women with disabilities are less likely to be employed than women without disabilities or men with and without disabilities. The magnitude of the differences in the studies reviewed ranged from 4 to 60 %, and over half the studies reported at least a 20–30 % lower employment rate for women with disabilities.
- Women with disabilities earn substantially less than men with disabilities, and the wage gap between women and men with disabilities increases as the time since exiting high school increases. Studies have shown that young women with disabilities earn up to 78 % less than young men with disabilities within the first 2 years after high school.

- Women with disabilities are more likely than men with disabilities to be found that women with disabilities were overrepresented in lower-skill occupations and underrepresented in higher-skill jobs.
- Women with disabilities are less likely to be engaged in full-time employment than their male peers. Studies reviewed found that, on average, women with disabilities were 11–49 % less likely than men with disabilities to be engaged in full-time employment (Doren and Benz 2001).

To further complicate the matter, there is a reciprocal relationship among gender, disability, and several other factors impacting equity in education, including socioeconomic status and poverty level, as well as race and ethnicity. For example, there is a reciprocal relationship between poverty and disability. Poverty can cause disability, particularly in women and girls, who in the face of limited resources are more likely than their male counterparts to be deprived of basic necessities, such as food and medicine (Groce 1997). Disability, in turn, can contribute to poverty, because of the additional expenses that it can entail or its impact on employment.

Third, around the globe, on every measure of educational, vocational, financial and social success, women and girls with disabilities fare less well than their non-disabled female or disabled male counterparts (Rousso and Wehmeyer 2001). Women with disabilities are often viewed as sick, childlike, dependent, asexual, or incompetent, and their talents and assets are overlooked (Asch et al. 2001).

Fourth, race and ethnicity can also be a compounding factor. In the U.S., for example, there are a disproportionate number of African American students receiving special education services, reflecting, in part, the intersection of race and disability bias, and thus affecting educational equity. A report from the U.S. Department of Education's Office of Special Education Programs showed that African-American students were over-represented in 9 of 13 disability categories, but particularly in the category of intellectual disability, in which African-American students represent more than twice the national population estimates (OSEP 2000).

Further, any discussion about disability and diversity issues must acknowledge that, fundamentally, there is no such thing as a unitary "disability identity." Indeed, it is difficult to generalize almost anything as applying to the group referred to as "people with disabilities" due in part to the sheer number of people in this category. According to a U.S. Census Bureau report (2010), there are 54 million people in the United States with disabilities, a large and diverse group in and of itself. Some of these people are born with a disability, and their identity emerges with that as part of how they think about themselves and how others think about them. Others experience injuries or are identified later in childhood or adolescence and must therefore accommodate this new aspect of themselves into their still forming identities (Wehmeyer 2008). Some disabilities are "hidden" and known only by the people who have them and those close to them, while others are openly discernible. Some disabilities impact cognitive development and performance, while others do not.

Not surprisingly, then, differences among and between people with disabilities are often as notable as differences between people with and without disabilities. Looking, once again, at data related to post-school outcomes for young adults with disabilities, there are stark differences as a function of type of disability. More than half of young people with impairments such as speech language (SLI), hearing (HI), visual (VI), orthopedic (OI), and other health impairments (OHI) including attention deficit and hyperactivity disorder, attend some postsecondary institution (Newman et al. 2009a). Slightly fewer than half of students with learning disabilities (47 %) attend postsecondary education. Youth with intellectual disability (ID) and EBD are also among the least likely to enroll in 4-year colleges (Newman et al. 2009a). Similar discrepancies exist when examining employment outcomes, independent living outcomes, and so forth.

12.3 Disability and Positive Psychology

Before reviewing the literature on positive psychology and disability, we would make one more observation. We have noted the complexities associated with the experience of disability. We have also acknowledged that within the disability literature, a positive psychological approach is still an emerging focus. We would also note, however, that the disability presence in the positive psychological literature must be characterized as limited. Recently, Shogren (2012) reviewed abstracts of articles published in *The Journal of Positive Psychology* since its inception in 2006 (through Volume 6, Issue 2) to determine the extent to which articles focused on any aspect of disability. Shogren determined that only 4 % of articles published in this journal over the past 5 years explicitly mentioned people with disabilities or people with health related issues associated with disability. It is fair to say that disability, as a construct, is not well integrated into the field of positive psychology.

12.3.1 Disability and Specific Positive Psychological Constructs

This section provides a brief summary of the limited research pertaining to disability and affective, cognitive, and interpersonal positive psychological constructs. It should be noted that there is no compelling reason to hypothesize that, in general, issues pertaining to affective, cognitive, or interpersonal positive psychological constructs differ among people with disabilities when compared to people without disabilities. What likely varies will be the type and frequency of interventions that are needed to promote optimal human functioning.

12.3.1.1 Affective Constructs

Among affective constructs, the *quality of life* concept has been most extensively applied to and studied in the field of disability, principally to provide a framework for organizations supporting people with disabilities in ways that promote optimal human functioning and life satisfaction. Schalock and colleagues (Brown et al. 2009) have defined quality of life as a multidimensional construct influenced by personal characteristics and environmental factors (as per a person-environment fit/interaction model) composed of a set of core dimensions, which include personal development, self-determination, interpersonal relations, social inclusion, rights, emotional well-being, physical well-being, and material well-being (Schalock and Verdugo 2012).

The application of the quality of life construct in disability research is best understood in disability contexts with reference to outcomes at a systemic or group level, and not at an individual level (Bramston et al. 2005). The majority of research articles in the field describe changes in quality of life dimensions (well-being, self-determination, etc.) as a function of organizational or service changes or structure. Measurement of quality of life remains a relatively contentious issue in the field, in part because of difficulties experienced by some people with disabilities in reliably completing self-report measures and, in light of this, bringing into question the validity of proxy measures of quality of life (e.g., using parents or staff to determine an individual's responses to a quality of life measure; Schalock et al. 2002).

There are limited comparative data examining differences in these domains between people with disability and their non-disabled peers. In addition, most such comparative studies examine differences among and between domains as a function of context or supports provided or among and between people with different disability types or behavioral issues (Beadle-Brown et al. 2009). Those studies that compare quality of life issues between people with and without disabilities generally find lower quality of life indicators for people with disabilities (Schalock and Verdugo 2012).

At the individual level, a limited number of studies examine relationships among positive psychological constructs and quality of life. For example, Smedema et al. (2010) examined relationships among coping variables and quality of life, as conceptualized by measures of life satisfaction and subjective well-being, for people with spinal cord injuries. Positive coping strategies (hope, proactive coping style, sense of humor) were positively associated with subjective well-being and positive self-worth. Shogren et al. (2007) conducted a study of positive psychological constructs that predict life satisfaction in adolescents with and without cognitive disabilities in which hope and optimism predicted life satisfaction for both groups (with and without disability). Engagement in meaningful work and the provision of workplace accommodations to support employment were positively related to life satisfaction for people with disabilities (Moore et al. 2011). Moore and colleagues also determined that factors differed in predicting life satisfaction as a function of whether the disability was of childhood onset or adult onset. Age predicted enhanced life satisfaction for people with adult-onset disabilities, but not for workers with childhood-onset disabilities, and the role of workplace accommodations on life satisfaction varied according to onset.

Other "life circumstances" (in addition to employment) are linked to life satisfaction and quality of life for people with disabilities. Miller and Chan (2008) determined that social supports and interpersonal skills predicated life satisfaction for people with intellectual disability. At the systemic level, research has linked such environmental factors as community integration, residence type and size, and choice making opportunities as predictive of better quality of life and well-being (Heller et al. 2002). O'Brien et al. (2001) documented that movement from living in a large congregate setting to one's community improved life satisfaction and quality of life, a finding that is consistent in the literature.

12.3.1.2 Cognitive Constructs

Among cognitive constructs, self-efficacy has been most frequently studied among people with disabilities. Most of the literature in the field has focused on changing self-efficacy and efficacy-expectations through environmental or instructional modifications (Schunk 1989). Further, there is evidence that the experience of disability, or more accurately the stigma associated with disability, actually influences self-efficacy beliefs, which mediate other outcomes. Jodrell (2010) studied social identity (e.g., self-concept derived from perceived membership in social groups) and self-efficacy for college students with dyslexia, and found that self-efficacy was influenced by the student's social identity.

In general, the limited research suggests that youth and adults with disabilities have lower self-efficacy and outcome expectations, but opportunity and interventions can enhance self-efficacy and outcome expectations. Wehmeyer (1994) found that youth with intellectual disability held less adaptive attributions of efficacy and expectancy than did non-disabled peers and that such attributions became less adaptive as the student got older, a trend not consistent with typical developmental functions for these attributes. Hall and Webster (2008) studied the self-efficacy of college students with learning disabilities and determined that self-efficacy in regard to coursework was significantly lower than for their non-disabled peers.

There are only a few studies examining the role of hope in the lives of people with disability. Smedema et al. (2010) and Shogren et al. (2006), determined that hope was a predictor of life satisfaction for people with spinal cord injuries and intellectual disability, respectively. Hammond (2004) found that hope was one of several psychosocial qualities (including self-esteem, self-efficacy, a sense of purpose, and social integration) that mediated protection against and recovery from mental health difficulties and the progression of chronic illness or disability.

Rand and Shea (2012) conducted a review of the literature pertaining to optimism and disability, and concluded that, in general, findings are consistent with the general literature in optimism, showing that optimism is an effective strategy for dealing with stress and adversity, is an effective coping strategy, and facilitates goal oriented action. Shogren et al. (2006) found that optimism and hope were the strongest predictors of life satisfaction for people with cognitive disabilities. Gruber-Baldini et al. (2009) associated optimism with improved quality of life for people with Parkinson's disease, and Dunn (1996) found that optimism contributed to fewer depressive symptoms and greater perceived control for people who had lost limbs due to amputation. Rand and Shea documented a number of studies, across various traumatic episodes resulting in functional loss and disability, from spinal cord injury to traumatic brain injury, in which higher levels of optimism mediated or mitigated better psychological functioning, including diminished experiences of posttraumatic stress, anxiety, and depression. Research with people with arthritis also documents the positive effects of optimism on better psychological well-being (Luger et al. 2009).

12.3.1.3 Interpersonal Constructs

People with disabilities often report high levels of social isolation and limited friendships, although this ranges across types of disability (Turnbull et al. 2013). Such social isolation can be a function of difficulties with social skills, issues of mobility or access, the disproportionate experience of segregation, and/or the general public's response to disability. There is a substantial literature base, albeit much of this not empirical, documenting the negative consequences, for example, of educating students with disabilities in segregated classrooms on friendship development, or the lack thereof (Janney and Snell 2006). Newman et al. (2009b) reported findings from a comprehensive longitudinal study of post-high school outcome of students with disabilities, and found that the percentage of young adults who saw friends outside of school or work at least weekly ranged from highs of 84.4 % (speech/language impairment), 82.5 % (learning disability) and 80 % (other health impairments) to lows of 48.2 % (autism), 52.8 % (multiple disabilities), 58.1 % (intellectual disability) and 62.3 (deaf/blindness).

There are only a few studies attempting to parcel out contributors to, for example, happiness of people with disabilities. Marini and Glover-Graf (2011) found that religiosity and spirituality among people with spinal cord injury contributed to greater happiness. Yu et al. (2002) found that people with severe cognitive and multiple disabilities showed more indicators of happiness during leisure activities than during other times.

12.3.1.4 Self-Determination

Promoting self-determination has become a best practice in the education of students with disabilities and in supporting adults with disabilities (Wehmeyer et al. 2003, 2007). Self-determination refers to self- (vs. other-) caused action—to people acting volitionally, based on their own will. Volition is the capability of conscious choice, decision, and intention. Self-determined behavior is defined as "volitional actions that enable one to act as the primary causal agent in one's life and to maintain or improve one's quality of life" (Wehmeyer 2005, p. 117). *Causal agency* implies that it is the individual who makes or causes things to happen in his or her life and that the individual acts with an eye toward causing *an effect* to *accomplish* a *specific end* or to *cause* or *create change*.

Wehmeyer and colleagues (Wehmeyer et al. 2003, 2007) proposed a *functional model of self-determination* in which self-determination is conceptualized as a dispositional characteristic (enduring tendencies used to characterize and describe differences between people) based on the *function* a behavior serves for an individual. Self-determination is a general psychological construct within the organizing structure of theories of human agency which refers to self- (vs. other-) caused action—to people acting volitionally, based on their own will. Human agency refers to the sense of personal empowerment involving both knowing and having what it takes to achieve goals. Human agentic theories share the meta-theoretical view that organismic aspirations drive human behaviors.

Self-determination emerges across the lifespan as children and adolescents learn skills and develop attitudes and beliefs that enable them to be causal agents in their lives. These are the *component elements* of self-determined behavior, and include choice making, problem solving, decision making, goal setting and attainment, self-advocacy, and self-management skills.

Abery and colleagues (Abery and Stancliffe 1996; Stancliffe et al. 2000) proposed an *ecological model of self-determination* that defines the self-determination construct as "a complex process, the ultimate goal of which is to achieve the level of personal control over one's life that an individual desires within those areas the individual perceives as important" (p. 27). The ecological model views self-determination as driven by the intrinsic motivation of all people to be the primary determiner of their thoughts, feelings, and behavior. Self-determination, accordingly, is the product of both the person and the environment—of the person using the skills, knowledge, and beliefs at his/her disposal to act on the environment with the goal of obtaining valued and desired outcomes. The ecological model within which people develop and lead their lives is viewed as consisting of four levels: the *microsystem*, *mesosystem*, *exosystem*, and *macrosystem* (See Wehmeyer et al. 2003 for more detail).

Research in the contexts of these models has documented that if provided instruction to promote self-determination, students with disabilities can acquire knowledge and skills pertaining to this construct and its component elements (Algozzine et al. 2001; Cobb et al. 2009). Also, self-determination status has been linked to the attainment of more positive academic (Konrad et al. 2007; Lee et al. 2010), adult (e.g., employment, independent living; Wehmeyer and Palmer 2003; Wehmeyer and Schwartz 1997), and quality of life and life satisfaction (Lachapelle et al. 2005; Nota et al. 2007; Shogren et al. 2006; Wehmeyer and Schwartz 1998) outcomes for people with disabilities.

Interventions in disability supports have focused on enabling youth and adults to self-regulate learning, using self-directed learning strategies (discussed in greater detail subsequently), to set and attain goals, to solve problems, to make choices, and to advocate for one's own needs. The *Self-Determined Learning Model of Instruction* (SDLMI; Wehmeyer et al. 2007) is an example of this type of intervention research. The SDLMI is a model of teaching based on the component elements of self-determination, the process of self-regulated problem solving, and research on student-directed learning. Teachers use the model to teach students to self-regulate problem solving, leading to student's setting educational goals, creating action plans to achieve those goals, and monitoring and evaluating their progress toward those goals, modifying their plan or goal as needed. There are more than a dozen studies investigating the efficacy of the SDLMI (see Wehmeyer et al. 2007).

12.3.2 *Positive Psychology and Disability Supports*

Although the research pertaining to disability and positive psychological is limited, there are a number of best practices in disability that embody the principles of positive psychology.

12.3.2.1 Positive Behavior Supports

Positive Behavior Supports (PBS) is a systems-level and evidence-based method for improving valued social and learning outcomes for all students, including students with disabilities. It is proactive, problem-solving-oriented, and data-based; it elicits appropriate behavior and contributes to academic, social, and communication outcomes throughout a school building (Dunlap et al. 2010; Janney and Snell 2008). PBS is based on values and principles in positive psychology because it emphasizes individual strengths, reducing problem behavior by teaching alternatives, addressing issues in the environment or context, and emphasizes student involvement and choice.

Because problem behavior often results from someone else's failure to provide individualized and comprehensive support (Janney and Snell 2008), positive behavior support seeks to tailor students' environments to their preferences, strengths, and needs. It rearranges school environments and changes school systems to discourage students [with disabilities, all students] from engaging in problem behaviors in the first place.

12.3.2.2 Self-Regulated Learning

The application of self-regulated learning has been studied extensively with students with disabilities (Schunk and Bursuck 2012; Schunk and Zimmerman 2008). Among the most commonly used strategies are picture cues and antecedent cue regulation strategies, self-instruction, self-monitoring, self-evaluation and self-reinforcement. Schunk and Bursuck (2012) noted that there is strong evidence, across disability types and tasks, for the efficacy of these interventions. Harris, Graham and colleagues (Harris et al. 2006) have evaluated, for example, the Self-Regulated Strategy Development (SRSD) intervention to teach students with learning disabilities academic content skills, particularly reading, writing, and mathematics. Wehmeyer and colleagues (2003) provided evidence of the efficacy of teaching self-regulated problem solving strategies to enable students with disabilities to achieve academic and functional goals, as discussed in the section on self-determination.

12.3.2.3 Supported Employment

Supported employment refers to a compilation of practices that support people with disabilities to work in typical work environments with their non-disabled peers (Wehman et al. 2012). The core values of supported employment draw from principles of positive psychology; that people have strengths that enable them to contribute to meaningful work, that environments can be modified to enable people with disabilities to be successful in real jobs with their non-disabled peers, and that such experiences enhance inclusion and individual perceptions of value and worth. There is now three decades worth of research establishing that supported employment strategies can enable people with even the most significant disabilities to engage in meaningful work (Wehman et al. 2012).

12.4 Conclusion

The knowledge base with regard to people with disability and positive psychology can best be described as emerging at this point. Historic ways of understanding disability in terms of deficit and disease have hindered progress in research and practice in positive psychology for this population. In addition, viewing those with disabilities as a homogenous populations, as opposed to recognizing the dynamic interplay between disability and other personal and cultural facets has limited understanding of this population. Nevertheless, there is a growing emphasis, particularly in providing disability supports but also in research, on promoting optimal human functioning for people with disability. Changing understandings of disability are facilitating this shift. There is no reason to believe that people with disability are, substantially, any different from anyone else with regard to the potential for a focus on positive attributes to benefit their lives, and research and practice should, and likely will, pursue such avenues aggressively.

References

Abery, B. H., & Stancliffe, R. J. (1996). The ecology of self-determination. In D. J. Sands & M. L. Wehmeyer (Eds.), *Self-determination across the life span: Independence and choice for people with disabilities* (pp. 111–145). Baltimore: Paul H. Brookes.

Algozzine, B., Browder, D., Karvonen, M., Test, D. W., & Wood, W. M. (2001). Effects of interventions to promote self-determination for individuals with disabilities. *Review of Educational Research, 71*, 219–277.

Asch, A., Rousso, H., & Jeffries, T. (2001). Beyond pedestals: The lives of girls and women with disabilities. In H. Rousso & M. L. Wehmeyer (Eds.), *Double jeopardy: Addressing gender equity in special education* (pp. 13–48). Albany: SUNY Press.
Beadle-Brown, J., Murphy, G., & DiTerlizzi, M. (2009). Quality of life for the Camberwell cohort. *Journal of Applied Research in Intellectual Disabilities, 22*, 380–390.
Bramston, P., Chipuer, H., & Pretty, G. (2005). Conceptual principles of quality of life: An empirical exploration. *Journal of Intellectual Disability Research, 49*, 728–733.
Brown, R. I., Schalock, R. L., & Brown, I. (2009). Quality of life: Its application to persons with intellectual disabilities and their families—introduction and overview. *Journal of Policy and Practice in Intellectual Disabilities, 6*, 2–6.
Cobb, B., Lehmann, J., Newman-Gonchar, R., & Alwell, A. (2009). Self-determination for students with disabilities: A narrative metasynthesis. *Career Development for Exceptional Individuals, 32*, 108–114.
Doren, B., & Benz, M. (2001). Gender equity issues in the vocational and transition services and employment outcomes experienced by young women with disabilities. In H. Rousso & M. Wehmeyer (Eds.), *Double jeopardy: Addressing gender equity in special education* (pp. 289–312). Albany: State University of New York Press.
Dunlap, G., Iovannone, R., Kincaid, D., Wilson, K., Christiansen, K., Strain, P., et al. (2010). *Prevent-Teach-Reinforce: The school-based model of individualized positive behavior support*. Baltimore: Paul H. Brookes.
Dunn, D. S. (1996). Well-being following amputation: Salutary effects of positive meaning, optimism, and control. *Rehabilitation Psychology, 41*, 285–302.
Groce, N. (1997). Women with disabilities in the developing world. *Journal of Disability Policy Studies, 8*, 178–192.
Gruber-Baldini, A. L., Ye, J., Anderson, K. E., & Shulman, L. M. (2009). Effects of optimism/pessimism and locus of control on disability and quality of life in Parkinson's disease. *Parkinsonism & Related Disorders, 15*, 665–669.
Hall, C. W., & Webster, R. E. (2008). Metacognitive and affective factors of college students with and without learning disabilities. *Journal of Postsecondary Education and Disability, 2*, 32–41.
Hammond, C. (2004). Impacts of lifelong learning on emotional resilience, psychological and mental health: Fieldwork evidence. *Oxford Review of Education, 30*(4), 551–568.
Harris, K. R., Graham, S., & Mason, L. H. (2006). Improving the writing, knowledge, and motivation of struggling young writers: Effects of self-regulated strategy development with and without peer support. *American Educational Research Journal, 43*, 295–340.
Heller, T., Miller, A. B., & Hsieh, K. (2002). Eight-year follow-up of the impact of environmental characteristics on well-being of adults with developmental disabilities. *Mental Retardation, 40*, 366–378.
Janney, R., & Snell, M. E. (2006). *Social relationships and peer support*. Baltimore: Paul H. Brookes Publishing Co.
Janney, R., & Snell, M. E. (2008). *Behavioral support*. Baltimore: Paul H. Brookes Publishing Co.
Jodrell, D. (2010). Social-identity and self-efficacy concern for disability labels. *Psychology Teaching Review, 16*, 111–121.
Konrad, M., Fowler, C. H., Walker, A. R., Test, D. W., & Wood, W. M. (2007). Effects of self-determination interventions on the academic skills of students with learning disabilities. *Learning Disabilities Quarterly, 30*, 89–113.
Lachapelle, Y., Wehmeyer, M. L., Haelewyck, M. C., Courbois, Y., Keith, K. D., & Schalock, R. (2005). The relationship between quality of life and self-determination: An international study. *Journal of Intellectual Disability Research, 49*, 740–744.
Lee, S. H., Wehmeyer, M. L., Soukup, J. H., & Palmer, S. B. (2010). Impact of curriculum modifications on access to the general education curriculum for students with disabilities. *Exceptional Children, 76*, 213–233.
Luger, T., Cotter, K. A., & Sherman, A. M. (2009). It's all in how you view it: Pessimism, social relations, and life satisfaction in older adults with osteoarthritis. *Aging & Mental Health, 13*, 635–647.

Marini, I., & Glover-Graf, N. M. (2011). Religiosity and spirituality among persons with spinal cord injury: Attitudes, beliefs, and practices. *Rehabilitation Counseling Bulletin, 54*, 82–92.

Miller, S. M., & Chan, F. (2008). Predictors of life satisfaction in individuals with intellectual disabilities. *Journal of Intellectual Disability Research, 52*, 1039–1047.

Moore, M. E., Konrad, A. M., Yang, Y., Ng, E. S. W., & Doherty, A. J. (2011). The vocational well-being of workers with childhood onset of disability: Life satisfaction and perceived workplace discrimination. *Journal of Vocational Behavior, 79*, 681–698.

Newman, L., Wagner, M., Cameto, R., & Knokey, A. M. (2009a). *The post-high school outcomes of youth with disabilities up to 4 years after high school: A report from the National Longitudinal Transition Study-2 (NLTS2)*. Menlo Park: SRI International.

Newman, L., Wagner, M., Knokey, A. M., Marder, C., Nasgle, K., Shaver, D., et al. (2009b). *The post-high school outcomes of young adults with disabilities up to 8 years after high school: A report from the National Longitudinal Transition Study-2 (NLTS2)*. Menlo Park: SRI International.

Nota, L., Ferrrari, L., Soresi, S., & Wehmeyer, M. L. (2007). Self-determination, social abilities, and the quality of life of people with intellectual disabilities. *Journal of Intellectual Disability Research, 51*, 850–865.

O'Brien, P., Thesing, A., Tuck, B., & Capie, A. (2001). Perceptions of change, advantage and quality of life for people with intellectual disability who left a long stay institution to live in the community. *Journal of Intellectual and Developmental Disability, 26*, 67–82.

Office of Special Education Programs. (2000). *Twenty-second annual report to Congress on the implementation of the individuals with Disabilities Education Act*. Washington, DC: Federal Printing Office.

Rand, K. L., & Shea, A. M. (2012). Optimism within the context of disability. In M. Wehmeyer (Ed.), *Handbook of positive psychology and disability* (pp. 48–59). Oxford, UK: Oxford University Press.

Rousso, H., & Wehmeyer, M. L. (Eds.). (2001). *Double jeopardy: Addressing gender equity in special education*. Albany: State University of New York Press.

Schalock, R. L., & Verdugo, M. A. (2012). The impact of the quality of life concept on the field of intellectual disability. In M. L. Wehmeyer (Ed.), *Handbook of positive psychology and disability* (pp. 37–47). Oxford, UK: Oxford University Press.

Schalock, R. L., Brown, I., Brown, R., Cummins, R. A., Felce, D., Matikka, L., et al. (2002). Conceptualization, measurement, and application of quality of life for persons with intellectual disabilities: Report of an international panel of experts. *Mental Retardation, 40*, 157–170.

Schalock, R., Borthwick-Duffy, S., Bradley, V., Buntinx, W., Coulter, D., Craig, E., et al. (2010). *Intellectual disability: Definition, classification, and systems of support* (11th ed.). Washington, DC: American Association on Intellectual and Developmental Disabilities.

Schunk, D. H. (1989). Self-efficacy and cognitive achievement: Implications for students with learning problems. *Journal of Learning Disabilities, 22*, 14–22.

Schunk, D. H., & Bursuck, W. (2012). Self-regulation and disability. In M. Wehmeyer (Ed.), *Handbook of positive psychology and disability* (pp. 265–278). Oxford, UK: Oxford University Press.

Schunk, D. H., & Zimmerman, B. J. (Eds.). (2008). *Motivation and self-regulated learning: Theory, research, and applications*. New York: Taylor & Francis.

Shogren, K. (2012). Positive psychology and disability: A historical analysis. In M. Wehmeyer (Ed.), *Handbook of positive psychology and disability* (pp. 19–35). Oxford, UK: Oxford University Press.

Shogren, K. A., Lopez, S. J., Wehmeyer, M. L., Little, T. D., & Pressgrove, C. L. (2006). The role of positive psychology constructs in predicting life satisfaction in adolescents with and without cognitive disabilities: An exploratory study. *The Journal of Positive Psychology, 1*, 37–52.

Shogren, K. A., Wehmeyer, M. L., Pressgrove, C. L., & Lopez, S. J. (2007). The application of positive psychology and self-determination to research in intellectual disability: A content analysis of 30 years of literature. *Research and Practice for Persons with Severe Disabilities, 31*, 338–345.

Smedema, S. M., Catalano, D., & Ebener, D. J. (2010). The relationship of coping, self-worth, and subjective well-being: A structural equation model. *Rehabilitation Counseling Bulletin, 53*, 131–142.

Stancliffe, R. J., Abery, B. H., & Smith, J. (2000). Personal control and the ecology of community living settings: Beyond living-unit size and type. *American Journal on Mental Retardation, 105*, 431–454.

Turnbull, A., Turnbull, H. R., Wehmeyer, M., & Shogren, K. (2013). *Exceptional lives: Special education in today's schools* (7th ed.). Upper Saddle River: Merrill/Prentice Hall.

U.S. Census Bureau. (2010). *Profile America: Facts for features*. Washington, DC: U.S. Printing Office. Accessed online July 6, 2012 at http://www.census.gov/newsroom/releases/archives/facts_for_features_special_editions/cb10-ff13.html

Wehman, P., Brookes, V., Lau, S., & Targett, P. (2012). Supported employment. In M. Wehmeyer (Ed.), *Handbook of positive psychology and disability* (pp. 338–364). Oxford, UK: Oxford University Press.

Wehmeyer, M. L. (1994). Perceptions of self-determination and psychological empowerment of adolescents with mental retardation. *Education and Training in Mental Retardation and Developmental Disabilities, 29*, 9–21.

Wehmeyer, M. L. (2005). Self-determination and individuals with severe disabilities: Reexamining meanings and misinterpretations. *Research and Practice for Persons with Severe Disabilities, 30*, 113–120.

Wehmeyer, M. L. (2008). The impact of disability on adolescent identity. In M. Sadowski (Ed.), *Adolescents at school: Perspectives on youth, identity, and education* (2nd ed., pp. 167–184). Cambridge, MA: Harvard Education Press.

Wehmeyer, M. L., & Palmer, S. B. (2003). Adult outcomes from students with cognitive disabilities three years after high school: The impact of self-determination. *Education and Training in Developmental Disabilities, 38*, 131–144.

Wehmeyer, M. L., & Schwartz, M. (1997). Self-determination and positive adult outcomes: A follow up study of youth with mental retardation or learning disabilities. *Exceptional Children, 63*, 245–255.

Wehmeyer, M. L., & Schwartz, M. (1998). The relationship between self-determination and quality of life for adults with mental retardation. *Education and Training in Mental Retardation and Developmental Disabilities, 33*, 3–12.

Wehmeyer, M. L., Abery, B., Mithaug, D. E., & Stancliffe, R. J. (2003). *Theory in self-determination: Foundations for educational practice*. Springfield: Charles C Thomas Publisher, LTD.

Wehmeyer, M. L., Agran, M., Hughes, C., Martin, J., Mithaug, D. E., & Palmer, S. (2007). *Promoting self-determination in students with intellectual and developmental disabilities*. New York: Guilford Press.

Wehmeyer, M. L., Buntinx, W. E., Lachapelle, Y., Luckasson, R., Schalock, R., Verdugo-Alonzo, M., et al. (2008). The intellectual disability construct and its relationship to human functioning. *Intellectual and Developmental Disabilities, 46*, 311–318.

World Health Organization. (1980). *International classification of impairments, disabilities, and handicaps. A manual of classification relating to the consequences of disease*. Geneva: Author.

World Health Organization. (2001). *International classification of functioning, disability, and health (ICF)*. Geneva: Author.

Yu, D. C. T., Spevack, S., Hiebert, R., Martin, T. L., Goodman, R., Martin, T. G., et al. (2002). Happiness indices among persons with profound and severe disabilities during leisure and work activities. *Education and Training in Mental Retardation and Developmental Disabilities, 37*, 421–426.

Chapter 13
Positive Psychology and LGBTQ Populations

Sharon G. Horne, Julia A. Puckett, Raphael Apter, and Heidi M. Levitt

In this chapter, we explore positive psychology as it relates to lesbian, gay, bisexual, transgender, and queer (LGBTQ) identities. It can be helpful to clarify a few terms at the outset of discussions of sex, gender and sexual orientation. *Sex* is a biological term referring to physical anatomy (APA 2011); the term *gender* is a social construct referring to the groupings of characteristics that are typically associated with the male and female sexes (e.g., strong, caring) (APA 2011). *Transgender* refers to people who identify their gender outside of the male-female binary (National Center for Transgender Equality 2009). *Queer* is a term used to encompass the identities of those who do not identify as heterosexual and may find the mainstream labels of LGBT confining (National Center for Transgender Equality 2009). "Sexual orientation" refers to attraction, and typically it connotes the sex(es) to which one is attracted, if any (APA 2011). Throughout the chapter, we use the acronym, "LGBTQ", to capture the diversity of sexual minority (e.g., people who have affectional, sexual, and/or romantic same-sex attractions, including gay, lesbian, and bisexual individuals), and gender minority lives and experiences (individuals who have a sense of themselves as a gender other than the gender associated with the biological sex they were born with, such as transgender individuals). LGBTQ, will be used to refer collectively to those who find themselves on the margins as either sexual or gender minorities. We begin with a narrative that sets the context for the importance of using a positive psychology lens in exploring LGBTQ issues.

In 2001, we (Horne & Levitt) produced and filmed a short documentary film of LGBTQ youth experiences in Memphis, Tennessee. It was shot with a basic

S.G. Horne, Ph.D. (✉) • R. Apter
Department of Counseling and School Psychology, University of Massachusetts Boston, 100 Morrissey Blvd., Boston, MA 02125, USA
e-mail: sharon.horne@umb.edu

J.A. Puckett • H.M. Levitt
Department of Psychology, University of Massachusetts Boston, 100 Morrissey Blvd., Boston, MA 02125, USA

J. Teramoto Pedrotti and L.M. Edwards (eds.), *Perspectives on the Intersection of Multiculturalism and Positive Psychology*, Cross-Cultural Advancements in Positive Psychology 7, DOI 10.1007/978-94-017-8654-6_13,

camcorder, and edited on an iMac, and given that we had absolutely no experience in film-making, *School's Out* did not receive critical acclaim. Although it was featured in the local LGBTQ film festival and continues to be shown by the local LGBTQ youth group, the intention of the film had been to highlight negative school experiences as part of a research program to determine the effectiveness of a training program for school professionals to increase their skills in working with LGBTQ youth.

The **youth** who participated in the film contributed heart-felt, stirring stories of school bullying, family rejection, suicide attempts, hospitalizations after beatings, dropping out of school, self-mutilation, and struggles with substance abuse. They presented a compelling case for greater attention to the needs of LGBTQ youth in schools and the desire for gay-straight alliances, which to this day still are not present in the area. However, at the end of our interviews, we asked the youth what was good about being LGBTQ. What occurred next was a complete surprise.

When we initiated the film, it was the beginning of public awareness of the challenges that many LGBTQ youth faced. We knew—and the youth knew—that the stories of betrayal, violence, and rejection were the ones most likely to catch the attention of authorities and parents, the ones who could have the most impact the school systems. But, when they answered the question about positive aspects of being LGBTQ, the answers tripped easily off their tongues: "more creative," "more compassionate," "more loving," "closer connections to my friends and family," "more giving," "peaceful and caring," and "better able to manage life challenges." "I'm truly myself and I'm proud of it," was the overarching message they shared. These answers were delivered with smiles and bashful grins, and although we knew the responses would challenge the popular representation of LGBTQ youth victimhood, we retained this segment and concluded with these responses as well as footage from the local LGBTQ prom. When we screened the film at the local film festival, the kids came to watch themselves on the big screen and they left the theater smiling, with the sense of empowerment, joy and mutual connection that we felt too. They had communicated that being LGBTQ in Southwestern Tennessee at the turn of this century certainly had its challenges, but there were many positives as well, and they wanted the audience, including their family and friends, teachers and neighbors, to know them. It is our hope, then, to bring to the fore positive experiences and strengths of LGBTQ-identified individuals and communities that have become more visible given changes to the present sociopolitical climate. Before addressing these significant shifts, it is necessary to understand the historical shift within psychology from pathologizing sexual and gender minorities to the more accepting views present today.

13.1 History of Psychological Research on LGBTQ Issues

Although it is indeed changing, the field of psychology has been slow to recognize the psychological strengths related to being LGBTQ. First, homosexuality and non-conforming gender identity have historically been considered mental illnesses.

Homosexuality was only removed from the *Diagnostic and Statistical Manual* (DSM) in 1973, although it persisted in milder forms until 1987 in the diagnoses of sexual orientation disturbance or ego-dystonic homosexuality). Gender identity disorder remains in the present version of the *DSM* (American Psychiatric Association 2000). Prior to 1973, psychologists primarily were invested in proving either that *homosexual* individuals and those with non-conforming gender identities should receive mental health treatment due to their sexual attractions and behaviors (e.g., Socarides 1968), or demonstrating that sexual minorities were not mentally ill and did not differ in degree of pathology from heterosexual individuals (e.g., Hooker 1957).

After 1973, research shifted to the issues that were relevant to LGBTQ individuals such as discrimination and heterosexism (e.g., Herek 1989), sexual identity development (e.g., Cass 1984), mistreatment by mental health professionals (e.g., Garnets et al. 1991), and LGBTQ-related stigma and the link to **minority stress** and health behaviors including substance abuse, suicide attempts, and depression (e.g., Bradford and Ryan 1988; Mays and Cochran 2001; Meyer 1995). During the 1980s, scholarship on HIV/AIDS was launched in the face of the health crisis; however, research did little to dispel negative characterizations of LGBTQ persons (Herek and Capitanio 1993). All in all, research in the 1980s, 1990s, and early 2000s was instrumental in providing an analysis of LGBTQ-related problems and concerns; however, on whole, it focused solely on the negative aspects of LGBTQ lives.

It is only within the past decade that positive aspects of LGBTQ identity have been the focus. This shift has occurred due to the recent resurgence of the field of positive psychology (Lopez and Snyder 2009), which emphasizes strengths and resilience; an increase in the numbers of counseling psychologists who research LGBTQ issues (a psychology specialization that emphasizes resilience and strengths rather than psychopathology); and finally, greater receptivity of LGBTQ research in mainstream academic publications. These changes in psychology occurred at the same time that significant strides were made in LGBTQ rights, including same-sex marriage in many states, the removal of the "Don't Ask, Don't Tell" federal policy from the military, and increased protections at the state and local levels for nondiscrimination in housing, accommodations, and employment for LGBTQ individuals. Consequently, the narratives about LGBTQ identity, family, and community have begun to broaden to include positive aspects.

Among these are the psychological strengths associated with LGBTQ identity, including increased confidence from self-disclosure and living an authentic life, as well as greater insight into and empathy for self and others (Levitt et al. 2013; Riggle et al. 2008; Rostosky et al. 2010); benefits from same-sex relationships and family life (Horne and Biss 2009; Mohr and Fassinger 2006); and positive psychological gains with engagement with LGBTQ community life (Cohen and Murray 2006). We will take this opportunity to summarize three main areas of LGBTQ positive psychology, and then make suggestions for expansion of research and theory.

13.2 Psychological Strengths Associated with LGBTQ Identity

LGBTQ people may have strengths that evolve from the complex understandings that they may develop of themselves, due to their minority sexual orientation and/or gender expressions. Although a heteronormative society may consider sexual and gender minorities to be non-conforming and a threat to traditional family norms of gender, sexual minority individuals tend to consider freedom from dichotomies as one of their strengths (Riggle et al. 2008). Research has shown that sexual identity may be somewhat fluid for some individuals, with women in particular reporting some shifts in their sexual identities and attractions over time (Diamond 2008). With minority sexual identity may come other strengths, such as sexual minority women reporting a strong capacity to handle strong degrees of ambiguity, an important coping strategy (Ohnstad 2009). Bisexual people may share this ability to view the world and other people in non-dichotomous ways because of their experience of resisting labels or categories that are restrictive and confining (Parker et al. 2007).

LGBTQ individuals have been expanding definitions of gender beyond a binary construct for decades (Hiestand and Levitt 2005). Gender itself can be viewed as a spectrum instead of a binary classification system and there are various ways that gender is enacted within the LGBTQ community. For instance, *butch* and *femme* gender identities are ways sexual minority women challenge heteronormative views of gender and desire (Eves 2004). Butch and femme genders are groupings of traits that lesbian communities have created that have social meaning and expectations and can be central to women's identities (e.g., Levitt et al. 2003). Although they share some similarities, these genders are not associated with all the same stereotypes within lesbian communities as mainstream masculinity and femininity—for instance, femme women are known for their assertiveness and self-confidence (Levitt et al. 2003) and butch women are associated with nurturance of others rather than aggression toward others (Hiestand and Levitt 2005; Levitt and Hiestand 2004). Based on interviews, Levitt and Hiestand (2004) identified many strengths, including butch-identified women describing freedom from mainstream gender stereotypes, self-acceptance, access to leadership roles, feeling powerful/attractive, a pride in challenging societal gender boundaries, and a camaraderie with men and other butch women. Femme-identified women reported an increased awareness of social injustices, feeling pride in themselves and their bodies, feeling empowered, and enjoying gender differences in their romantic lives without the accompanying power differences that they attributed to heterosexual intimate relationships (Levitt et al. 2003). Like the reconstruction of gender in heterosexual contexts, gender identities can be generated by LGBTQ communities and they may offer different benefits.

Gender expressions can be shaped by communities to reflect distinct values held by that community and the organization around those values might lead to different strengths. For example, masculinity has been associated with specific meanings, signifiers, and values within different communities of gay men (Taywaditep 2002), such as with *bear-identified* men (i.e., gay men who emphasize masculinity through their physical appearance, including their dress and body hair) (Manley et al. 2007) and *leathermen* culture (i.e., gay men who emphasize masculinity) (Mosher et al. 2006). Among the strengths identified by members of bear communities were the appreciation of a natural aesthetic and maturity, and a valuing of nurturance and intimacy between men. Leathermen reported a sense of pride with their community and emphasized the development of trust and loyalty between men.

The organization of a community to develop and support a particular LGBTQ identity may enhance positive self-perception. Transgender-identified individuals report feeling positively about their transgender identities (72 % report feeling extremely positive and 25 % report feeling somewhat positive), with the development and acceptance of a transgender identity giving them a means for understanding and conceptualizing their experiences (Riggle et al. 2011). Developing transgender identities also is perceived by these individuals as a catalyst for growth, with changes in their gender expression providing them with particular insights into both sexes and genders (Levitt and Ippolito 2013). This experience reportedly enables some transgender individuals to gain a better understanding of systems of oppression.

Youth who identify as queer and/or trans are faced with the challenge of living in a society that "deprives them of a sense of self, self-value, and a recognized social existence" by attempting to force them into gender categories and to use language that does not match their experience or identities" (Saltzburg and Davis 2010, p. 95). However, these youth appear able to move beyond the binary views held within society and find meaning in their experiences, including rising above the limitations of binary categories and gaining a greater understanding about themselves (Saltzburg and Davis 2010).

Many LGBTQ individuals face obstacles such as discrimination, harassment, rejection from their families of origin, and being the victims of hate crimes (Herek et al. 1997). Within the United States, cultural heterosexism has been institutionalized (as manifested by the denial of legislative protections and rights for sexual minority individuals; Herek 1989). Cultural heterosexism and *transphobia* (prejudice against people whose gender identity or gender expression does not conform to societal expectations) are evident in the lack of a federal nondiscrimination policy that includes sexual orientation and gender identity/expression, and by the fact that only 21 states and the District of Columbia have state nondiscrimination policies (Human Rights Campaign, September 2009). Currently, LGBTQ individuals cannot file employment grievances with the Equal Employment Opportunity Commission because there is no federal law against discrimination for LGBT individuals (Van Den Berghe 2003). In addition, it is estimated that 3.1 million LGBTQ people reside in states that do not have workplace nondiscrimination policies (Ramos et al. 2008).

Some qualitative research has identified strengths that have resulted from LGBTQ movements to halt anti-LGBTQ amendments. When Colorado passed a bill banning LGB individuals from claiming a minority status or discrimination based on sexual orientation, Russell's (2000) participants spoke about the personal strengths that developed as a result of developing ties with others in their LGBTQ community. Levitt et al. (2009) interviewed LGBTQ people during the period when a state marriage amendment to the constitution was preparing for passage in TN. Their participants also reported developing a closer sense of community, as well as developing leadership skills, learning to understand heterosexist perspectives while accepting themselves, and finding outlets for activism.

Transgender individuals have fewer legal protections than other sexual minorities, increased rates of poverty and unemployment, and higher rates of homelessness than the general population (Grant et al. 2011). Transgender individuals also face having their identities regulated by state policies, impacting their ability to marry, change their sex on documents, and other rights. Despite these stressors, transgender individuals report identifying as transgender contributes to an authentic sense of self, assists with developing coping tools, and increases the capacity for resilience in the face of adversity (e.g., Devor 1997).

Indeed, coming out (the act of disclosing one's minority sexual or gender identity to others) has been shown to be associated with psychological growth for sexual minority women (Oswald 2000). Women were able to find support and build connections that ultimately enabled them to build a LGBTQ community and strengthen their sexual identity. Oswald states that the act of disclosing gave the people on the receiving end of the disclosure an opportunity for growth because they were able to evaluate and potentially change the ways they thought about sexual minority groups. Coming out also can improve the self-perception of the person disclosing as well as how positively they perceive other LGBTQ individuals (Vaughan and Waehler 2010). Coming out as trangender has been linked to improved interpersonal relationships and more positive self- perceptions (Riggle et al. 2011).

Psychological growth as a result of coming out may have other benefits. Cochran et al. (2009) investigated the altruistic and empathic characteristics of heterosexual and sexual minority participants, finding that sexual minority men and women reported engaging in greater altruistic behaviors than heterosexual men and women, although they did not differ on empathic concern. Common narratives in the literature include LGBTQ individuals describing themselves as attuned to others, able to engage in other-perspective taking and able to appreciate differences (e.g., Riggle et al. 2008, 2011; Rostosky et al. 2010).

13.3 Strengths of LGBTQ Relationships and Families

Literature about gay and lesbian relationships, particularly those of cohabitating couples, predates the more recent national debate about same-sex marriage. As early as 1987, Schmitt and Kurdek found positive correlates between gay identity and relationship stability in same-sex couples. Mohr and Fassinger (2006) studied how sexual identity impacted the quality of romantic relationships in same-sex couples, finding that perceived identity similarity between partners actually helped to increase overall relationship satisfaction. Roisman et al. (2008) reported similar findings of same-sex couple happiness in their study, and suggested that gender similarity may be as important a factor in these couples' satisfaction as sexual orientation.

Coming out as a couple to one's partner's family of origin has been shown to strengthen relationships for gay male couples by increasing inclusion in each of the partner's families, decreasing the need to hide the relationship, and validating the relationship (LaSala 2000). Even when these gay couples received hostile or negative reactions from their families, they were able to sustain their communication and continued to strengthen their bonds in spite of the challenges they were facing with their families. Thus, despite negative societal and family reactions these couples remained resilient and satisfied.

Patterson's (2000) summary of family relationships of lesbian and gay men also paints a positive portrait of same-sex couples who report as much relationship satisfaction as heterosexual couples, low rates of separation in relationships of over ten years (Kurdek 1995), and more equal division of household chores than that of heterosexual couples. In their study of conflict interactions of gay, lesbian, and heterosexual couples, Gottman et al. (2003) found that same-sex couples were more positive than other-sex couples in both how they approach and how they cope with dispute resolution. They hypothesized that this optimism may be the result of the strong value placed on relationship equality in same-sex relationships (e.g., Horne and Biss 2009). Though more research is necessary, these findings suggest that same-sex relationships may have a number of strengths.

LGBTQ parents can encounter additional challenges, such as discrimination when seeking to have or adopt children and issues around legal rights within their roles as parents. The social context for LGBTQ parents can influence the experience of parents and children within these families; for example, parents who live in states that have hostile environments for LGBTQ parents report higher levels of depression and anxiety than their counterparts in less hostile states (Goldberg and Smith 2011). However, despite the difficulties these families face, they are able to provide loving and caring environments for their children and have been shown to possess a number of strengths, including low rates of parenting stress, and high parenting efficacy (Reeves and Horne 2012). In addition, in Gartrell and Bos's (2010) longitudinal study of lesbian planned families, the now 17-year-old offspring were found to be "significantly higher in social, school/academic, and total competence and significantly lower in social problems, rule-breaking, aggressive, and externalizing problem behavior" in comparison to age-matched counterparts (p. 28). Gay- and lesbian-headed families characterize themselves as being warm and caring, with high levels of family functioning (Johnston et al. 2010).

LGBTQ parents may have a lot to offer in helping children understand and negotiate difference. For example, Ausbrooks and Russell (2011) provided a framework for the strengths lesbian and gay parents have that may assist them in raising transracial adoptees, including passing on coping skills from dealing with their own experiences of heterosexism and transphobia, as well as exposure to interpersonal differences. LGBTQ parents can prepare their children for encountering experiences where they may be faced with the decision to disclose having LGBTQ family members to others. For transracial adoptees, the racial differences in their families may prompt others to question whether they are adopted, which can ultimately lead to conversations about LGBTQ parenting relationships (Gianino et al. 2009).

While these disclosures can be anxiety provoking, children report having closer friendships after the disclosures; parents can provide them with language to describe their experiences, and model acceptance and feelings of pride (Gianino et al. 2009). When parents have these important conversations with their biological or adopted children it can create a sense of openness and support within the family (Lynch and Murray 2000). These disclosures may challenge societal notions of the meaning and definitions of family (Goldberg 2007). For example, children of LGBTQ parents who come out can provide opportunities for other children to discuss many variations on family structure (e.g., single parent, step-families).

In addition, children of LGBTQ parents have been shown to benefit from belonging to these families in various ways. For example, children of lesbian and bisexual parents have reported feeling that having sexual minority mothers enabled them to think about their own sexuality and gender in broader terms than traditional heterosexual views of a dichotomous sexual orientation or gender expression (Kuvalanka and Goldberg 2009). Having sexual minority parents provided youth with support in their own identity exploration while also providing them with positive role models who challenge prevailing negative societal views. LGBTQ parents can address the discrimination their families experience in ways that increase levels of awareness in children and further facilitate their growth. For example, gay fathers have been shown to emphasize the importance of understanding and respecting differences in others, as well as understanding the ways homophobia and heterosexism can impact LGBTQ individuals (Bigner 1999). Children of same-sex parents have been found to have an increased level of awareness of prejudice and acceptance of diversity (Lynch and Murray 2000).

LGBTQ individuals have a long history of forming inclusive, tight-knit communities (Weston 1991). LGBTQ individuals may experience rejection by or distance from their families of origin when they disclose their identity, and given this reality, LGBTQ individuals have been shown to rely more on friends for support instead of family members (Dewaele et al. 2011). These groups can develop into what is characterized as a *family of choice*, a network of LGBTQ-identified individuals who accept, support, and care for one another like a family (Weston 1991). Families of choice can take a variety of forms and have many purposes. For example, these family networks might include lesbian, bisexual, and heterosexual women who have come together to care for each other while aging (Ariel 2008), gay men in rural areas (Cody and Welch 1997), or lesbian-identified nuns seeking a place of belonging (Hunyady 2008). Shippy (2007) conducted a study of LGBTQ adults to assess the extent of caring for both biological families and families of choice, finding that 41 % of participants were caring for individuals living with HIV/AIDS, while the other 59 % were caring for individuals dealing with general illnesses found in older adult populations.

13.3.1 "House" Culture

Another type of family of choice is created when individuals form a *house* or a *gay family*. While these networks vary somewhat in terms of structure and purpose, they are a means for LGBTQ individuals to have connection to each other within a supportive and accepting group. Houses are typically networks of people of color, usually African American or Latino, who are LGBTQ-identified and often are in need of support after being rejected by their families of origin (Phillips et al. 2011). For these individuals who may face multiple forms of oppression due to their minority identities, these constructed family networks serve to build community, protect members, and support the development of a positive LGBTQ identity (Horne et al. 2013; Phillips et al. 2011).

Houses are organized in ways that can be similar to some family of choice networks (in some regions of the US they are called gay families), with members taking part as mothers and/or fathers or children (often young men just coming out) in each house. House mothers are typically there for the children of the house when they are in crisis, and provide food, nurturance, and housing when needed (Arnold and Bailey 2009). Typically, house fathers take on a mentor role and are seen as authority figures within the family (Arnold and Bailey 2009). These gendered constructions of the roles of mothers and fathers provide the children of the house with relationships and support that they might not receive from their families of origin including HIV awareness and prevention (Horne et al. 2013).

13.3.2 Virtual Community: It Gets Better/Make It Better

In the fall of 2010, there were a number of LGBTQ teens (e.g., Tyler Clementi, Billy Lucas, and Asher Brown, among others) who took their own lives reportedly due to the harassment and bullying they were encountering as sexual and/or gender minorities. Reactions throughout the country varied. Movements started to build and efforts were made to provide youth with positive messages to counter the discrimination and harassment they were experiencing in their lives. One action that started in response to these suicides was the *It Gets Better* project, which is a video blog initiated by journalist and author Dan Savage (September 21, 2010). In his initial video, Savage and his partner shared their experiences of being bullied during adolescence and the lack of a productive response from the administrators they informed of the mistreatment they were experiencing. The video emphasizes that life gets better after high school and encourages teens to wait out the difficulties they are facing. The video was followed by a massive response from people in the community, with individuals creating videos to share their stories and provide words of encouragement. Currently, there are more than 20,000 videos on the *It Gets Better* YouTube page and the channel has received over 2,500,000 views.

Since its launch, the *It Gets Better* campaign has been critiqued for its emphasis on tolerating heterosexism until it gets easier later in life. In response, *Make It Better* (http://www.makeitbetterproject.org/) was initiated to provide youth with resources to better their school climates and empower them to immediate action as opposed to waiting for something external to change. This website includes videos of teens who are making strides in creating more welcoming and responsive environments in their schools and communities. Such programs engender strength and resiliency in LGBTQ youth from an early age and help them develop positive and affirming LGBTQ identities. Both initiatives aim to reach racially and ethnically diverse youth, as well as youth living in rural areas, although it remains to be seen how effective these programs are in empowering LGBTQ youth.

13.3.3 Community Engagement

Research exploring volunteerism or **social activism** in the LGBTQ community (Omoto and Synder 2002; Ramirez-Valles et al. 2005; Ramirez-Valles et al. 2010) has found this work beneficial to an individual's mental health. Ramirez-Valles et al. (2005, 2010) found that Latino LGBTQ people reported that reductions in maladaptive coping mechanisms occurred after working with HIV/AIDS outreach organizations. Reviewing several of their longitudinal studies of AIDS volunteers, Omoto and Snyder (2002) reported that LGBTQ volunteers indicated a stronger association between their volunteer work and the furthering of community concerns than that of non-LGBTQ volunteers. These kinds of mental health benefits are not only reserved for LGBTQ adults. In their study of gay-straight alliances, Herdt et al. (2007) found that engagement in youth activism has been critical to both LGBTQ youth and straight allies in terms of identity formation, educating young people on the issues facing the LGBTQ community and as an important affirmation of other realities and alternatives to heterosexuality. Transgender individuals also have identified the development of empathy and engagement in activism as one of their strengths, which also increases their connection to LGBTQ communities (Riggle et al. 2011). LGBTQ identity may provide individuals with more opportunities for activism and volunteering, which may be beneficial to mental health overall.

13.4 Multi-level Strengths and Resiliency

LGBTQ individuals exhibit many strengths, including personal growth experiences from the coming out process, a sense of altruism and large-scale community engagement. There are now LGBTQ role models on primetime television, in many of our schools, and in the U. S. Congress. LGBTQ couples and families have been found to be resilient and appear to have strengths when it comes to conflict resolution and parenting healthy kids. LGBTQ community involvement and activism has a long history, and LGBTQ people continue to receive benefit from engagement with issues and concerns.

There is much that is positive to focus on, and much more to be developed within positive psychology with LGBTQ populations. For example, it would be helpful to know how incorporating positive narratives and positive psychology into therapy might benefit the coming out process, instead of utilization of common models based on loss or bereavement. More research needs to be done on the mainstreaming of LGBTQ communities and what impact these changes will have on the salience of sexual and gender identity and the impact it may have on gender roles and expectations. Families of choice and support networks should be explored further for their potential role in positive self-perception, and preventing health risk behaviors. . Finally, research into the potential for stigma to have an impact on cognitive flexibility, altruistic behaviors and self-acceptance should be further explored. Despite the ongoing challenges to the safety and civil liberties of LGBTQ individuals, research suggests that LGBTQ people have considerable strengths in terms of self-definition, self-determination, perspective-taking, community building, and creating family networks and communities.

References

American Psychological Association (APA). (2011). Definition of terms: Sex, gender, gender identity, sexual orientation. In *Excerpt from: The guidelines for psychological practice with lesbian, gay, and bisexual clients, adopted by the APA Council of Representatives*, February 18–20, 2011. Retrieved November 11, 2012, from http://www.apa.org/pi/lgbt/resources/sexuality-definitions.pdf

American Psychiatric Association. Task Force on DSM-IV. (2000). *Diagnostic and statistical manual of mental disorders: DSM-IV-TR*. Washington, DC: American Psychiatric Association.

Ariel, J. (2008). Women aging together in community. *Journal of Lesbian Studies, 12*, 283–292.

Arnold, E. A., & Bailey, M. M. (2009). Constructing home and family: How the ballroom community supports African American GLBTQ youth in the face of HIV/AIDS. *Journal of Gay and Lesbian Social Services, 21*, 171–188.

Ausbrooks, A. R., & Russell, A. (2011). Gay and lesbian family building: A strengths perspective of transracial adoption. *Journal of GLBT Family Studies, 7*, 201–216.

Bigner, J. J. (1999). Raising our sons: Gay men as fathers. *Journal of Gay & Lesbian Social Services: Issues In Practice, Policy & Research, 10*(1), 61–77. doi:10.1300/J041v10n01_04.

Bradford, J., & Ryan, C. (1988). *The national lesbian health care survey: Final report*. Washington, DC: National Lesbian and Gay Health Foundation.

Cass, V. C. (1984). Homosexual identity formation: Testing a theoretical model. *Journal of Sex Research, 20*, 143–167.

Cochran, S. D., Mays, V., Corliss, H., Smith, T. W., & Turner, J. (2009). Self-reported altruistic and reciprocal behaviors among homosexually and heterosexually experienced adults: Implications for HIV/AIDS service organizations. *AIDS Care, 21*(6), 675–682. doi:10.1080/09540120802511919.

Cody, P. J., & Welch, P. L. (1997). Rural gay men in northern New England. *Journal of Homosexuality, 33*, 51–67.

Cohen, H. L., & Murray, Y. (2006). Older lesbian and gay caregivers. *Journal of Human Behavior in the Social Environment, 14*, 275–298.

Devor, A. H. (1997). *FTM: Female-to-male transsexuals in society*. Bloomington: Indiana University Press.

Dewaele, A., Cox, N., van den Berghe, W., & Vincke, J. (2011). Families of choice? Exploring the supportive networks of lesbians, gay men, and bisexuals. *Journal of Applied Social Psychology, 41*, 312–331.

Diamond, L. M. (2008). *Sexual fluidity: Understanding women's love and desire*. Cambridge, MA: Harvard University Press.

Eves, A. (2004). Queer theory, butch/femme identities and lesbian space. *Sexualities, 7*, 480–496. doi:10.1177/1363460704047064.

Garnets, L., Hancock, K., Cochran, S. D., Goodchilds, J., & Peplau, L. A. (1991). Issues in psychotherapy with lesbians and gay men: A survey of psychologists. *American Psychologists, 46*, 964–972.

Gartrell, N., & Bos, H. (2010). US National longitidunal lesbian family study: Psychological adjustment of 17-year-old adolescents. *Pediatrics, 126*, 1–11.

Gianino, M., Goldberg, A., & Lewis, T. (2009). Family outings: Disclosure practices among adopted youth with gay and lesbian parents. *Adoption Quarterly, 12*, 205–228.

Goldberg, A. E. (2007). Talking about family: Disclosure practices of adults raised by lesbian, gay, and bisexual parents. *Journal of Family Issues, 28*, 100–131.

Goldberg, A. E., & Smith, J. Z. (2011). Stigma, social context, and mental health: Lesbian and gay couples across the transition to adoptive parenthood. *Journal of Counseling Psychology, 58*, 139–150.

Gottman, J. M., Leveson, R. W., Gross, J., Fredrickson, B. L., McCoy, K., Rosenthal, L., Yoshimoto, D. (2003). Correlates of gay and lesbian couples' relationship satisfaction and relationship dissolution. *Journal of Homosexuality, 45*(1), 23–43.

Grant, J. M., Mottet, L. A., Tanis, J., Harrison, J., Herman, J. L., & Keisling, M. (2011). *Injustice at every turn: A report of the national transgender discrimination survey*. Washington, DC: The National Gay and Lesbian Task Force and the National Center for Transgender Equality.

Herdt, G., Russell, S. T., Sweat, J., & Marzullo, M. (2007). Sexual inequality, youth empowerment, and the GSA: A community study in California. In N. Teunis & G. Herdt (Eds.), *Sexual inequalities and social justice* (pp. 233–251). Berkeley: University of California Press.

Herek, G. M. (1989). Hate crimes against lesbians and gay men. *American Psychologist, 44*, 948–955.

Herek, G. M., & Capitanio, J. P. (1993). Public reactions to AIDS in the United States: A second decade of stigma. *American Journal of Public Health, 83*(4), 574–577.

Herek, G. M., Gillis, J. R., Cogan, J. C., & Glunt, E. K. (1997). Hate crime victimization among lesbian, gay, and bisexual adults: Prevalence, psychological correlates, and methodological issues. *Journal of Interpersonal Violence, 12*, 195–215.

Hiestand, K. R., & Levitt, H. M. (2005). Butch identity development: The formation of an authentic gender. *Feminism and Psychology, 15*, 61–85.

Horne, S. G., & Biss, W. (2009). Equality discrepancy between women in same-sex relationships: The mediating role of attachment in relationship satisfaction. *Sex Roles: A Journal of Research, 60*, 721–730.

Horne, S. G., Levitt, H. M., Puckett, J., & Sweeney, K. (2013). *Family networks as a point of entry for HIV prevention and intervention among African American young men.* Unpublished manuscript.

Hooker, E. (1957). The adjustment of the male overt homosexual. *Journal of Projective Techniques, 21*, 18–31.

Hunyady, M. K. (2008). We are family: I got all my sisters with me! *Journal of Lesbian Studies, 12*, 293–300.

Johnston, L. B., Moore, B. A., & Judd, R. (2010). Gay and lesbian households' perceptions of their family functioning: Strengths and resiliency. *Journal of GLBT Family Studies, 6*, 315–325.

Kurdek, L. A. (1995). Lesbian and gay couples. In A. R. D'Augelli & C. J. Patterson (Eds.), *Lesbian, gay, and bisexual identities over the lifespan: Psychological perspectives* (pp. 243–261). New York: Oxford University Press.

Kuvalanka, K. A., & Goldberg, A. E. (2009). "Second generation" voices: Queer youth with lesbian/bisexual mothers. *Journal of Youth and Adolescence, 38*, 904–919.

LaSala, M. C. (2000). Gay male couples: The importance of coming out and being out to parents. *Journal of Homosexuality, 39*, 47–71.

Levitt, H. M., & Hiestand, K. R. (2004). A quest for authenticity: Contemporary butch gender. *Sex Roles, 50*, 605–621.

Levitt, H. M., & Hiestand, K. (2005). Enacting a gendered sexuality: Butch and femme perspectives. *Journal of Constructivist Psychology, 18*, 39–51.

Levitt, H. M., & Ippolito, M. R. (2013). Being transgender: Navigating minority stressors and developing authentic self-presentation. *Psychology of Women Quarterly*. OnlineFirst at http://pwq.sagepub.com/content/early/recent. doi:10.1177/0361684313501644.

Levitt, H. M., Gerrish, E. A., & Hiestand, K. R. (2003). The misunderstood gender: A model of modern femme identity. *Sex Roles, 48*, 99–113.

Levitt, H. M., Ovrebo, E., Anderson-Cleveland, M. B., Leone, C., Jeong, J. Y., Arm, J. R., Horne, S. G. (2009). Balancing dangers: GLBT experience in a time of anti-GLBT legislation. *Journal of Counseling Psychology, 56,* 67–81.

Levitt, H. M., Horne, S. G., Ippolito, M., Reeves, T., Baggett, L., Dunavant, B., Geiss, M., Maxwell, D., & Huang, Q. (2013). *An in-depth exploration of minority stress reflective of GLB experience*. Unpublished manuscript.

Lopez, S. J., & Snyder, C. R. (Eds.). (2009). *Oxford handbook of positive psychology*. New York: Oxford University Press.

Lynch, J. M., & Murray, K. (2000). For the love of the children: The coming out process for lesbian and gay parents and stepparents. *Journal of Homosexuality, 39,* 1–24.

Manley, E., Levitt, H. M., & Mosher, C. M. (2007). Understanding the bear movement in gay male culture: Redefining masculinity. *Journal of Homosexuality, 53*(4), 89–112.

Mays, V. M., & Cochran, S. D. (2001). Mental health correlates of perceived discrimination among lesbian, gay, and bisexual adults in the United States. *American Journal of Public Health, 91,* 1869–1876.

Meyer, I. H. (1995). Minority stress and mental health in gay men. *Journal of Health and Social Behavior, 36,* 38–56.

Mohr, J. J., & Fassinger, R. E. (2006). Sexual orientation identity and romantic relationship quality in same-sex couples. *Personality and Social Psychology Bulletin, 32,* 1085–1099.

Mosher, C. M., Levitt, H. M., & Manley, E. (2006). Layers of leather: The identity formation of leathermen as a process of transforming meanings of masculinity. *Journal of Homosexuality, 51,* 93–123.

National Center for Transgender Equality. (2009). Transgender terminology. Retrieved November 12, 2012, from http://transequality.org/Resources/NCTE_TransTerminology.pdf

Ohnstad, A. (2009). If I am not straight or gay, who am I? *Clinical Social Work Journal, 37,* 357–367. doi:10.1007/s10615-009-0210-8.

Omoto, A. M., & Synder, M. (2002). Considerations of community: The context and process of volunteerism. *American Behavioral Scientist, 45*(5), 846–867.

Oswald, R. (2000). Family and friendship relationships after young women come out as bisexual or lesbian. *Journal of Homosexuality, 38*(3), 65–83.

Parker, B. A., Adams, H. L., & Phillips, L. D. (2007). Decentering gender: Bisexual identity as an expression of a non-dichotomous worldview. *Identity: An International Journal of Theory and Research, 7,* 205–224.

Patterson, C. J. (2000). Family relationships of lesbians and gay men. *Journal of Marriage and the Family, 62*(4), 1052–1069. doi:10.1111/j.1741-3737.2000.01052.x.

Phillips, G., Peterson, J., Binson, D., Hidalgo, J., & Magnus, M. (2011). House/ball culture and adolescent African-American transgender persons and men who have sex with men: A synthesis of the literature. *AIDS Care, 23,* 515–520.

Ramirez-Valles, J., Fergus, S., Reisen, C. A., Poppen, P. J., & Zea, M. (2005). Confronting stigma: Community involvement and psychological well-being among HIV-positive Latino gay men. *Hispanic Journal of Behavioral Sciences, 27*(1), 101–119. doi:10.1177/0739986304270232.

Ramirez-Valles, J., Kuhns, L. M., Campbell, R. T., & Diaz, R. M. (2010). Social integration and health: Community involvement, stigmatized identities, and sexual risk in Latino sexual minorities. *Journal of Health and Social Behavior, 51*(1), 30–47. doi:10.1177/0022146509361176.

Ramos, C., Badgett, M. V. L., & Sears, B. (2008). *Evidence of employment discrimination on the basis of sexual orientation and gender identity: Complaints filed with state enforcement Agencies 1999–2007*. University of California, Los Angeles: The Williams Institute. Retrieved from: http://escholarship.org/uc/item/7j0413pd

Reeves, T., & Horne, S. G. (2012). *The impact of legal rights on parental stress and efficacy among LGBT parents.* Unpublished manuscript.

Riggle, E. D. B., Whitman, J. S., Olson, A., Rostosky, S. S., & Strong, S. (2008). The positive aspects of being a lesbian or gay man. *Professional Psychology: Research and Practice, 39*(2), 210–217.

Riggle, E. D. B., Rostosky, S. S., McCants, L. E., & Pascale-Hague, D. (2011). The positive aspects of a transgender self-identification. *Psychology & Sexuality, 2,* 147–158.

Roisman, G. I., Clausell, E., Holland, A., Fortuna, K., & Elieff, C. (2008). Adult romantic relationships as contexts of human development: A multimethod comparison of same-sex couples with opposite-sex dating, engaged, and married dyads. *Developmental Psychology, 44*(1), 91–101. doi:10.1037/0012-1649.44.1.91.

Rostosky, S. S., Riggle, E. D. B., Pascale-Hague, D., & McCants, L. E. (2010). The positive aspects of a bisexual self-identification. *Psychology & Sexuality, 1*, 131–144. doi:10.1080/19419899.2010.484595.

Russell, G. M. (2000). *Voted out: The psychological consequences of anti-gay politics*. New York: New York University Press.

Saltzburg, S., & Davis, T. S. (2010). Co-authoring gender-queer youth identities: Discursive telling and retellings. *Journal of Ethnic and Cultural Diversity in Social Work, 19*, 87–108.

Schmitt, J., & Kurdek, L. A. (1987). Personality correlates of positive identity and relationship involvement in gay men. *Journal of Homosexuality, 13*(4), 101–109. doi:10.1300/J082v13n04_06.

Shippy, R. A. (2007). We cannot go it alone: The impact of informal support and stressors in older gay, lesbian and bisexual caregivers. *Journal of Gay and Lesbian Social Services, 18*, 39–51.

Socarides, C. W. (1968). *The overt homosexual*. Northvale: Jason Aronson, Inc.

Taywaditep, K. J. (2002). Marginalization among the marginalized. *Journal of Homosexuality, 42*, 1–28.

Van Den Berghe, N. (2003). Getting a piece of the pie: Cultural competence for GLBT employees at the workplace. *Journal of Human Behavior in the Social Environment, 8*, 55–73. doi:10.1300/J137v08n02_04.

Vaughan, M. D., & Waehler, C. A. (2010). Coming out growth: Conceptualizing and measuring stress-related growth associated with coming out to others as a sexual minority. *Journal of Adult Development, 17*, 94–109. doi:10.1007/s10804-009-9084-9.

Weston, K. (1991). *Families we choose: Lesbians, gays, kinship*. New York: Columbia University Press.

Part IV
Applications of Positive Psychology in Multicultural Contexts

Chapter 14
Positive Psychological Practices in Multicultural School Settings

Casey A. Holtz and Michael J. Martinez

Schools are increasingly diverse with regard to variety of racial and ethnic groups (Aud et al. 2010), socioeconomic status (Kahlenburg 2006), level of ability (Olszewski-Kubilius et al. 2004), worldviews (Lonborg and Bowen 2004), and sexual orientation (Espelage et al. 2008). With increased diversity in schools, school professionals are charged with the task of providing culturally appropriate services to a broad range of students. That challenge is great given that the role of school is much more than academic instruction (Greenberg et al. 2003). Schools have the responsibility to help children engage in safe, positive, and healthy behaviors and to ensure students possess social-emotional competencies, strong work habits, and an ethical framework. Unfortunately, many schools have yet to find effective solutions to long-standing problems including academic underachievement, student-to-student conflict, drug and alcohol abuse, and development of unhealthy social relationships (Wiehe et al. 2005). Diversity in schools makes the identification of a sole solution to the problems in schools more complex because there is no panacea to address the needs of all students.

Interestingly, a major part of the "problem" is that schools are often too focused on problems and problem solution. Schools often ineffectively address their primary problems because they rely on fragmented programs designed to target such diverse issues as HIV/AIDS, alcohol and drug abuse, delinquency, dropout, family life, morals, multiculturalism, and violence (Greenberg et al. 2003). Although school-based targeted programs have demonstrated effectiveness at decreasing harmful behaviors in children already engaged in drug and alcohol abuse (O'Leary-Barrett et al. 2010),

C.A. Holtz, Ph.D. (✉)
Psychology Department, Wisconsin Lutheran College,
8800 W. Bluemound Road, Milwaukee, WI 53226, USA
e-mail: Casey.holtz@wlc.edu

M.J. Martinez, M.A.
Department of Counseling and Eductational Psychology,
Marquette University, Milwaukee, WI, USA

J. Teramoto Pedrotti and L.M. Edwards (eds.), *Perspectives on the Intersection of Multiculturalism and Positive Psychology*, Cross-Cultural Advancements in Positive Psychology 7, DOI 10.1007/978-94-017-8654-6_14,

violent behaviors (Flannery et al. 2003), risky sexual behaviors (Kirby et al. 2004), and delinquency (Hawkins et al. 2009), these programs do not appear to consistently thwart future problem occurrences (Thomas and Perera 2006).

Educational experts who advocate for improved provision of school-based services suggest a shift in philosophy from a focus on problem remediation toward a mindset of prevention (Adelman and Taylor 2010; Greenberg et al. 2003). Theoretically, if schools shift their focus to prevention-based services, providing children the opportunities to develop skills (e.g., communication, social, emotional, cognitive, behavioral, moral competence, and positive identity) and strengths (e.g., belief in the future, resilience, prosocial behavior), they likely will address the root causes of the problems they strongly desire to eliminate (Greenberg et al. 2003; Weissberg and Greenberg 1998). The education reformation, and its push to increase prevention and focus on positive skill development, suggests positive psychology has great merit when applied to educational settings.

14.1 Positive Psychology in Multicultural Schools

Schools are the ideal institution and place in the community to provide excellent role models and developmentally appropriate activities and resources for helping children develop a sense of importance, values, and direction (Adelman and Taylor 2010). Schools best serve their students when they embrace the role of supporting positive social, emotional, and academic achievement. Research suggests this is critically important for children from racial and ethnic minority backgrounds and lower socioeconomic status families because they historically have had inadequate educational opportunities (Kuh et al. 2006; Lee 2005a) and/or have experienced social inequalities (Noguera 2003) that have contributed to the continued academic achievement gap. A shift in focus toward optimal student development is especially applicable for students from racial and ethnic minority backgrounds because past models of human functioning (deficit models) have neglected strengths and the influence of the environment (e.g., discrimination), and have viewed behavior from these groups as deficient (Sue and Constantine 2003).

The change toward positive psychology in schools, however, has been slow and, at times, difficult because teachers are under the pressure of educational standards, and the accountability of schools related to academic achievement often undermines teachers' desires to focus on social, emotional, and psychological competencies. Also, a shift toward positive psychology in schools means changing a philosophy that has been in place since the infancy of psychology and a philosophy that remains in other fields (e.g., medicine) and society, in general.

The goal of changing schools, especially diverse schools, toward a focus on strengths and strengths development is well worth the effort. In order to reap these rewards, however, schools with a high degree of diversity must recognize and foster these strengths within youth from diverse backgrounds (Dahlsgaard et al. 2005; Constantine and Sue 2006). The next section of this chapter provides research on the positive effects of a focus on strengths, while acknowledging cultural differences, to provide a rationale for practitioners who would like to provide school-based services that target multicultural strengths.

14.2 Positive Psychology's Effect on Students of All Cultures

School-based research on programs designed to optimize student development has largely focused on prevention-minded programs that coordinate social, emotional, and academic learning. Programs that target social-emotional learning (SEL; Elias et al. 1997) integrate the development of children's social skills (e.g., appreciate perspective of others, effective management of interpersonal situations) and emotional skills (e.g., emotional management, sustaining hope, development of positive goals) into their academic curriculum. Programs that focus on strength development have demonstrated it is necessary to focus on strengths and skill development for future negotiation of diverse contexts and challenges throughout child development (Weissberg and Greenberg 1998). Research also suggests students from all backgrounds and cultures benefit from a focus on student strengths as demonstrated by improved academic (Nickerson 2007), social (Lyubomirsky et al. 2005), and interpersonal (Lee 2005b) functioning (Bray and Kehle 2011).

14.2.1 Research Related to Academic Success

Professionals working in multicultural school settings are often focused on academic achievement and on closing the achievement gap. Therefore, it is appropriate to first help professionals understand how a focus on development of student strengths also facilitates improved academic functioning in students from all backgrounds. Durlak et al. (2011) completed a meta-analysis of 213 studies that occurred in Urban (47 %), Suburban (16 %), and Rural areas (15 %). This meta-analysis included studies on school-based, universal social and emotional learning programs (focused on strength development) found that students within these programs, compared to controls, demonstrated significantly improved social and emotional skills, attitudes, behavior, and academic performance. A review paper by Catalano et al. (2002) highlighted a number of prevention programs that demonstrated significant effects on student cognitive and academic achievement with students from racial and ethnic minority groups. For example, the PATHS program (Greenberg 1996) had a significant effect on academic achievement for students of all ethnic groups. The Social Competence Program for Young Adolescents is another program that was found to have a significant effect on academic achievement in a large sample of students from racial and ethnic minority backgrounds (Caplan et al. 1992). These findings demonstrate that programs designed to foster certain positive characteristics can assist students in successfully navigating the social-emotional aspects of school, due to their strengths and competencies, and render them more able to fully reach their academic potential. Insight into the effectiveness of programs that focus on strengths and positive psychology can also be found within research on educational motivation that demonstrates that students who are self-aware and confident in their ability to navigate academic and social challenges also try harder in their academic efforts (Zins et al. 2004).

Students from minority racial and ethnic backgrounds have much to gain from schools that focus on cultural strengths (Edwards et al. 2007). When schools focus on nurturance of culturally specific strengths (e.g., ethnic identity, biculturalism), they allow students from multicultural backgrounds to view their cultural and familial background as strengths rather than a barrier to their education. The focus on multiculturally-relevant strengths is beneficial for many reasons. First, strong ethnic identity development protects youth from believing negative stereotypes regarding poor academic achievement and risky behaviors (Fuligni et al. 2005). Additionally, schools that stress maintenance of ethnic identity rather than assimilation positively impact student's success in school (Phinney et al. 2001). School and home settings that support students in their attempts to embrace their ethnic identity, while also navigating mainstream culture, foster biculturalism. Biculturalism, the ability to internalize two cultures, contributes to higher academic achievement and lower drop-out rates (Feliciano 2001). Culturally specific strengths, such as ethnic identity and biculturalism, are important characteristics of students from minority racial backgrounds that can contribute to improved academic performance. Thus helping to facilitate and enhance these types of characteristics should be a primary goal for schools working with students from many backgrounds.

14.2.2 Research Related to Social Functioning

Students live in a social world that is increasingly complex with the emergence of social networking and constant communication through the use of cell phones and social media. Although academic achievement is often the focus of education, children rate social skills as the most important aspect of development. Students who have challenges socially are at risk for a variety of negative outcomes including school avoidance, school drop-out, and academic underachievement (Lopez and Dubois 2005). Positive psychology is one important avenue to optimal development of student social abilities. A review of 161 positive youth development programs designed to support the development of strengths (e.g., self-efficacy, competence, bonding, hope) in students from diverse racial and ethnic backgrounds demonstrated many of these programs (e.g., Success for All, Slavin et al. 1996; Growing Healthy Program, Smith et al. 1992) improved student peer and adult relationships, and interpersonal skills in students from racial and ethnic minority cultures through a focus on strengths (Catalano et al. 2002). Within these programs, children from all backgrounds learned skills to recognize and manage their emotions, appreciate the perspective of others, establish positive goals, make responsible decisions, and handle interpersonal situations effectively (Lemerise and Arsenio 2000). Caplan et al. (1992) found students from racial and ethnic minority backgrounds living in urban areas benefitted from stress management training, self-esteem building, and problem solving skills through the Positive Youth Development Program (Weissberg et al. 1997). Another important factor related to social ability is the development of a school community that encourages "belonging" and cooperation. Educational research suggests programs designed to strengthen student social-emotional competencies enhance student connectedness to school (McNeeley et al. 2002; Osterman 2000). Connection to school and an experience of school as a community has a significant positive effect on students from diverse racial and ethnic backgrounds. Research on culturally specific strengths (e.g., bicultural identity, ethnic/cultural pride) has also demonstrated a focus on these strengths can provide a buffer against the influence of negative peers and negative peer influences (e.g., drug and alcohol abuse; Kulis et al. 2002). Programs such as those mentioned above that focus on the development of these types of strengths may have important impact for multicultural student bodies.

14.3 Role of School Professionals

It is apparent that changing schools from problem-focused institutions toward institutions focused on strengths is a worthy goal. Unfortunately, there are various school-level and individual-level barriers (Clonan et al. 2004). While barriers must be acknowledged, it is also necessary to reenergize, refocus on the positive possibilities, and realize school professionals remain in an ideal position to have a positive effect on students from diverse backgrounds. The remainder of this chapter provides recommendations for school-based practitioners on how to begin to initiate healthy changes within the school setting that will appropriately shift the focus from the long-standing deficit models toward a model of strength-based child development, in a multiculturally competent way. Recommendations begin with broad overviews of ways to strive toward cultural competence and healthier conceptualizations of students and conclude with specific recommendations for professionals within their respective roles.

14.3.1 Understanding Self and Others – Cultural Competence

As the student population becomes increasingly diverse (National Center for Educational Statistics 2008), school professionals are called upon to develop and strengthen their cultural competence (Boyle et al. 1999; Dessel 2010; Ullucci and Battey 2011). In fact, within the last two decades, national professional organizations have published documents formally identifying competencies, guidelines, or position statements regarding working with culturally diverse individuals (American School Counselor Association [ASCA] 2009; American Psychological Association [APA] 2003;

Arredondo et al. 1996; National Education Association [NEA] 2008). Central to each of these documents is acknowledgement of the importance for school professionals to develop both an awareness of their own cultural identity and an understanding and appreciation of others' culture and worldview. To meet this need, school professionals are encouraged to seek out and engage in training opportunities that focus on increasing cultural sensitivity. One example of a training program is the Racial and Ethical Sensitivity Training (REST; Rogers-Sirin and Sirin 2009). In this workshop, participants are exposed to relevant research, self-reflection exercises, and examination of school policies. Key to the training is the development of an ethical decision making model to specifically use when school staff are confronted with a dilemma involving cultural issues. The training provides a space for school professionals to view videos of sample ethical dilemmas and role-play/rehearse potential responses. Another example of a proposed method to increase cultural awareness is through storytelling and folklore. Carter-Black (2007) suggests that through cultural fables, parables, and proverbs, social work students showed an increased sensitivity, understanding, and appreciation of diverse cultures. Specifically, Carter-Black argues that discussion of cultural topics can feel safer to all groups when done in the context of storytelling – a medium that is fairly universal across cultures. Increased safety can facilitate dialogue about potentially charged, challenging and personal topics such as worldviews, biases, values, and societal inequities. Additionally, she points out that the sharing of cultural stories or folklore creates opportunities for individuals to identify how they are both different and similar to each other, thus contributing to increased awareness of both self and other.

However, some contend that for professionals in education and psychology, broadly speaking, a significant component of cultural competence also includes work beyond individual encounters with students/clients/patients. For instance, Vera and Speight (2003) indicated a need for multicultural competence to also include advocacy, prevention, and outreach as part of a social justice mission – thus encouraging a more systemic view to include work with families, communities and even the greater society. Indeed, this sentiment has been reiterated in research and recommendations specific to school professionals, indicating they should be agents of change who work within the system to promote social justice and equity (APA 2003; ASCA, 2009; Day-Vines and Terriquez 2008). One way to adopt this social justice mission is to actively work toward challenging the current, predominate deficit model (Walker 2011). The following section describes several models or frameworks that advocate a more positive, strengths-based approach in how school-based professionals interact with and even conceptualize students of diverse cultures in their schools.

14.3.2 *Conceptualizing Diverse Youth Based on Their Strengths*

Perhaps the largest drawback of using a deficit thinking paradigm is that it contains the idea that something is inherently 'wrong' with the student (or their family, culture, environment) and therefore improvement is beyond the influence of school professionals (Walker 2011). Saleebey (2008) emphatically notes that every student, family, community, and school has assets and resources to consider. He continues stating that, "Even the most downtrodden, or most angry, or most defeated of us, there are strengths to be found and nurtured…everyone has a basic faculty for health and self-righting" (p. 69). Cultural background is a source of strength for students and their families, in that it consists of values, traditions, and pride (Saleebey 2008). Several recent frameworks that can be implemented by a variety of school professionals, intend to challenge the deficit-focused paradigm by alternatively conceptualizing traditionally disenfranchised students from a strengths-based, positive, healthy perspective. These frameworks are briefly discussed in the following paragraphs to provide an initial paradigm for professionals.

14.3.2.1 Strength-Based Frameworks

There are multiple approaches that offer school professionals who utilize assessment a more balanced approach than traditional assessment approaches which tend to emphasize negative aspects of client functioning and minimize or ignore positive aspects (Magyar-Moe 2009). The Four-Front Approach (Wright 1991), and other approaches modeled after it (e.g., Snyder et al. 2006) attend to the individuals internal psychological strengths, internal psychological weaknesses, environmental assets/resources, and environmental weaknesses/challenges. Hays' (1996) ADDRESSING model also aims to increase clinician's sensitivity and responsiveness to the many different aspects of students' identities. Specifically, it outlines a strategy for the interviewer to assess multiple identity domains including: age, developmental issues, disabilities, religion/spirituality, ethnicity, socioeconomic status, sexual orientation, indigenous origins, and gender. Hays clearly points out that using this framework provides the interviewer with multiple opportunities to assess for client strengths related to these cultural identities which otherwise, if using a different assessment model, might be overlooked. (For further discussion of these frameworks please refer to Chap. 2 of this volume.)

14.3.2.2 Culturally Relevant Pedagogy

Culturally relevant teachers "create learning environments that support, develop, and draw from the students' cultural and ethnic identities" (Bales and Saffold 2011, p. 961) because they are developing students academically, supporting their own cultural competence, and developing a "sociopolitical or critical consciousness" (Ladson-Billings 1995, p. 483). The model views students' cultures as knowledge to be owned and shared within the classroom. Central to the spirit of *culturally relevant pedagogy* is the teachers' genuine belief that all students can be educated and can succeed. Ladson-Billings noted rather than incorporating a "language of lacking" (referring to single-parent households, welfare, or psychological deficiencies), a *culturally relevant teacher* highlights student expertise and makes clear an expectation that all students will "excel at something" (p. 480). In these classrooms, learning collaboratively is encouraged, with the intent of creating a community of learning where individual successes are celebrated by the entire classroom (or school). A classroom/school community implementing this approach is simultaneously actively identifying and applying students' cultures and strengths.

14.4 Specific Recommendations to Promote Strengths Among Diverse Students

14.4.1 School Counselors, School Social Workers and School Psychologists

The shift from problem reduction to strengths promotion is possible, though no school professional will be able achieve it alone. For school counselors, psychologists and social workers especially, with their demanding student to clinician ratio, collaboration is not only beneficial but necessary. In applying this collaboration, school counselors are uniquely positioned, based on their training and expertise, to establish or develop unique programs that acknowledge student culture as strength. For instance, in one high school with predominately African American and Latina/o students, an innovative disciplinary process was established (Day-Vines and Terriquez 2008). In that school, students worked together with teachers, administrators and counselors in making decisions about disciplinary cases. Students of all cultural backgrounds helped create policy and felt empowered by drawing on their own strengths to help negotiate conflict successfully. Collaborating with and empowering parents as part of the educational team is important because it can demystify a school setting that may appear intimidating, cold, or disinterested (Matthews and Mahoney 2005).

While collaborating with families and other school staff is important, school counselors need also to create relationships with individuals and institutions in the greater community in which the school resides (Day-Vines and Terriquez 2008). One promising example of this type of systemic collaboration is The Boston Connects Program. The Boston Connects program resides in 14 public elementary schools sponsored by a local university, in diverse, low-income neighborhoods (Walsh et al. 2008). Through this program, school counselors identify strengths and weaknesses of all students, collaborate with other school staff to develop a plan, engage with student families, establish partnerships with community agencies, and refer students/families to appropriate resources. Results indicate an increase in the range of resources/services to which students are referred as well as a shift to services that build strengths as opposed to offering remedial services.

Another intervention area where collaboration from multiple school stakeholders is possible is group work. In one group developed by school counselors, middle-school male students participated in a 12-session strengths-based group with the objective of increasing academic motivation, decreasing discipline referrals, identifying/developing strengths, and increasing knowledge related to post-secondary education (Clark et al. 2008). Participants included students of low socioeconomic status, students of color, and students receiving exceptional education services. Group content included motivational guest speakers from the community and strength-building sessions (health, organization, mediation). Results showed that discipline referrals decreased, attitudes toward school became more positive, and they had more focused future goals. Not only do these programs acknowledge and seek out individual strengths within the students, it simultaneously recognizes the internal and external resources within the school's/students' surrounding community, and from their diverse cultural backgrounds and uses these to improve academic and behavioral outcomes thus working to close the achievement gap.

14.4.2 Teachers

Any teacher choosing to teach in a multicultural school community must realize that success, for both teacher and student, will require a willingness to critically examine their own beliefs about teaching and learning and how students' cultures interact with classroom instruction (Bales and Saffold 2011). In one study, teachers were found to lack knowledge about the environment in which their students live, and therefore of available cultural resources (Matthews and Mahoney 2005). Alternatively, when teachers physically make themselves a part of the (geographic) community in which the school is, it sends the message to students and their families that the environment is worthwhile and that the teacher wants to be, or is, a part of that community (Ladson-Billings 1995).

Garcia's (2002) pedagogy of empowerment emphasizes the importance of respecting and integrating students' beliefs, histories, and experiences into their learning opportunities. It recognizes the importance of building new knowledge on a foundation of current knowledge and experiences. The framework calls teachers and other service providers to acknowledge and challenge preconceived, negative beliefs about students from diverse cultures – particularly those from lower socio-economic status or cultures in which English is not the primary/first language. In following these guidelines, students and families become empowered and the role of the teacher is redefined.

14.4.3 Administrators and Policy

School administrators must remember that each school professional has unique training, experience, and cultural background. Therefore, within one school staff it is likely there will exist a broad range of developmental levels of multicultural competence. As such, administrators are encouraged to be supportive and aware of this continuum while also recognizing the importance of providing ongoing continuing education or training opportunities for school staff (Walker 2011). Administrators can tailor these trainings to fit the unique needs of their school's stakeholders. In determining how to implement such programs, school administrators may find benefit in recognizing the strengths and resources within the school staff itself.

School administrators and policy makers are encouraged to consider assessments of cultural sensitivity to district policies and trends that affect all groups of students, specifically those from traditionally underserved groups. For instance, when establishing a school's crisis intervention plan, administration can seek input from families and students, especially those from diverse groups and assess resources present in the greater community (Annandale et al. 2011). Additionally, when evaluating a staff person's effectiveness, administration is encouraged to consider the individual's cultural competence in addition to student achievement outcome data (Walker 2011).

Finally, school administrators are encouraged to develop new or identify existing training opportunities to increase cultural competence and raise cultural awareness (of self and others). In support of this sentiment, Rogers-Sirin and Sirin (2009) argue that currently, cultural competence is a personal choice though it should be a professional ethical requirement. They developed a training workshop (Racial and Ethical Sensitivity Training KIT) with the objective to "increase school professionals' ability to recognize discrimination and racism in their schools and to equip them with basic skills for handling these situations" (p. 21). Facilitators use multiple teaching techniques (lecture, video, discussion, role-plays) to allow opportunities for discourse and rehearsal. Results indicated that participants increased their ethical sensitivity towards issues of racial intolerance and their ability to recognize when ethical violations (regarding discrimination and racism) occur. Participants also increased their knowledge and awareness about racism in schools and the impact it has in their own lives.

14.5 Conclusion

Diversity is increasing within schools and, while diversity contributes strength to schools in many ways, school professionals are challenged with the responsibility to provide educational and adjunctive programming to support the broad variety of students within their schools. Because school has such a profound effect on student development and because student success within school has such a profound effect on their access to higher education (and subsequent employment), this challenge must not be taken lightly. This chapter provided research and theory that suggests schools should consider using student strengths as a conduit to improving student outcomes. Specifically, a focus on strengths within schools will benefit students from culturally diverse backgrounds and provide them with the opportunity to succeed within the school setting.

References

Adelman, H., & Taylor, L. (2010, September). *Turning around, transforming, and continuously improving schools: Federal proposals are still based on a two- rather than a three- component blueprint*. Center for Mental Health in Schools. [Online]. Available: http://smhp.psych.ucla.edu/pdfdocs/turning.pdf

American Psychological Association. (2003). Guidelines on multicultural education, training, research, practice, and organizational change for psychologists. *American Psychologist, 58*, 377–402. http://www.apa.org/pi/oema/resources/policy/multicultural-guidelines.aspx

American School Counselor Association. (2009). *The ASCA national model: A framework for school counseling programs* (3rd ed.). Alexandria: ASCA.

Annandale, N. O., Heath, M. A., Dean, B., Kemple, A., & Takino, Y. (2011). Assessing cultural competency in school crisis plans. *Journal of School Violence, 10*, 16–33.

Arredondo, P., Toporek, M. S., Brown, S., Jones, J., Locke, D. C., Sanchez, J., & Stadler, H. (1996). *Operationalization of the multicultural counseling competencies*. Alexandria: AMCD. http://www.counseling.org/resources/competencies/multcultural_competencies.pdf

Aud, S., Fox, M., & KewalRamani, A. (2010). Status and trends in the education of racial and ethnic groups (NCES 2010–015), Indicators 23–24. In US Department of Education, National Center for Education Statistics (Ed.). Washington, DC: Government Printing Office.

Bales, B. L., & Saffold, F. (2011). A new era in the preparation of teachers for urban schools: Linking multiculturalism, disciplinary-based content, and pedagogy. *Urban Education, 46*, 953–974.

Boyle, D. P., Nackerud, L., & Kilpatrick, A. (1999). The road less traveled: Cross cultural, international experiential learning. *International Social Work, 42*, 201–214.

Bray, M. A., & Kehle, T. J. (2011). *The Oxford handbook of school psychology*. New York: Oxford University Press.

Caplan, M., Weissberg, R. P., Grober, J. S., Sivo, P. J., Grady, K., & Jacoby, C. (1992). Social competence promotion with inner-city and suburban young adolescents: Effects on school adjustment and alcohol use. *Journal of Consulting and Clinical Psychology, 60*(1), 56–63. doi:10.1037/0022-006X.60.1.56.

Carter-Black, J. (2007). Teaching cultural competence: An innovative strategy grounded in the universality of storytelling as depicted in African and African American storytelling traditions. *Journal of Social Work Education, 43*, 31–50.

Catalano, R. F., Berglund, M. L., Ryan, J. A. M., Lonczak, H. S., & Hawkins, J. D. (2002). Positive youth development in the United States: Research findings on evaluations of positive youth development programs. *Prevention and Treatment, 5*(15). http://journals.apa.org/prevention/volume5/pre0050015a.html. Accessed 12 Nov 2012.

Clark, M. A., Flower, K., Walton, J., & Oakley, E. (2008). Tackling male underachievement: Enhancing a strengths-based learning environment for middle school boys. *Professional School Counseling, 12*, 127–132.

Clonan, S. M., Chafouleas, S. M., McDougal, J. L., & Riley-Tillman, T. C. (2004). Positive psychology goes to school: Are we there yet? *Psychology in the Schools, 41*(1), 101–110.

Constantine, M., & Sue, D. W. (2006). Factors contributing to optimal human functioning of people of color in the United States. *The Counseling Psychologist, 34*, 228–244.

Dahlsgaard, K., Peterson, C., & Seligman, M. E. P. (2005). Shared virtue: The convergence of valued human strengths across culture and history. *Review of General Psychology, 9*, 203–213.

Day-Vines, N. L., & Terriquez, V. (2008). A strengths-based approach to promoting prosocial behavior among African American and Latino students. *Professional School Counseling, 12*, 170–175.

Dessel, A. (2010). Prejudice in schools: Promotion of an inclusive culture and climate. *Education and Urban Society, 42*, 407–429.

Durlak, J. A., Weissberg, R. P., Dynmicki, A. B., Taylor, R. D., & Schellinger, K. B. (2011). The impact of enhancing students' social and emotional learning: A meta-analysis of school-based universal interventions. *Child Development, 82*, 405–432.

Edwards, L. M., Holtz, C. A., & Green, M. B. (2007). Promoting strengths among culturally diverse youth in schools. *School Psychology Forum, 2*, 39–49.

Elias, M. J., Zins, J. E., Weissberg, K. S., Greenberg, M. T., Haynes, N. M., Kessler, R., et al. (1997). *Promoting social and emotional learning: Guidelines for educators*. Alexandria: Association for Supervision and Curriculum Development.

Espelage, D. L., Aragon, S. R., Birkett, M., & Koenig, B. W. (2008). Homophobic teasing, psychological outcomes, and sexual orientation among high school students: What influence do parents and schools have? *School Psychology Review, 37*, 202–216. http://www.nasponline.org/publications/spr/pdf/spr372espelage.pdf

Feliciano, C. (2001). The benefits of biculturalism: Exposure to immigrant culture and dropping out of school among Asian and Latino youths. *Social Science Quarterly, 82*(4), 865–879.

Flannery, D. J., Vazsonyi, A. T., Liau, A. K., Guo, S., Powell, K. E., Atha, H., Vesterdal, W., & Embry, D. (2003). Initial behavior outcomes for the PeaceBuilders universal school- based violence prevention program. *Developmental Psychology, 39*, 292–308. http://www.ncbi.nlm.nih.gov/pubmed/12661887

Fuligni, A. J., Witkow, M., & Garcia, C. (2005). Ethnic identity and the academic adjustment of adolescents from Mexican, Chinese, and European backgrounds. *Developmental Psychology, 41*, 799–811. http://www.ncbi.nlm.nih.gov/pubmed/16173876

Garcia, E. (2002). *Student cultural diversity*. Boston: Houghton Mifflin Company.

Greenberg, M. T. (1996). *The PATHS project: Preventive intervention for children: Final report to NIMH*. Seattle: University of Washington, Department of Psychology.

Greenberg, M. T., Weissberg, R. P., Obrien, M. U., Zins, J. E., Fredericks, L., Resnik, H., & Elias, M. J. (2003). Enhancing school-based prevention and youth development through coordinated social, emotional, and academic learning. *American Psychologist, 58*, 466–474. http://casel.org/wpcontent/uploads/2011/04/AmericanPsychologist2003.pdf

Hawkins, J. D., Oesterle, S., Brown, E. C., Arthur, M. W., Abbott, R. D., Fagan, A. A., & Catalano, R. F. (2009). Results of a type 2 translational research trial to prevent adolescent drug use and delinquency. *Archives of Pediatric and Adolescent Medicine, 163*, 789–798. http://www.ncbi.nlm.nih.gov/pubmed/19736331

Hays, P. A. (1996). Culturally responsive assessment with diverse older clients. *Professional Psychology: Research and Practice, 27*, 188–193.

Kahlenburg, R. D. (2006). Helping children move from bad schools to good ones. The Century Foundation. Retrieved from http://www.tcf.org/Publications/Education/kahlenbergsoa6-15-06.pdf

Kirby, D. B., Baumler, E., Coyle, K. K., Basen-Engquist, K., Parcel, G. S., Harrist, R., & Banspach, S. W. (2004). The "Safer Choices" intervention: Its impact on the sexual behaviors of different subgroups of high school students. *Journal of Adolescent Health, 35*, 442–452. http://www.ncbi.nlm.nih.gov/pmc/articles/PMC1913682/

Kuh, G. D., Kinzie, J., Buckley, J. A., Bridges, B. K., & Hayek, J. C. (2006). *What matters to student success: A review of the literature*. Retrieved October 8, 2011, from http://nces.ed.gov/npec/pdf/kuh_team_report.pdf

Kulis, S., Marsiglia, F. F., & Hecht, M. L. (2002). Gender labels and gender identity as predictors of drug use among ethically diverse middle school students. *Youth and Society, 33*, 442–475.

Ladson-Billings, G. (1995). Toward a theory of culturally relevant pedagogy. *American Educational Research Journal, 32*, 465–491. doi:10.3102/00028312032003465.

Lee, C. C. (2005a). *Multicultural issues in counseling*. Alexandria: American Counseling Association.

Lee, R. M. (2005b). Resilience against discrimination: Ethnic identity and other-group orientation as protective factors for Korean Americans. *Journal of Counseling Psychology, 52*, 36–44. doi:10.1037/0022-0167.52.1.36.

Lemerise, E. A., & Arsenio, W. F. (2000). An integrated model of emotion processes and cognition in social information processing. *Child Development, 71*, 107–118.

Lonborg, S. D., & Bowen, N. (2004). Counselors, communities, and spirituality: Ethical and multicultural considerations. *Professional School Counseling, 7*, 318–325.

Lopez, C., & DuBois, D. L. (2005). Peer victimization and rejection: Investigation of an integrative model of effects on emotional, behavioral, and academic adjustment in early adolescence. *Journal of Clinical Child and Adolescent Psychology, 34*, 25–36.
Lyubomirsky, S., King, L., & Diener, E. (2005). The benefits of frequent positive affect: Does happiness lead to success? *Psychological Bulletin, 131*, 803–855.
Magyar-Moe, J. L. (2009). Four-Front assessment approach. In S. J. Lopez (Ed.), *The encyclopedia of positive psychology*. Hoboken: Wiley-Blackwell Publishing.
Matthews, M., & Mahoney, A. (2005). Facilitating a smooth transitional process for immigrant Caribbean children: The role of teachers, social workers, and related professional staff. *Journal of Ethnic & Cultural Diversity in Social Work, 14*, 69–92.
McNeeley, C. A., Nonnemaker, J. M., & Blum, R. W. (2002). Promoting school connectedness: Evidence from the National Longitudinal Study of Adolescent Health. *Journal of School Health, 72*, 138–146.
National Center for Educational Statistics. (2008). Retrieved August 15, 2010, from http://nces.ed.gov/programs/coe/2010/section1/table-1er-1.asp
National Education Association. (2008). *Rankings and estimates: Rankings of the states 2008*. Retrieved from www.nea.org
Nickerson, A. (2007). The use and importance of strengths-based assessment. *School Psychology Forum: Research in Practice, 2*, 15–25.
Noguera, P. A. (2003). *City schools and the American dream*. New York: Teachers College Press.
O'Leary-Barrett, M., Mackie, C. J., Castellanos-Ryan, N., Al-Khudhairy, N., & Conrod, P. J. (2010). Personality-targeted interventions delay uptake of drinking and decrease risk of alcohol-related problems when delivered by teachers. *Journal of the American Academy of Child and Adolescent Psychiatry, 49*, 954–963. http://www.ncbi.nlm.nih.gov/pubmed/20732631
Olszewski-Kubilius, P., Lee, S., Ngoi, M., & Ngoi, D. (2004). Addressing the achievement gap between minority and nonminority children by increasing access to gifted programs. *Journal for the Education of the Gifted, 28*, 127 158. http://www.davidsongifted.org/db/Articles_id_10670.aspx
Osterman, K. F. (2000). Students' need for belonging in the school community. *Review of Educational Research, 70*, 323–367.
Phinney, J. S., Horenczyk, G., Liebkind, K., & Vedder, P. (2001). Ethnic identity, immigration, and well-being: An interactional perspective. *Journal of Social Issues, 57*, 493–510.
Rogers-Sirin, L., & Sirin, S. R. (2009). Cultural competence as an ethical requirement: Introducing a new educational model. *Journal of Diversity in Higher Education, 2*, 19–29.
Saleebey, D. (2008). Commentary on the strengths perspective and potential applications in school counseling. *Professional School Counseling, 12*, 68–75.
Slavin, R. E., Madden, N. A., Dolan, L. J., Wasik, B. A., Ross, S., Smith, L., & Dianda, M. (1996). Success for all: A summary of research. *Journal of Education for Students Placed at Risk, 1*(1), 41–76.
Smith, D. W., Redican, K. J., & Olsen, L. K. (1992). The longevity of growing healthy: An analysis of the eight original sties implementing the School Health Curriculum Project. *Journal of School Health, 62*(3), 83–87.
Snyder, C. R., Ritschel, L. A., Rand, K. L., & Berg, C. J. (2006). Balancing psychological assessments: Including strengths and hope in client reports. *Journal of Clinical Psychology, 62*, 33–46. http://www.ncbi.nlm.nih.gov/pubmed/16273519
Sue, D. W., & Constantine, M. G. (2003). Optimal human functioning in people of color in the United States. In B. W. Walsh (Ed.), *Counseling psychology and optimal human functioning* (pp. 151–169). Hillsdale: Lawrence Erlbaum Associates.
Thomas, R., & Perera, R. (2006). School-based programmes for preventing smoking. *Cochrane Database of Systematic Reviews, 3*, 1–30.
Ullucci, K., & Battey, D. (2011). Exposing color blindness/grounding color consciousness: Challenges for teacher education. *Urban Education, 46*, 1195–1295.
Vera, E. M., & Speight, S. L. (2003). Multicultural competence, social justice, and counseling psychology: Expanding our roles. *The Counseling Psychologist, 31*, 253–272.

Walker, K. L. (2011). Deficit thinking and the effective teacher. *Education and Urban Society, 43*, 576–597.
Walsh, M. E., Kenny, M. E., Wieneke, K. M., & Harrington, K. R. (2008). The Boston connects program: Promoting learning and healthy development. *Professional School Counseling, 12*, 166–169.
Weissberg, R. P., & Greenberg, M. T. (1998). Prevention science and collaborative community action research: Combining the best from both perspectives. *Journal of Mental Health, 7*(5), 479–492.
Weissberg, R. P., Barton, H. A., & Shriver, T. P. (1997). The social competence promotion program for young adolescents. In G. W. Albee & T. P. Gullotta (Eds.), *Primary prevention works* (pp. 268–290). Thousand Oaks: Sage.
Wiehe, S. E., Garrison, M. M., Christakis, D. A., Ebel, B. E., & Rivara, F. P. (2005). A systematic review of school-based smoking prevention trials with long-term follow-up. *Journal of Adolescent Health, 36*, 162–169. www.rwjf.org/publichealth/product.jsp?id=14464
Wright, B. A. (1991). Labeling: The need for greater person-environment individuation. In C. R. Snyder & D. R. Forsyth (Eds.), *Handbook of social and clinical psychology: The health perspective* (pp. 469–487). New York: Pergamon Press.
Zins, J. E., Weissberg, R. P., Wang, M. C., & Walberg, H. J. (Eds.). (2004). *Building academic success on social and emotional learning: What does the research say?* New York: Teachers College Press.

Chapter 15
A Positive Approach to Multiculturalism and Diversity Management in the Workplace

Carolyn M. Youssef-Morgan and James Hardy

Today, the global economy is allowing companies both large and small to compete in ways unheard of in the past. Competitive advantage is no longer gained solely through better logistics, reducing costs of production or adding new technology. The United States workforce is becoming increasingly diverse in terms of race, gender, culture, age, religion and sexual orientation, as well as personalities, work ethic, mental models, goals and aspirations. Along with the economic challenges of this decade, this multifaceted diversity is now a driving force for changes in how organizations leverage human capital to realize and maintain a sustainable competitive edge. Organizations are now learning to seek out change in unique ways that can lead to a human-based competitive advantage that competitors cannot readily copy or imitate (Luthans and Youssef 2004).

Moreover, in light of the present economic uncertainty, global insecurity and social value deterioration, many sources report that the current business world seems to be dominated by ineffective leaders, abusive supervision, unethical behaviors, discrimination, stress and burnout, and dysfunctional systems in general (e.g., Brown and Trevino 2006). Meanwhile, in the middle of this prevalent negativity, the workplace is craving for *positivity*. Positive organizational scholars define positivity in terms of elevating processes and outcomes, intentional behaviors that depart from the norm of a reference group in honorable ways, exceptional outcomes that dramatically exceed common or expected performance, and "an affirmative bias in change, or toward an emphasis on strengths, capabilities, and possibilities rather than problems, threats, and weakness" (Cameron 2008, p. 8). The workplace has moved beyond just being a source of income to also giving a diverse workforce meaning, personal value, and opportunities to flourish (Keyes and Haidt 2003).

C.M. Youssef-Morgan, Ph.D. (✉) • J. Hardy
College of Business, Bellevue University,
1000 Galvin Road South, Bellevue, NE 68005, USA
e-mail: Carolyn.youssef@bellevue.edu

J. Teramoto Pedrotti and L.M. Edwards (eds.), *Perspectives on the Intersection of Multiculturalism and Positive Psychology*, Cross-Cultural Advancements in Positive Psychology 7, DOI 10.1007/978-94-017-8654-6_15,

In this chapter, we make the case for the value of and the critical contributions positivity can make in leveraging diversity and multiculturalism in the workplace. Since this is the only chapter in this volume that focuses on the interface between work and multiculturalism, we start with an overview of diversity as it is manifested, influences, and is influenced by the workplace. We then introduce workplace positivity in general, and more specifically several work-related positive constructs and approaches that emerged as offshoots of the positive psychology movement. The term "diversity" as a demographic differentiator across groups in the workplace has been marked by a history of prejudice and an inferiority perspective (Ramarajan and Thomas 2012) that can lead to a deficit approach to multiculturalism and diversity management. We distinguish this deficit approach from a positive approach, which we propose should go beyond reducing, neutralizing, or even overcoming the negative, to also challenge the status quo and find new ways to understand, appreciate and leverage the full potential of a diverse workforce. Linkages between diversity, multiculturalism and positivity are then proposed, and future directions for the research and practice of multiculturalism in the workplace are offered.

15.1 Diversity in the Workplace

Thomas and Ely (1996) define diversity as "the varied perspectives and approaches to work that members of different identity groups bring" (p. 80). Large scale changes in the demographic makeup of the U.S. have led to its labor force being the most diverse in history.

15.1.1 Racial and Ethnic Diversity

Between 2010 and 2050, the U.S. population is projected to grow from 310 to 439 million, an increase of 42 % (Vincent and Velkoff 2010). The nation will also become more racially and ethnically diverse. By 2042, the U.S. population will be more non-White than White, resulting in Whites becoming a majority minority (Grieco and Trevelyan 2010). Over the last 40 years, the foreign-born population of the United States has also continued to increase in relation to the total population. In 1970, the percentage of foreign-born residents was 9.6 million or 4.7 %. By the year 2009, some estimates were around 38.5 million or 12.5 % of the total United States population (Grieco and Trevelyan 2010). This explosion in growth has come from all corners of the globe and has shown no signs of slowing down. Grieco and Trevelyan observe that the growth in foreign-born population has come from Latin America (53 %), Asia (28 %), Europe (13 %), Africa (4 %), with the remaining 3 % coming from other regions. These cross-cultural differences (i.e., between people coming from different countries) contribute to the unique multicultural makeup of the United States.

One of the challenges with these demographic shifts is the potential impact on the educational experience of the workers. For example, Hispanic workers currently have the lowest education attainment of any other major ethnic group in the United States, while they are also the fastest growing major ethnic group (Thomas and Ely 1996). If the educational attainments of Hispanics entering the workforce do not increase at a higher rate, the United States will see a challenge in meeting the skill demands that the knowledge economy requires.

15.1.2 Age Diversity

In 2050, the number of individuals in the United States aged 65 or older is projected by the U.S. Census Bureau to reach over 88 million, which is double the number of seniors in 2011. Over the coming decade, substantial growth will occur among the population of 65- to 69-year-olds. This group is expected by the U.S. Census Bureau to increase by another 37 % from 2010 to 2020. The increase in the age group 70 and over is anticipated to be almost 40 %, from 24.6 to 31.8 million during the same period of time (Grieco and Trevelyan 2010; Vincent and Velkoff 2010).

Four generations are currently represented in the workplace (Meister and Willyerd 2010): the Silent generation (born between 1925 and 1945), the Baby Boomers (born between 1946 and 1964), Generation Xers (born from 1965 to 1980) and the Millennials (born between 1981 and 1999). The Silent generation was the first to be grouped by age. Before this generation, the expectation for young adults was to work or start a family prior to finishing a secondary education, and most never completed a secondary education (Meister and Willyerd 2010). The Baby Boomers were born just after World War II. They witnessed the social changes brought by the Civil Rights movement and the Vietnam War, great technological changes and an unprecedented accumulation of wealth. The Baby Boomers, currently the largest generation, were raised on hard work and stayed with one company for the majority of their careers (Cennamo and Gardner 2008; Dries et al. 2008).

Generation X was raised on television and the increased access and exposure to world events. They witnessed societal changes such as the collapse of the Berlin Wall and Communism, and watched the Challenger Disaster and Desert Storm from their living rooms (Twenge and Campbell 2008). Generation Y or the Millennial Generation witnessed the Y2K event. For this generation, reality television, school shootings, and the war on terrorism are in full swing (Cennamo and Gardner 2008; Dries et al. 2008). Generation Y has seen the devastation of unethical organizational actions such as Enron, TYCO and Arthur Anderson to families and careers. According to Greenberg (2008), this generation desires to leverage morality and revolutionary change to make the world a better place.

Each of the four generations brings its own set of values, experiences, perspectives and ethics to the workplace, forcing society to look at life and work through a different lens, and resulting in key changes to workplace policies and procedures. For example, the Traditionalist Generation is influencing the design of retirement and savings programs and seasonal work. Baby Boomers and Generation X are changing how health and wellness, women in the workplace, and work life balance are tackled by major employers in order to recruit and retain key associates that value these changes. The Millennial Generation is changing how the workplace integrates technology through facets such as social media.

15.1.3 Gender and Sexual Orientation

The twenty-first century has lived up to previous expectations of more women and employees with different racial and ethnic backgrounds, sexual orientations, and intergenerational differences than in the past. For example, Griffith and Hebl (2002) noted that gay and lesbian employees accounted for between 10 and 14 % of the workforce. However, the research and data has been limited on this group even though gay employees constitute a larger proportion of the workforce than many other minority groups (Ragins et al. 2003).

With regard to gender, in 2009, 59.2 % of women, or 60 million, were in the workforce, compared to approximately 30 million in 1970 (U.S. Bureau of Labor 2009). This research additionally states that of the 60 million, 26 % are the primary wage earners of their families, and that figure has almost doubled over the last 25 years. It has been well documented that there has been an underrepresentation of women in leadership roles. Eagly and Chin (2010) note that this trend is starting to change with the beginning of the second decade of the twenty-first century. According to the U.S. Bureau of Labor Statistics (2009), 23 % of chief executives of all U.S. organizations in the public and private sectors are now women.

15.1.4 Research Findings on Diversity in the Workplace

As the workforce in the United States becomes increasingly diverse, organizations that desire to attract and retain the best talent need to find ways to attract individuals from a wide range of backgrounds. Diversity is important because demographically diverse groups have been shown to outperform homogeneous groups on problem solving and creativity tasks due to their diverse perspectives (Konrad 2003). Recent research demonstrates a relationship between diversity and organizational performance. For example, firms that are more open to traditionally underrepresented groups have been shown to significantly outperform others in the same industry (Von Bergen et al. 2005). In addition, research supports a relationship between gender diversity and organizational performance, but this relationship has been shown to be moderated by the organization's culture and strategic orientation (Dwyer et al. 2003). The moderating effect of business strategy has also been supported in the relationship between racial diversity and organizational performance (Richard 2000). For example, in the banking industry, studies show that racial diversity has a positive effect on organizational performance in banks pursuing an innovation strategy, but a negative effect on those low on innovation (Richard et al. 2003).

Moreover, a number of studies show that the relationship between diversity and organizational performance is curvilinear and industry-specific. For example, the relationships between gender and racial diversity, and organizational performance have been shown to be curvilinear and moderated by two dimensions of the organization's strategy, namely entrepreneurial orientation and risk-taking (Richard et al. 2004). Specifically, in firms with innovative orientations there was a u-shaped relationship between diversity and performance. In high-risk-taking firms, an inverted u-shaped relationship was found between gender diversity and performance.

Finally, recent meta-analytical findings shed additional light on the nature of the relationship between diversity and organizational performance. Culturally diverse teams realize gains through increased creativity and satisfaction, but at the same time incur losses due to increased task conflict and decreased social integration. The relative gains and losses are contingent on a myriad of contextual factors (Stahl et al. 2010). For example, white individuals' information processing has been shown to improve in heterogonous groups, which is inconsistent with the common notion that the primary gains from diversity are attributable to the novel contributions of racial or ethnic minority members (Sommers et al. 2008). Group dynamics and organizational processes have also been supported as important moderators for important outcomes such as satisfaction and turnover (Kochan et al. 2003).

15.2 Positive Psychology in the Workplace

Similar to the field of psychology as a whole, until recently the emphasis of organizational practitioners and scholars has excessively focused on addressing the negative attributes and weaknesses of individuals and organizations as the best approach to improve performance and effectiveness. However, several positively oriented approaches have shifted the emphasis to the positive attributes of individuals and organizations, such as their strengths, capabilities, potential, wellbeing, and contributions to the greater good (Keyes and Haidt 2003). Approaches such as these can be beneficial in creating positive environments in the workplace that are supportive of diversity. Two of these, Positive Organizational Behavior and Positive Organizational Scholarship, will be discussed here in general before moving to their potential use within a multicultural environment.

15.2.1 Positive Organizational Behavior and Psychological Capital

Luthans (2002a) defines positive organizational behavior (POB) as "the study and application of positively oriented human resources strengths and psychological capacities that can be measured, developed, and effectively managed for performance improvement in today's workplace" (p. 59). For a positive psychological capacity to qualify for inclusion in POB, it must have sufficient theory and research foundations and valid measures (Luthans and Youssef 2007). The inclusion criterion of theory, research, and measurement is what separates POB from the popular, positively-oriented personal development literature (Youssef and Luthans 2009). It also must be state-like (as opposed to trait-like), which would make it malleable and thus open to development and manageable for performance improvement, also a criteria for inclusion in POB. Positive states that meet the POB definitional criteria are self-efficacy, hope, optimism and resilience, which are primarily researched, measured, developed, and managed at the individual, micro level (Luthans 2002a, b; Youssef and Luthans 2007).

The four psychological resources of self-efficacy, hope, optimism and resilience have been shown to form a higher-order construct that has been termed Psychological Capital, or PsyCap (Luthans et al. 2007a). PsyCap is defined as: "an individual's positive psychological state of development and is characterized by: (a) having confidence (self-efficacy) to take on and put in the necessary effort to succeed at challenging tasks; (b) making a positive attribution (optimism) about succeeding now and in the future; (c) persevering toward goals and, when necessary, redirecting paths to goals (hope) in order to succeed; and (d) when beset by problems and adversity, sustaining and bouncing back and even beyond (resiliency) to attain success" (Luthans et al. 2007b, p. 3).

PsyCap has been demonstrated conceptually and empirically to be a valid and reliably measurable higher-order core construct. The underlying theoretical mechanism for PsyCap, shared across its four constituent psychological resources, is a cognitive, agentic, developmental capacity representing "one's positive appraisal of circumstances and probability for success based on motivated effort and perseverance" (Luthans et al. 2007a, p. 550). Avey et al. (2011) note that those higher in PsyCap expect positive things to happen at work, believe they create their own sense of accomplishment, and are more resistant to setbacks when compared with those lower in PsyCap. They are more committed to their organizations due to the buildup of self-efficacy and accomplishment which drives worker engagement. Psychological capital also goes beyond human capital and social capital in that it focuses on what individuals can become now and in the future, rather than whom or what an individual currently knows (Luthans and Youssef 2004).

Beside this theoretical foundation, PsyCap as a higher-order construct also meets the POB inclusion criterion of malleability and developmental potential. Several successful interventions have been implemented to increase PsyCap in work settings (Luthans et al. 2010), including online interventions (Luthans et al. 2008b). The state-like, developmental quality of PsyCap presents management researchers and practitioners with a new potential source of human-based competitive advantage. Finally, in terms of performance impact, recent meta-analytical findings support PsyCap as a predictor of job performance, as well as several other desirable attitudinal and behavioral outcomes directly related to performance such as job satisfaction, organizational commitment, psychological well-being, cynicism, turnover intentions, job stress, anxiety, and employee deviance (Avey et al. 2011).

Thus, PsyCap can have a substantial impact in terms of both employee and organizational performance and wellbeing. Particularly relevant for this chapter is the emerging evidence for the external validity and applicability of PsyCap cross-culturally. Consistent with research findings in the U.S., recent studies in other countries also demonstrate significant relationships between PsyCap and desirable outcomes in the workplace (Badran and Youssef 2011; Luthans et al. 2008a; Story et al. 2013; Tatiukoskula et al. 2010). Though research studies with multicultural populations within one context (e.g., the U.S. or another country) have yet to be done, it may be that PsyCap can benefit in these situations as well.

15.2.2 Positive Organizational Scholarship

Another application of positive psychology in the workplace is positive organizational scholarship (POS), which has been defined as the scientific investigation of positive, life-giving phenomena in organizations. This includes elevating processes, outcomes, interpersonal and structural dynamics, and other factors that can create a positive environment for flourishing (Cameron and Caza 2004). Of particular relevance here would be an environment that is open to and appreciative of multiculturalism.

The positivity literature in general, and especially its applications to the workplace, have specifically emphasized cross-cultural differences and the possibility for positivity to be culturally-based (Lopez and Snyder 2009). Thus, the potential for positivity to enhance the management of a multicultural workforce is there, but largely remains unexplored. The balance of this chapter is a step in that direction. In the next section, we distinguish between deficit and positive approaches to diversity management and multiculturalism and propose linkages between multiculturalism and positivity in the workplace.

15.3 Toward a More Positive Multicultural Workplace

Positive psychology received increased attention when Martin Seligman, former president of the American Psychological Association, called psychologists to redirect their focus away from the "disease model" that emphasizes healing mental illness, and toward psychology's other two "forgotten missions" of helping healthy people become happier and more productive and actualizing human potential. To date, despite the increasing interest in and recognition of the positive outcomes of diversity, the prevalent paradigm for managing diversity in the workplace (and many other contexts) seems to be consistent with the same "disease model" that guided the field of psychology since World War II. In this model, diversity is managed through a deficit approach, as a problem to be solved, rather than an opportunity to be pursued and leveraged. In contrast, positive psychology needs to move away from "inferiority" and "deficit" models of diversity, and toward recognizing the strengths of cultural pluralism in general (Pedrotti et al. 2009), and particularly the untapped potential of a multicultural workplace.

15.3.1 *From a Deficit to a Positive Approach*

Diversity has been defined as "a characteristic of a group (of two or more people) that refers to demographic differences among group members in race, ethnicity, gender, social class, religion, nationality, sexual orientation, or other dimensions of social identity that are marked by a history of intergroup prejudice, stigma, discrimination, or oppression ... diversity as variety" (Ramarajan and Thomas 2012, p. 553). This definition clearly highlights an inferiority perspective, and would promote a deficit approach to the management of diversity and multiculturalism in the workplace.

Unfortunately, the diversity literature for the most part has been dominated by this deficit approach. For example, in their comprehensive review of over a decade of diversity research, Ramarajan and Thomas (2012) found that only about 25 % of articles dealt with positive aspects of diversity such as equality, positive relationships, and positive outcomes, while the rest emphasized the reduction or minimization of negative outcomes (e.g., prejudice, stigma, discrimination, oppression, conflict). There is now substantial support to the notion that positive and negative constructs and processes are not necessarily polar opposites on the same continuum, but may represent different continuums, with unique antecedents, underlying mechanisms and outcomes (Cacioppo and Berntson 1994; Dunlop and Lee 2004; Sackett et al. 2006; Taylor 1991). Eliminating or reducing negative or dysfunctional beliefs, attitudes and behaviors may be necessary to achieve a neutral, equilibrium state, but not sufficient for the positive outcomes of diversity to materialize (Pittinsky et al. 2011).

A positive approach to multiculturalism and diversity management should go beyond reducing, neutralizing, or even overcoming the negative, to also challenge the status quo and find new ways to understand, appreciate and leverage the full potential of a diverse workforce. This is also consistent with what Luthans and Avolio (2009) call an *inquiry perspective*, rather than the *advocacy* perspective that dominates most problem-oriented models, including many of the diversity management programs and initiatives to-date. It also aligns with what positive organizational scholars refer to as *appreciative inquiry*, where the emphasis is on phenomena of excellence, exceptional performance, and the art of asking the right questions to better understand the mechanisms toward revolutionary, strengths-based change (Cooperrider and Whitney 2005).

Importantly, the goal should not be to eliminate or neutralize cultural differences. In fact, Chen et al. (2009) challenge the emphasis of cross-cultural research on cultural differences as the most effective way to advance knowledge in this area.

They make the case for theoretical frameworks that go beyond cross-cultural differences (or similarities), toward innovative, "frame-breaking" (Chen et al. 2009, p. 220) models that can inform research and practice, even in culturally homogenous contexts. Thus, the value of pluralism should become the primary emphasis, where cultural differences are viewed as unique resources and strengths that can positively contribute to and promote the overall healthy functioning of individuals, groups, organizations and societies. This perspective stands in stark contrast with the common notion of the U.S. culture as a "melting pot" where diverse groups are to blend in and produce a homogenous culture over time (Pedrotti et al. 2009). Instead, cultural differences are viewed here as value-adding mechanisms, rather than problems or "errors" to be eliminated. In the workplace, it is those differences that bring added value to an organization through life experiences, which help shape a varied viewpoint on work related issues. These unique perspectives help organizations achieve new goals and promote innovative ideas and new techniques for problem solving. In addition, heterogeneity can promote a broadened perspective and higher performance among majority groups as well (Sommers et al. 2008).

We propose that positivity may engender the dynamic mechanisms that can help leverage diversity, create long-term competitive advantage, and in the process shape a clearer vision for what constitutes optimal functioning in a multicultural workplace. Two specific sets of mechanisms are proposed next: one at the individual-level, and the other at the organizational level.

15.3.2 Contributions of Individual-Level Positivity to Multiculturalism in the Workplace

At the individual level, PsyCap represents an agentic resource that can be voluntarily mobilized to create positive appraisals of current events and situations and a positive outlook toward the future. In turn, this positivity can generate the motivation to pursue challenging goals, the ability to generate ways to achieve those goals, and the staying power when faced with obstacles (Luthans et al. 2007a, b). PsyCap can leverage multiculturalism in the workplace through several mechanisms. First, managers and employees with high PsyCap, whether members of the majority or a minority group, are more likely to view and cognitively appraise the presence of diversity in the workplace as an opportunity to be pursued, rather than a problem or a threat to be avoided. As a result, they are more likely to interact with their "different" colleagues. Contact theory of diversity, which has received significant support (Pettigrew and Tropp 2006), implies that this increased contact alone can help diminish intergroup prejudice. However, positivity can also expand the impact of contact into finding common interests, developing deeper relationships, and collaboration toward common goals. For example, PsyCap hope can promote the pursuit of a broadened set of pathways toward goals, which would likely be more inclusive of multicultural individuals, perspectives and experiences.

Second, research shows that members of both majority and minority groups would like to have more interactions with each other, but that fear of rejection and perception of other group's disinterest in interaction are some of the primary barriers of interracial interaction (Shelton and Richeson 2005). Positivity can help resolve these self-other biases. PsyCap triggers agentic actions and motivated goal pursuit. In the context of a multicultural workplace, this would mean a stronger desire to interact with those who are different from oneself, and being more proactive to do so despite personal biases or social barriers. Once sufficient interaction has been initiated, the biases of other members of both groups are expected to diminish (Turner et al. 2008). More importantly, beyond just no longer avoiding others who are different, over time mutual reciprocity and *allophelia* (liking of members of other groups) can trigger distinct positive outcomes such as intentionally seeking collaboration with and being more generous toward others. These types of outcomes cannot be explained only through deficit perspectives such as reduced prejudice (Pittinsky et al. 2011).

Third, the positive nature of PsyCap might yield what Barbara Fredrickson (2001, 2009) calls a "broaden-and-build" effect. In this theory, positivity can "broaden" one's thought action repertoires, allowing for a wider range of perceived choices and action tendencies. In terms of multiculturalism, PsyCap may expand perceptions and beliefs of what is possible when culturally diverse individuals and groups are integrated. It may also facilitate the development of creative approaches or pathways to leverage diversity, for example through increased collaboration and communication. On the other hand, negativity has a narrowing effect. It triggers a fight-or-flight mode that limits one's thoughts and actions to tried-and-true habitual tendencies. In the context of a deficit approach, this would be comparable to stereotypes and other perceptual biases that hinder effective interaction, reciprocity and liking across diverse groups.

Positivity can also "build" physical, social, and psychological inventories of resources, which can be drawn upon in times of negativity (Fredrickson 2001, 2009). In the context of multiculturalism, people from different backgrounds have been found to utilize similar cognitive and behavioral coping mechanisms in relation to adversities, despite differences in adaptive mechanisms and outcomes (Shaw et al. 1997). Thus, we propose that members of majority and minority groups who have higher PsyCap may be more likely to overcome the obstacles and setbacks of prejudice, stigma, discrimination, oppression, and conflict. They are more likely to resiliently bounce back from these situations, and confidently, hopefully and optimistically continue to assert their unique identities and contributions and those of the other groups represented in their workplace.

This is not to say that these problems and biases will completely give way to higher tolerance or more inclusion, nor do we believe that this is necessary. If positivity can drive sufficient positive, appreciative, respectful and genuinely inclusive interactions to balance prejudiced, discriminatory or oppressive encounters, an optimal medium can be created for leveraging multiculturalism. This is also consistent with the recent meta-analytical findings cited earlier (Stahl et al. 2010) supporting the outcomes of workplace diversity as the balance between the realized gains (e.g., increased creativity) and losses (e.g., conflict), as determined by a wide range of contextual factors. We propose positivity as one of those critical intervening factors in the dynamic process of balancing the benefits and costs of diversity and multiculturalism. It is important to note that the presence of the negative is also necessary to challenge the status quo, confront inequities, and provide a force social change (Cameron 2008; Ramarajan and Thomas 2012), all of which have been critical for the strides made to-date in managing diversity. Indeed, positivity can facilitate organizational change (Avey et al. 2008).

15.3.3 *Contributions of Organizational-Level Positivity to Multiculturalism*

Organizational-level theories in diversity research also exhibit the same distinctions between advocacy and inquiry. According to Ely and Thomas (2001), organizations may hold one of three distinct perspectives on diversity in the workplace. The first is the *discrimination-and-fairness perspective*, in which the emphasis is on the moral obligation to restore equity and justice. The second is the *access-and-legitimacy perspective*, which emphasizes the utilitarian value of diversity in facilitating the organization's access to and giving it a legitimate image in a diverse marketplace. The third is the *integration-and learning perspective* in which diversity is viewed as a resource for learning, development, adaptation and change.

Interestingly, only the third perspective was shown to relate to sustainable positive outcomes (Ely and Thomas 2001). It can be argued that the other two perspectives are narrower and more deficit-oriented. For example, the discrimination-and-fairness perspective may be motivated by the fear of negative legal and social consequences. The access-and-legitimacy perspective may be motivated by the avoidance of negative reputational and economic consequences. Research grounded in a deficit perspective blames the victims of established oppression for their own victimization by referring to negative stereotypes and assumptions regarding certain groups or communities. This perspective overlooks the root causes of oppression by localizing the issue within individuals and their communities (Bourdieu 1997).

On the other hand the integration-and learning perspective is motivated by respect for the uniqueness of diverse groups and appreciation for what they can offer, which can be more instrumental toward the pursuit of excellence and striving toward the realization of full human and organizational potential. Indeed, positivity has been shown to mediate the relationship between a supportive organizational climate and employee performance (Luthans et al. 2008c). This would imply that positivity can accelerate the positive outcomes of an integration-and-learning perspective.

15.4 Conclusion and Future Directions

The business environment is characterized by constant and revolutionary change. In order to remain competitive, organizations are in need for a multicultural workforce that can adaptively capitalize on both the similarities and differences of diverse groups, within a framework of appreciation and respect for human individuality and uniqueness. Positivity offers a new perspective for leveraging multiculturalism in the workplace. Future research and practice should explore this notion.

First, most of the literature approaches diversity from a deficit perspective, as a problem, rather than as an opportunity. New conceptual models that emphasize the positive dimensions of multiculturalism and their distinct antecedents, mechanisms and outcomes are needed (Ramarajan and Thomas 2012). In practice, organizations should approach diversity from an integration-and-learning perspective in order to realize its full benefits and leverage it as a source of sustainable, human-based competitive advantage (Ely and Thomas 2001).

Second, the diversity literature in general seems to be fragmented across levels of analysis. Multi-level research can facilitate the understanding of positivity across individual, group, organizational and societal boundaries. In application to practice, organizations need to assess the fit of potential positive diversity initiatives with the various internal and external environmental contingencies (Richard 2000; Richard et al. 2003, 2004).

Third, similar to many psychosocial phenomena, positive approaches to multiculturalism in the workplace are more likely to be understood, appreciated and leveraged through longitudinal research designs and long term implementation and evaluation. Organizations that truly want to realize the benefits of a multicultural work environment should be willing to sustain their investment in appreciative inquiry, integration-and-learning, and other positive initiatives until optimal functioning and flourishing can be manifested.

References

Avey, J. B., Wernsing, T. S., & Luthans, F. (2008). Can positive employees help positive organizational change? *The Journal of Applied Behavioral Science, 44*, 48–70.

Avey, J. B., Reichard, R. J., Luthans, F., & Mhatre, K. H. (2011). Meta-analysis of the impact of positive psychological capital on employee attitudes, behaviors, and performance. *Human Resource Development Quarterly, 22*, 127–152.

Badran, M. A., & Youssef, C. M. (2011). *West meets middle-east: Psychological capital and job satisfaction*. Paper presented at the National Academy of Management, San Antonio, TX.

Bourdieu, P. (1997). The forms of capital. In A. Halsey, H. Lauder, P. Brown, & A. Wells (Eds.), *Education: Culture, economy, and society* (pp. 40–58). Oxford: Oxford University Press.

Brown, M. E., & Trevino, L. K. (2006). Ethical leadership: A review and future directions. *Leadership Quarterly, 17*, 595–616.

Cacioppo, J. T., & Berntson, G. G. (1994). Relationship between attitudes and evaluative space: A critical review, with emphasis on the separability of positive and negative substrates. *Psychological Bulletin, 115*, 401–423.

Cameron, K. S. (2008). Paradox in positive organizational change. *Journal of Applied Behavioral Science, 44*, 7–24.

Cameron, K. S., & Caza, A. (2004). Contributions to the discipline of positive organizational scholarship. *American Behavioral Scientist, 47*, 731–739.

Cennamo, L., & Gardner, D. (2008). Generational differences in work values, outcomes and person-organisation values fit. *Journal of Managerial Psychology, 23*, 891–906.

Chen, Y., Leung, K., & Chen, C. (2009). Bringing national culture to the table: Making a difference with cross-cultural differences and perspectives. *Academy of Management Annals, 3*, 217–249.

Cooperrider, D. L., & Whitney, D. (2005). *Appreciative inquiry: A positive revolution in change*. San Francisco: Berrett-Koehler.

Dries, N., Pepermans, R., & De Kerpel, E. (2008). Exploring four generations' beliefs about career: Is "satisfied" the new "successful"? *Journal of Managerial Psychology, 23*, 907–928.

Dunlop, P. D., & Lee, K. (2004). Workplace deviance, organizational citizenship behavior, and business unit performance: The bad apples do spoil the whole barrel. *Journal of Organizational Behavior, 25*, 67–80.

Dwyer, S., Richard, O. C., & Chadwick, K. (2003). Gender diversity in management and firm performance: The influence of growth orientation and organizational culture. *Journal of Business Research, 56*, 1009–1019.

Eagly, A. H., & Chin, J. L. (2010). Diversity and leadership in a changing world. *American Psychologist, 65*, 216–224.

Ely, R. J., & Thomas, D. A. (2001). Cultural diversity at work: The moderating effects of work group perspectives on diversity. *Administrative Science Quarterly, 46*, 229–273.

Fredrickson, B. L. (2001). The role of positive emotions in positive psychology: The broaden-and-build theory of positive emotions. *American Psychologist, 56*, 218–226.

Fredrickson, B. L. (2009). *Positivity*. New York: Crown/Random House.

Greenberg, E. H. (2008). *Generation we*. Emeryville: Pachatusan.

Grieco, E. M., & Trevelyan, E. N. (2010, October). *Place of birth of the foreign-born population: 2009*. American Community Survey Briefs. Retrieved from United States Census Bureau website: http://www.census.gov/prod/2010pubs/acsbr09-15.pdf

Griffith, K. H., & Hebl, M. R. (2002). The disclosure dilemma for gay men and lesbians: "Coming Out" at work. *Journal of Applied Psychology, 87*, 1191–1199.

Keyes, C., & Haidt, J. (Eds.). (2003). *Flourishing: Positive psychology and the life well-lived*. Washington, DC: American Psychological Association.

Kochan, T., Bezrukova, K., Ely, R., Jackson, S., Joshi, A., Jehn, K., Leonard, J., Levine, D., & Thomas, D. (2003). The effects of diversity on business performance: Report of the diversity research network. *Human Resource Management, 42*(1), 3–21.

Konrad, A. (2003). Defining the domain of workplace diversity scholarship. *Group & Organizational Management, 28*, 4–17.

Lopez, S. J., & Snyder, C. R. (Eds.). (2009). *Oxford handbook of positive psychology* (2nd ed.). New York: Oxford University Press.

Luthans, F. J. (2002a). The need for and meaning of positive organizational behaviour. *Journal of Organizational Behavior, 23*, 695–706.

Luthans, F. (2002b). Positive organizational behavior: Developing and managing psychological strengths. *Academy of Management Executive, 16*, 57–72.

Luthans, F., & Avolio, B. J. (2009). The 'point' of positive organizational behavior. *Journal of Organizational Behavior, 30*, 291–307.

Luthans, F., & Youssef, C. M. (2004). Human, social, and now positive psychological capital management: Investing in people for competitive advantage. *Organizational Dynamics, 33*, 143–160.

Luthans, F., & Youssef, C. M. (2007). Emerging positive organizational behavior. *Journal of Management, 33*, 321–349.

Luthans, F., Avolio, B. J., Avey, J. B., & Norman, S. M. (2007a). Psychological capital: Measurement and relationship with performance and satisfaction. *Personnel Psychology, 60*, 541–572.

Luthans, F., Youssef, C. M., & Avolio, B. J. (2007b). *Psychological capital: Developing the human competitive edge*. Oxford, UK: Oxford University Press.

Luthans, F., Avey, J. B., Clapp-Smith, R., & Li, W. (2008a). More evidence on the value of Chinese workers' psychological capital: A potentially unlimited competitive resource? *The International Journal of Human Resources Management, 19*, 818–827.

Luthans, F., Avey, J. B., & Patera, J. L. (2008b). Experimental analysis of a web-based training intervention to develop positive psychological capital. *Academy of Management Learning and Education, 7*, 209–221.

Luthans, F., Norman, S. M., Avolio, B. J., & Avey, J. B. (2008c). The mediating role of psychological capital in the supportive organizational climate-employee performance relationship. *Journal of Organizational Behavior, 29*, 219–238.

Luthans, F., Avey, J. B., Avolio, B. J., & Peterson, S. J. (2010). The development and resulting performance impact of positive psychological capital. *Human Resource Development Quarterly, 21*, 41–67.

Meister, J. C., & Willyerd, K. (2010). *The 2020 workplace*. New York: HarperCollins.

Pedrotti, J. T., Edwards, L. M., & Lopez, S. J. (2009). Putting positive psychology into a multicultural context. In S. J. Lopez (Ed.), *Oxford handbook of positive psychology* (2nd ed., pp. 49–57). New York: Oxford University Press.

Pettigrew, T., & Tropp, L. R. (2006). A meta-analytic test of intergroup contact theory. *Journal of Personality and Social Psychology, 90*, 751–783.

Pittinsky, T. L., Rosenthal, S., & Montoya, R. M. (2011). Liking is not the opposite of disliking: The functional separability of positive and negative attitudes toward minority groups. *Cultural Diversity and Ethnic Minority Psychology, 17*, 134–143.

Ragins, B. R., Cornwell, J. M., & Miller, J. S. (2003). Heterosexism in the workplace. *Group & Organization Management, 28*, 45–74.

Ramarajan, L., & Thomas, D. (2012). A positive approach to studying diversity in organizations. In K. Cameron & G. Spreitzer (Eds.), *Oxford handbook of positive organizational scholarship* (pp. 552–565). New York: Oxford University Press.

Richard, O. C. (2000). Racial diversity, business strategy, and firm performance: A resource based view. *Academy of Management Journal, 43*, 164–177.

Richard, O. C., McMillan, A., Chadwick, K., & Dwyer, S. (2003). Employing an innovation strategy in racially diverse workforces. *Group & Organization Management, 28*, 107–126.

Richard, O. C., Barnett, T., Dwyer, S., & Chadwick, K. (2004). Cultural diversity in management, firm performance, and the moderating role of entrepreneurial orientation dimensions. *Academy of Management Journal, 47*, 255–266.

Sackett, P. R., Berry, C. M., Wiemann, S. A., & Laczo, R. M. (2006). Citizenship and counterproductive behavior: Clarifying relations between the two domains. *Human Performance, 19*, 441–464.

Shaw, W. S., Patterson, T. L., Semple, S. J., Grant, I., Yu, E. S. H., Zhang, M. Y., He, Y., & Wu, W. Y. (1997). A cross-cultural validation of coping strategies and their associations with caregiving distress. *Gerontologist, 37*, 490–504.

Shelton, J. N., & Richeson, J. A. (2005). Intergroup contact and pluralistic ignorance. *Journal of Personality and Social Psychology, 88*, 91–107.

Sommers, S. R., Warp, L. S., & Mahoney, C. C. (2008). Cognitive effects of racial diversity: White individuals' information processing in heterogeneous groups. *Journal of Experimental Social Psychology, 44*, 1129–1136.

Stahl, G. K., Maznevski, M. L., Voigt, A., & Jonsen, K. (2010). Unraveling the effects of cultural diversity in teams: A meta-analysis of research on multicultural work groups. *Journal of International Business Studies, 41*, 690–709.

Story, J. S., Youssef, C. M., Luthans, F., Barbuto, J. E., & Bovaird, J. (2013). Contagion effect of global leaders' positive psychological capital on followers: Does distance and quality of relationship matter? *International Journal of Human Resource Management, 24*, 2534–2553.

Tatiukoskula, S., Luthans, B. C., & Luthans, F. (2010). *Empirical evidence of the value of an unrecognized resource for economic development in Southeast Asia: The psychological capital of Thai entrepreneurs*. Paper presented at Pan Pacific Conference, Bali, Indonesia.

Taylor, S. E. (1991). Asymmetrical effects of positive and negative events: The mobilization-minimization hypothesis. *Psychological Bulletin, 110*, 67–85.

Thomas, D. A., & Ely, R. J. (1996). Making differences matter: A new paradigm for managing diversity. *Harvard Business Review, 74*, 79–91.

Turner, R. N., Hewstone, M., Voci, A., & Vonofakou, C. (2008). A test of the extended contact hypothesis: The mediating role of intergroup anxiety, perceived ingroup and outgroup norms, and inclusion of the outgroup in the self. *Journal of Personality and Social Psychology, 95*, 843–860.

Twenge, J. M., & Campbell, S. M. (2008). Generational differences in psychological traits and their impact on the workplace. *Journal of Managerial Psychology, 23*, 862–877.

U.S. Bureau of Labor Statistics. (2009). *Household data annual averages: Employed persons*. Retrieved October 13, 2011, from http://www.bls.gov/cps/cpsaat10.pdf

Vincent, G. K., & Velkoff, V. A. (2010, May). *The next four decades – The older population in the United States: 2010–2050 – Population estimates and projections*. Retrieved November 30, 2012, from United States Census Bureau website: http://www.census.gov/prod/2010pubs/p25-1138.pdf

Von Bergen, C. W., Soper, B., & Parnell, J. A. (2005). Workforce diversity and organizational performance. *Equal Opportunities International, 24*, 1–16.

Youssef, C. M., & Luthans, F. (2007). Positive organizational behavior in the workplace. The impact of hope, optimism and resilience. *Journal of Management, 33*, 774–800.

Youssef, C. M., & Luthans, F. (2009). An integrated model of psychological capital in the workplace. In A. Linley, S. Harrington, & N. Garcea (Eds.), *Oxford handbook of positive psychology and work* (pp. 277–288). New York: Oxford University Press.

Chapter 16
Infusing Multiculturalism and Positive Psychology in Psychotherapy

Jeana L. Magyar-Moe

Research on applications of positive psychology to the practice of counseling and psychotherapy has proliferated over the past decade. Indeed, there may be no better fit for positive psychology than within the therapy room. More specifically, research supports the notion that client conceptualizations and the incorporation of therapeutic models and exercises informed by positive psychology can provide lasting positive outcomes for therapy clients (Duckworth et al. 2005; Seligman et al. 2005, 2006). However, a major criticism of therapeutic applications of positive psychology is the lack of consistent focus upon cultural considerations, with many scholars seemingly promoting more of a one-size-fits-all approach to positive psychological applications. Indeed, Lopez and colleagues (2002) note that most positive psychology research has studied predominantly White populations versus understanding positive psychology within a multicultural context in which diverse meanings of the good life and optimal functioning are valued (Pedrotti et al. 2009). In this chapter, a brief history of the lack of focus on culture within therapeutic applications of positive psychology is explored, followed by information on how to incorporate existing positive psychological theories and therapies in a multiculturally informed manner.

J.L. Magyar-Moe, Ph.D. (✉)
UWSP Psychology Department, University of Wisconsin – Stevens Point,
D240 Science Building, Stevens Point, WI 54481, USA
e-mail: Jeana.Magyar-Moe@uwsp.edu

J. Teramoto Pedrotti and L.M. Edwards (eds.), *Perspectives on the Intersection of Multiculturalism and Positive Psychology*, Cross-Cultural Advancements in Positive Psychology 7, DOI 10.1007/978-94-017-8654-6_16,

16.1 The Absence of Culture Within Therapeutic Applications of Positive Psychology

Examination of the scholarly literature on positive psychology reveals several weaknesses of this field that need to be addressed to ensure that positive psychology is applicable to the lives of *all* people. More specifically, the reported areas of weakness include the largely individualistic, ethnocentric, one-size-fits-all nature of positive psychology that seems to neglect the cultural embeddedness of all human activities (Becker and Marecek 2008a; Christopher and Hickinbottom 2008; Christopher et al. 2008; D'Andrea 2005; Held 2004; Lopez et al. 2002; Pedrotti et al. 2009; Sandage and Hill 2001). Indeed, Becker and Marecek (2008a) contend that individualism pervades positive psychology as evidenced by "the movement's endorsement of self-fulfilment as the ultimate life goal, its promotion of self-improvement via personal effort, and its narrow sense of the social" (p. 1751). They further argue that "the bounded, autonomous self that strides through a positive life is an illusion, as is the notion that human flourishing and happiness are readily available to all" (p. 1751).

D'Andrea (2005) similarly notes that failure to define and control for race and ethnicity in positive psychology research has resulted in incomplete information and understandings of people from different racial and ethnic groups, thereby serving to inadvertently perpetuate a scientific form of racism. Likewise, Christopher et al. (2008) state that many positive psychology scholars endorse mental health ideals of the dominant United States-based ideals of personal autonomy and individual definitions of happiness and fulfilment. Furthermore, they note that "positive psychology overly hastily and somewhat naively universalizes its particular cultural preferences and ideals as good for or applicable to all human communities" (Christopher et al. 2008, p. 557).

Finally, Sandage and Hill (2001) contend that in order for positive psychology to be culturally relevant, scholars must ask questions that acknowledge multicultural awareness of *difference*. Such questions must include consideration of whose view of strengths, well-being, and happiness will be privileged, who will benefit from certain definitions of positive psychological constructs, how multiple definitions of the good life can be placed in a cultural context, and which cultural views of human strength, resilience, or virtue risk being overlooked or ignored (Christopher and Hickinbottom 2008; Sampson 1993; Sandage and Hill 2001). Indeed, Ryff and Singer (1998) have called for an awareness of multiple pathways to positive health and "diverse enactments of wellness" (p. 7) and Christopher and Hickinbottom (2008) endorse the importance of alternate interpretations of the meaning of values, strengths, and well-being. Becker and Marecek (2008b) further suggest that considering the individual within the context of his or her social environment and broadening definitions of happiness and virtue will serve to make positive psychology more relevant to the many.

Downey and Chang (2012) acknowledge that positive psychological research is becoming more culturally relevant, however, they also note that although such information and knowledge is being gathered that there are still many who are worried that appropriate application of these findings remains a challenge for practitioners (Conway Madding 2000; Orsi et al. 2010; Stuart 2004). In addition, rates of application of knowledge about race, culture, and development in the clinical realm are not progressing at similar rates for different groups (Downey and Chang 2012).

Downey and Chang (2012) propose that changes in clinical training will help to create multiculturally relevant therapeutic applications of positive psychology. Indeed, these scholars note that training of practitioners to date has not sufficiently, regularly, or explicitly incorporated positive psychology, multiculturalism, and lifespan perspectives. In response to this problem, Downey and Chang (2012) propose the concept of *multidimensional clinical competence*, defined as "the ability to work collaboratively and constructively with clients of diverse groups, cultures, developmental stages, and levels of functioning, to recognize, utilize, and develop their existing and potential strengths in the service of reducing existing or potential dysfunction in themselves or within their social systems" (p. 373). The remainder of this chapter will focus upon potential ways in which practitioners can enact multidimensional clinical competence through incorporation of positive psychological theories and therapies in a clinical context.

16.2 Multiculturally-Infused Positive Psychological Counseling and Psychotherapy

There are a multitude of potential applications of positive psychology within the practice of counseling and psychotherapy. The applications of positive psychology to client assessment and conceptualization and treatment planning and implementation are explored in the following sections, with special focus upon cultural considerations of such applications.

16.2.1 Client Assessment and Conceptualization

16.2.1.1 Seven-Axis System of Culturally Informed Positive Psychological Assessment

The first order of business when clients present for therapy is to engage in assessment for the purposes of accurately conceptualizing the client and his or her functioning and then formulating an appropriate treatment plan. Research from positive psychology can be used to inform this assessment process in order to balance out the deficit perspective or illness ideology that tends to pervade psychotherapy. Indeed, the current five-axis assessment system of the Diagnostic and Statistical Manual of Mental Disorders, Fourth Edition – Text Revision (DSM-IV-TR;

American Psychiatric Association 2000) encourages practitioners to focus on pathology while failing to hold therapists accountable for finding strengths and resources as well. In particular, Axes I (clinical syndromes and other conditions that may be a focus of clinical attention) and II (personality disorders and mental retardation) provide ample opportunities for therapists to document the weaknesses of clients, while Axis IV allows for psychosocial and environmental problems to be noted. Axis V, the Global Assessment of Functioning Scale (GAF), is focused exclusively on pathology with a score of 1 representing extremely severe pathology while the highest score of 100 simply indicates the absence of symptomology (American Psychiatric Association 2000). Given that the absence of symptomology is not equivalent to the presence of mental health, the GAF scale falls short in terms of mental health assessment.

A few basic changes or additions to the current DSM 5-Axis assessment system could assist clinicians in conceptualizing clients in a more balanced and culturally relevant way (Lopez et al. 2003; Magyar-Moe 2009; Snyder et al. 2003; Sue et al. 2006). More specifically, broadening Axis IV to include not only psychosocial and environmental problems but also psychosocial and environmental resources would require practitioners to attend to all aspects of their clients' environmental influences. The developers of the DSM note that Axis IV is included because the nine categories of psychosocial and environmental problems that are assessed on this Axis might contribute to or exacerbate the various disorders listed on Axes I and II. If such problems can exacerbate pathology, it is logical to assume that psychosocial and environmental resources might serve as protective factors that could potentially minimize the impact of disorders and therefore should be assessed as well (Snyder et al. 2003).

Broadening Axis V to include two global assessment of functioning scales with one focused on symptoms of mental illness and the other on symptoms of well-being would also make for a more complete assessment model (Magyar-Moe 2009). To broaden Axis V, therapists can utilize the current Global Assessment of Functioning Scale provided in the DSM, in which they rate clients on a scale of 1 (severely impaired functioning) to 100 (absence of symptomology) and then complete a second Global Assessment of *Positive* Functioning Scale (Magyar-Moe 2009) with anchors of 1 representing a complete absence of well-being symptoms and 100 representing optimal functioning.

Sue et al. (2006) recommend the addition of an Axis VI that focuses therapist attention to the cultural contexts of client's lives. Indeed, failure to attend to the cultural background and context that impacts so much of who clients are can completely override the utility of all of the other data that is collected. Furthermore, attending to strengths as well as struggles that may be associated with one's various cultural identities is essential. (Additional information on ways to assess the cultural contexts of clients is provided in a following section.)

Finally, adding an additional axis, Axis VII, in which the personal strengths and facilitators of growth of clients are documented is also recommended (Snyder et al. 2003). Through these changes to the current DSM-assessment system, therapists and clients become more aware of not only problems or areas of concern, but also of strengths and resources within a cultural context that can be utilized in sound treatment planning (Magyar-Moe 2009).

Given that the revised 7-Axis System (Magyar-Moe 2009) is not currently a part of the DSM, most mental health agencies and insurance companies do not require this information to be provided. This does not mean, however, that practitioners should not or could not include this information in their work with clients. The extra time it takes to gather and share this information with clients is well worth the benefits garnered from a more complete conceptualization. For example, when clients feel understood as whole people within a cultural context, the working alliance between therapist and client is strengthened and clients also may become more motivated to work in therapy. This contrasts sharply with being equated solely with their problems and seen only from the dominant cultural perspective. When the treatment plan incorporates building from culturally appropriate client strengths, clients may have more hope that things really can change. These are just a few examples of how a balanced conceptualization can lead to positive therapeutic outcomes (Magyar-Moe 2009).

16.2.1.2 The Process of Culturally-Sensitive Positive Psychological Assessment

In order to gather information to complete the 7-Axis Assessment model, practitioners must begin with self-awareness of their own biases and by taking the stance that all people have strengths and weaknesses as well as environmental deficits and resources that can be identified and utilized in the process of therapy (Wright and Lopez 2002). Culturally sensitive positive psychological assessment is multidimensional and begins with such therapist self-awareness as well an understanding of Multicultural Counseling Competencies (Sue et al. 1992), the Guidelines on Multicultural Education, Training, Research, Practice, and Organizational Change for Psychologists (American Psychological Association 2003), and the meaning of positive constructs among people of diverse cultures. Based on this foundation, culturally encompassing information should be gathered utilizing culturally appropriate tests and means of assessment, followed by providing culturally appropriate interpretations of the assessment results (Flores and Obasi 2003).

Culturally-Encompassing Data Gathering

Culturally-encompassing data gathering includes an examination of a client's sociocultural context, cultural identity, and worldview (Flores and Obasi 2003). Optimal human functioning can be appropriately assessed for people of diverse backgrounds by studying the cultural values, beliefs, and practices that moderate racial stress, such as collectivism, racial and ethnic pride, spirituality, religion, holistic health, and family and community importance. In addition, attending to client skills and strengths that have developed through overcoming adversity such as racism, prejudice, or oppression can also lead to important discoveries about culturally sensitive optimal human functioning (Constantine and Sue 2006).

Sue (2003) has noted that some of the skills or strengths that may develop for clients who overcome racial or cultural adversity include heightened perceptual wisdom (i.e., the ability to correctly perceive underlying motives, intentions, and meanings of others; to see beyond the obvious, or to 'read between the lines'), the ability to rely on non-verbal or contextual meanings (i.e., the ability to accurately read communication by attending to non-verbal behavior), and bicultural flexibility (i.e., openness to multiple worldviews, sensitivity to other's viewpoints, and behavioral flexibility). Indeed, Constantine and Sue (2006) point out that since we live in a multicultural context, bicultural flexibility is a major advantage for people of color in the U.S. that also positively affects them on an individual level. Sue (2003) also notes that such flexibility often leads to a broadened worldview, an appreciation for the strengths and weaknesses of all people, comfort with cultural differences and better effectiveness in relating to those of diverse backgrounds, an enhanced sense of self-fulfilment, and a sense of connection and commitment to better citizenship and social responsibility. Several methods for assessing cultural identities follow.

The ADDRESSING Model of Cultural Assessment

A useful tool that can be utilized to better ensure that all aspects of a client's cultural identity are assessed is the ADDRESSING model by Hays (2007). This model was designed to help therapists conceptualize individual's identities across multiple life domains. ADDRESSING is an acronym, with each of the ten letters representing one aspect of culture to be explored in a complementary manner in which both strengths and weaknesses associated with each of these cultural identities are explored. Please see Hays (2007) or Chap. 2, this volume, for more details regarding the ADDRESSING framework.

The RESPECTFUL Counseling Framework

The RESPECTFUL counseling framework consists of ten factors considered to be central to understanding cultural diversity (D'Andrea and Daniels 2001). RESPECTFUL in an acronym with each letter representing a key aspect of cultural identity as follows: **R**eligion and spirituality; **E**conomic/class background; **S**exual identity; **P**ersonal style; **E**thnicity/racial identity; **C**hronological/lifespan challenges; **T**rauma; **F**amily background; **U**nique physical characteristics; and **L**ocation of residence and language. Use of the RESPECTFUL framework in a therapeutic context can be used to focus on both the demands and resources as well as stressors and strengths for clients in order to empower them to take action to reduce stress and strengthen their resources and personal power (D'Andrea and Daniels 2001).

The Community Genogram

The community genogram is another useful tool for gathering culturally encompassing client data (Ivey and Ivey 1999). The goal for using such a genogram is to bring cultural issues to the forefront in the assessment process and to focus on the positive resources that come from understanding the multiple components of one's cultural experiences. Ivey and Ivey (1999) explicitly recommend that when helping clients construct community genograms, therapists should focus on stories of strength, rather than on problems. Such a focus often leads to client recollections of useful strategies they had relied upon in the past that can be implemented to help solve current issues.

Selection and Interpretation of Culturally Appropriate Tests and Measures

Many self-report measures are available to assist practitioners in the identification of client strengths and symptoms of well-being. Most of the measures are available free of charge, are quick to administer and score, and many are available on-line. The instruments available are related to the measure of character strengths, personal talents, life satisfaction, positive emotions, positive coping, and a host of other positive psychology constructs such as gratitude, forgiveness, empathy, hope, optimism, creativity, and more. Utilizing such measures in a culturally appropriate manner requires that a clinician understand the development and norming samples of each measure, and make decisions about the measure's equivalence (e.g., construct, semantic, measurement, etc.) for a given population. In some cases, a clinician may decide the measure is not appropriate, while in other situations she might choose to adapt the measure but contextualize interpretations of findings.

The Values in Action Inventory of Character Strengths (VIA-IS; Peterson and Seligman 2004) is among the most popular of all available positive psychological measures. This survey is based upon the Values in Action Classification System developed by Peterson and Seligman (2004). The VIA Classification System was created in order to be an adjunct or alternative to the DSM. Just as the DSM was designed to provide useful information about psychological disorders and a common lexicon for therapists to use in describing pathology, the VIA Classification System was designed to provide important information and a common lexicon for therapists to use in describing strengths (Peterson and Seligman 2004).

When utilizing the VIA-IS (Peterson and Seligman 2004) with clients of diverse backgrounds, one must be sure to consider the cultural appropriateness of the survey. Although the developers of this survey report that the 24 character strengths are ubiquitous or recognized and valued by virtually all people and cultures (Peterson and Seligman 2004), they also note that the strengths are not universal (Seligman et al. 2005). Furthermore, as previously noted, one of the biggest criticisms of positive psychology in general, and of the VIA Classification system in particular, centers around what many scholars view as the largely individualistic, ethnocentric, one-size-fits-all nature of these approaches that seem to neglect the cultural embeddedness of all human activities (Lopez et al. 2002; Held 2004; D'Andrea 2005; Becker and Marecek 2008a; Christopher and Hickinbottom 2008; Christopher et al. 2008; Sandage and Hill 2001).

Given these criticisms, it is highly imperative that use of measures such as the VIA-IS with diverse populations includes a thorough understanding of the ways in which cultural and individual differences impact the test results. In order to do so, practitioners should always discuss the outcomes of such measures with clients in order to understand how the findings may or may not actually be serving as strengths or positive indicators for each individual, as well as to note which cultural strengths or positive indicators may be missing from the particular measure being used. In addition, practitioners should actively seek out research related to strengths and optimal functioning related to the cultural identities of the clients with whom they are working in order to see what, if any, alternate interpretations may be supported by empirical data. For example, Chang (1996) has found that in comparison to Caucasian Americans, Asian Americans tend to be more pessimistic and this pessimism serves them well, as it is related to positive problem-solving behaviors and does not contribute to depression within this population. This is important information, as it appears that pessimism, rather than optimism, is a strength in this context. The VIA-IS (Peterson and Seligman 2004) includes only optimism as a strength, thereby leading one to conclude that pessimism is a weakness. While pessimism may be a weakness for some, it clearly is not the case for all. Furthermore, these findings make clear that the VIA-IS values optimism as a strength despite that fact that in some cultures, optimism may not be valued as a strength at all.

Similarly, Norem and Cantor (1986) have researched a type of pessimism, called defensive pessimism, which works very well for some people. More specifically, defensive pessimism occurs when people set their expectations low as they think through possible future outcomes (Norem and Cantor 1986; Norem and Illingworth 1993). They set these low expectations in order to prepare themselves for potential failure while at the same time motivating themselves to try to avoid that failure. People who are defensive pessimists initially feel anxious and out of control when faced with future challenges, even though they have previously performed well on such tasks (Norem and Cantor 1986). For defensive pessimists, being optimistic can actually be detrimental (Norem and Cantor 1986). Contrary to logic, the low expectations of defensive pessimists do not become self-fulfilling prophecies and in fact, when guiding defensive pessimists to think more like optimists, their performance declines (Norem and Illingworth 1993; Rich and Dahlheimer 1989).

The preceding examples highlight that the results of the VIA-IS (Peterson and Seligman 2004), as well as all other positive psychological assessment measures, must always be considered within the cultural contexts of the individuals with whom one is working. Of course, whenever possible, positive psychological measures that have been designed for use with the specific population should be utilized with clients from that group. Until more research is conducted in order to validate more positive psychology measures with diverse populations, utilization of currently available measures in a culturally sensitive manner is recommended.

16.2.2 Treatment Planning and Implementation

Treatment planning and implementation follows client assessment. Research to date reveals a number of positive psychological approaches to therapy and specific activities and exercises based on the principles of positive psychology that therapists can utilize in their treatment of clients (Duckworth et al. 2005; Frisch 2006; Lopez et al. 2004; Rashid 2008; Seligman et al. 2005, 2006; Smith 2006; Wong 2006). In the following sections, several models of therapy informed by positive psychology are reviewed with a focus upon the cultural components that are either inherent in these approaches or that can readily be infused by practitioners with multidimensional clinical competence.

16.2.2.1 Strengths-Based Counseling

Strengths-Based Counseling (Smith 2006) is a model for conducting therapy based on the premises of positive psychology, counseling psychology, prevention, positive youth development, social work, solution-focused therapy, and narrative therapy (Smith 2006). The model is based on 12 propositions that outline the basic principles of Strength-Based Counseling. Five of the 12 propositions are related to multiculturalism. More specifically, propositions related to culture include: (a) The strength-based counselor assumes that race, class, and gender are organizing elements in every counseling interaction; (b) Strengths develop as a result of internal and external forces and as part of the human driving force to meet basic psychological needs; (c) Humans are self-righting organisms who are constantly working to adapt to their environments. Strengths develop as people try to right themselves; (d) All people have the capacity for strength development and for growth and change. Strength development is a lifelong process that is influenced by the interaction of individual's heredity and the cultural, social, economic, and political environments in which they find themselves; and (e) All people have a reservoir of strengths, some of which have been tapped and others of which have been left unexplored and unrecognized (Smith 2006, pp. 34–38).

Strengths-Based Counseling (Smith 2006) is carried out in a series of ten stages, with the first three stages focused on the creation of a strong therapeutic alliance via helping clients to identify and use their strengths and competencies to confront their struggles. At the same time, a thorough assessment of client perceptions of their problems is to take place. During these stages, practitioners are also encouraged to help their clients uncover strengths at the biological, psychological, social, cultural, economic, and political levels (Smith 2006).

In stage four, therapists set out to encourage and instill a sense of hope in clients by focusing on and providing feedback to clients based upon their efforts or improvements, rather than the outcomes of their efforts (Smith 2006). In stage five, therapists help clients to frame solutions to their problems via solution-building conversations. The principles of solution-focused interviewing are key at this stage of the Strengths-Based Counseling process. (For a more detailed review of solution-focused therapy, see De Jong and Berg 2002.)

Stage six, building strength and competence, fosters the development of internal and external client assets by helping clients to realize that they have the power to effect important changes in their lives. This is accomplished via building upon and fostering personal strengths and environmental resources throughout the therapeutic process. Stages seven through nine, empowering, changing, and building resilience, are designed to promote agency and facilitate goal pursuits. Major components of these stages are to: (a) help clients develop an awareness of how their problems do not necessarily reside within them; (b) to help them see that change is a process, not an isolated event; (c) to utilize strengths to facilitate change; and (d) to view mistakes that occur en route to change as opportunities for learning, rather than as failures. Although not noted by Smith (2006), an important consideration in this stage is to recognize the multiple different ways in which a failure may be interpreted due to cultural context. For example, the process of reframing a mistake or error as an opportunity for learning would be very different for a client from an individualistic culture where the needs of the individual take priority versus a collectivistic culture where the needs of the family are prominent. For those from collectivistic backgrounds, a mistake or failure by the individual will affect the client as well as his or her family, making a reframe of the situation more challenging given all of the others who are involved.

Finally, stage ten consists of evaluating and terminating. This stage allows the therapist and client to identify the strengths that were most valuable to the change process and to honor the progress that has been made (Smith 2006).

Although the Strengths-Based Counseling model (Smith 2006) is lacking a bit in terms of specific strengths-enhancing techniques, it does provide therapists with a guiding framework for practicing from a strengths-based perspective that is also sensitive to culture.

16.2.2.2 Hope Therapy

Hope consists of one's perceptions of his or her abilities to create clear goals, to develop plans for reaching those goals (pathways thinking), and to find and maintain the energy and motivation necessary for following through with goal pursuits (agency thinking, Snyder 1994). Goals can be anything clients desire to experience, create, get, do, or become; hence, they may be major, lifelong goals or more minor, short-term goals. In order for clients to achieve their goals, both pathways and agency thinking are necessary (Lopez et al. 2004).

Hope Therapy (Lopez et al. 2004) is designed to capitalize upon hope in the therapy process, as hope seems to be a malleable strength that can indeed serve as an important therapeutic change agent. Therapists who practice Hope Therapy help clients to conceptualize clearer goals, to learn how to produce multiple pathways to reach goals, and to generate the mental energy needed to sustain goal pursuits in order to positively change client self-perceptions regarding their abilities to engage in goal-directed and agentic thinking (Lopez et al. 2000a).

There are multiple principles that undergird Hope Therapy, including the fact that Hope Therapy is designed to be a brief, semi-structured form of therapy in which the primary focus is upon current goals. In addition, in order to enhance hope, therapists help clients to focus on goals, possibilities, and past successes rather than on problems or failures (Lopez et al. 2000a).

As with all positive psychological interventions, it is important for therapists to be sensitive to the cultural contexts in which clients exist when implementing Hope Therapy. Although there is evidence that hope is prevalent across cultures and ethnic groups (Chang and Banks 2007), it has also been reported that barriers arise more often in the goal pursuits for some members of minority groups (Lopez et al. 2000b). Indeed, all people come across obstacles in the process of working towards their life goals and those who are high in hope are able to perceive these obstacles as challenges to be overcome. However, members of non-privileged religious backgrounds, ethnic and racial groups, immigrants, and gender and sexual minority groups are prone to experiencing larger impediments to their goals on a more frequent basis due to such factors as prejudice, racism, sexism, stereotyping, poverty, acculturation stress, language barriers, lack of privilege, and more. These obstacles exist on various levels, including the interpersonal, societal, and institutional (Lopez et al. 2000b).

Practitioners who want to be sure that they conduct Hope Therapy in a culturally appropriate manner are advised to be aware of the fact that various obstacles are more likely to be encountered by members of diverse groups, but to also realize that some marginalized racial or ethnic minority groups have shown equal and higher hope levels than European Americans (Chang and Banks 2007). Indeed, it appears that early experiences or expectancies of goal-related obstacles for some minorities may serve as opportunities for developing higher levels of hope and greater pathways thinking later in life. This research suggests that helping clients to develop goals within the context of their cultural frameworks and examining factors that are likely to make goals more or less available or attainable is critical. Finally, providing culture-specific examples of hope during the narrative work of the hope finding phase of Hope Therapy is recommended (Lopez et al. 2000a).

Hope Therapy practitioners should also be aware of the findings of Chang and Banks (2007) which indicate that although hope is a universally valid positive expectancy variable that functions similarly across different racial/ethnic groups, that cultivation of hope appears to differ based upon one's cultural make-up. More specifically, being satisfied with one's life served as a source of agentic hope thinking for European Americans, Latinos, and African Americans, but not for Asian Americans. Positive affect was found to be predictive of pathways hope thinking for European, African, and Asian-Americans but not for Latinos. Based upon these findings, Chang and Banks (2007) suggest that fostering hope in European Americans may be best achieved via using interventions that target the promotion of greater life satisfaction and positive affect in this group. For African Americans, lack of a negative problem orientation was the best predictor of agentic thinking, whereas positive problem orientation was the strongest predictor of pathways thinking. Therefore, increasing hope for African Americans might best be achieved through interventions that aim to reduce negative problem orientation and aim to increase positive problem orientation. For Latinos, rational problem solving was found to be the strongest predictor of agentic thinking and life satisfaction was found to be the only predictor of pathways thinking. Increasing hope for Latinos, therefore, might be best achieved through interventions that promote greater rational problem solving and life satisfaction. Finally, for Asian Americans, positive affect was the strongest predictor of agentic thinking and positive problem orientation was the best predictor of pathways thinking. Higher hope levels with Asian Americans might be accomplished through interventions which target the promotion of positive affect and positive problem orientation.

16.3 Conclusion

As noted throughout this chapter, positive psychological interventions in psychotherapy must be designed around the various cultural identities and the environmental contexts that make up the backdrop for each client with whom one works. Consideration of the appropriateness, meaning, and utility of each of the measures and activities provided to clients must be done in a thoughtful and thorough fashion. When possible, adjusting the activities to better fit the needs of clients is recommended. For example, when engaging in Hope Therapy, practitioners may find that some clients from collectivistic cultures may struggle to create goals on their own, as their goals are that of the larger family or social group. In such instances, having clients develop their goals within the context of and with assistance from these family members or social groups may serve to make the assignment more relevant. Likewise, capitalizing upon strengths that are identified through one's cultural experiences, rather than relying solely upon results of such strength measures as the VIA Strengths Inventory may be more meaningful for some. Finally, allowing clients to choose what their goals are in terms of desired therapy outcomes is also recommended. What complete mental health looks and feels like for some will not be the same for others. Indeed, using a cookie-cutter type approach to incorporating positive psychology into clinical practice is not only likely to be futile, but could even serve to make clients worse (Magyar-Moe 2009).

As research in positive psychology continues to proliferate, so too will the information relevant to the multicultural applications of positive psychology to psychotherapy. Perhaps someday, culturally competent positive psychology will become such an integral part of the training and work of all clinicians, that there will be no such thing as therapy that is not strengths-based and inclusive of client cultural identities and environmental factors delivered by providers who exhibit multidimensional clinical competence (Downey and Chang 2012).

References

American Psychiatric Association. (2000). *Diagnostic and statistical manual of mental disorders, fourth edition, text revision*. Washington, DC: American Psychiatric Association.

American Psychological Association. (2003). Guidelines on multicultural education, training, research, practice, and organizational change for Psychologists. *American Psychologist, 58*(5), 377–402. doi:10.1037/0003-066X.58.5.377.

Becker, D., & Marecek, J. (2008a). Dreaming the American dream: Individualism and positive psychology. *Social and Personality Psychology Compass, 2*(5), 1767–1780.

Becker, D., & Marecek, J. (2008b). Positive psychology: History in the remaking? *Theory and Psychology, 18*, 591–604.

Chang, E. C. (1996). Cultural differences in optimism, pessimism, and coping: Predictors of subsequent adjustment in Asian American and Caucasian American college students. *Journal of Counseling Psychology, 43*, 113–123.

Chang, E. C., & Banks, K. H. (2007). The color and texture of hope: Some preliminary findings and implications for hope theory and counseling among diverse racial/ethnic groups. *Cultural Diversity and Ethnic Minority Psychology, 13*(2), 94–103.

Christopher, J. C., & Hickinbottom, S. (2008). Positive psychology, ethnocentrism, and the disguised ideology of individualism. *Theory and Psychology, 18*, 563–589.

Christopher, J. C., Richardson, F. C., & Slife, B. D. (2008). Thinking through positive psychology. *Theory and Psychology, 18*, 551–561.

Constantine, M. G., & Sue, D. W. (2006). Factors contributing to optimal human functioning in people of color in the United States. *The Counseling Psychologist, 34*, 228–244.

Conway Madding, C. (2000). Maintaining focus on cultural competence in early intervention services to linguistically and culturally diverse families. *Infant-Toddler Intervention, 10*, 9–18.

D'Andrea, M. (2005, January). *Reclaiming positive psychology from a multicultural perspective: Combating new forms of racism and ethnocentrism in psychology*. Paper presented at the 2005 National Multicultural Summit, Hollywood, CA.

D'Andrea, M., & Daniels, J. (2001). RESPECTFUL counseling: An integrative model for counselors. In D. Pope-Davis & H. Coleman (Eds.), *The interface of class, culture and gender in counseling* (pp. 417–466). Thousand Oaks: Sage.

De Jong, P., & Berg, I. K. (2002). *Interviewing for solutions* (2nd ed.). Belmont: Thomson Brooks/Cole Publishing Co.

Downey, C. A., & Chang, E. C. (2012). Multidimensional clinical competence: Considering racial group, development, and the positive psychology movement in clinical practice. In E. C. Chang & C. A. Downey (Eds.), *Handbook of race and development in mental health* (pp. 335–382). New York: Springer.

Duckworth, A. L., Steen, T. A., & Seligman, M. E. P. (2005). Positive psychology in clinical practice. *Annual Review of Clinical Psychology, 1*, 629–651.

Flores, L. Y., & Obasi, E. M. (2003). Positive psychological assessment in an increasingly diverse world. In S. J. Lopez & C. R. Snyder (Eds.), *Positive psychological assessment: A handbook of models and measures* (pp. 443–458). Washington, DC: American Psychological Association.

Frisch, M. B. (2006). *Quality of life therapy: Applying a life satisfaction approach to positive psychology and cognitive therapy*. Hoboken: Wiley.

Hays, P. A. (2007). *Addressing cultural complexities in practice, second edition: Assessment, diagnosis, and therapy*. Washington, DC: American Psychological Association.

Held, B. S. (2004). The negative side of positive psychology. *Journal of Humanistic Psychology, 44*, 9–46.

Ivey, A. E., & Ivey, M. B. (1999). *Intentional interviewing and counseling: Facilitating client development in a multicultural society* (4th ed.). Pacific Grove: Brooks/Cole Publishing Company.

Lopez, S. J., Floyd, R. K., Ulven, J. C., & Snyder, C. R. (2000a). Hope therapy: Helping clients build a house of hope. In C. R. Snyder (Ed.), *Handbook of hope* (pp. 123–150). New York: Academic.

Lopez, S. J., Gariglietti, K. P., McDermott, D., Sherwin, E. D., Floyd, R. K., Rand, K., & Snyder, C. R. (2000b). Hope for the evolution of diversity: On leveling the field of dreams. In C. R. Snyder (Ed.), *Handbook of hope* (pp. 223–242). New York: Academic.

Lopez, S. J., Prosser, E. C., Edwards, L. M., Magyar-Moe, J. L., Neufeld, J. E., & Rasmussen, H. N. (2002). Putting positive psychology in a multicultural context. In C. R. Snyder & S. J. Lopez (Eds.), *Handbook of positive psychology* (pp. 700–714). New York: Oxford University Press.

Lopez, S. J., Snyder, C. R., & Rasmussen, H. N. (2003). Striking a vital balance: Developing a complementary focus on human weakness and strength through positive psychological assessment. In S. J. Lopez & C. R. Snyder (Eds.), *Positive psychological assessment: A handbook of models and measures* (pp. 3–20). Washington, DC: American Psychological Association.

Lopez, S. J., Snyder, C. R., Magyar-Moe, J. L., Edwards, L. M., Pedrotti, J. T., Janowski, K., Turner, J. L., & Pressgrove, C. (2004). Strategies for accentuating hope. In P. A. Linley & S. Joseph (Eds.), *Positive psychology in practice* (pp. 388–404). Hoboken: Wiley.

Magyar-Moe, J. L. (2009). *Therapist's guide to positive psychological interventions*. San Diego: Elsevier Academic Press.

Norem, J. K., & Cantor, N. (1986). Defensive pessimism: "Harnessing" anxiety as motivation. *Journal of Personality and Social Psychology, 52*, 1208–1217.

Norem, J. K., & Illingworth, K. S. S. (1993). Strategy-dependent effects on reflecting on self and tasks: Some implications of optimism and defensive pessimism. *Journal of Personality and Social Psychology, 65*, 822–835.

Orsi, J. M., Margellos-Anast, H., & Whitman, S. (2010). Black-white health disparities in the United States and Chicago: A 15-year progress analysis. *American Journal of Public Health, 100*, 349–356.

Pedrotti, J. T., Edwards, L. M., & Lopez, S. J. (2009). Positive psychology within a cultural context. In S. J. Lopez (Ed.), *Handbook of positive psychology* (2nd ed., pp. 49–58). New York: Oxford Press.

Peterson, C., & Seligman, M. E. P. (2004). *Character strengths and virtues: A handbook and classification*. New York: Oxford University Press.

Rashid, T. (2008). Positive psychotherapy. In S. J. Lopez (Ed.), *Positive psychology: Exploring the best in people (4)* (pp. 187–217). Westport: Praeger Publishers.

Rich, A. R., & Dahlheimer, D. (1989). The power of negative thinking: A new perspective on 'irrational' cognitions. *Journal of Cognitive Psychotherapy, 3*, 15–30.

Ryff, C. D., & Singer, B. (1998). The contours of positive human health. *Psychological Inquiry, 9*, 1–28.

Sampson, E. E. (1993). Identity politics: Challenges to psychology's understanding. *American Psychologist, 48*, 1219–1230.

Sandage, S. J., & Hill, P. C. (2001). The virtues of positive psychology: The rapprochement and challenges of an affirmative postmodern perspective. *Journal for the Theory of Social Behaviour, 31*, 241–260.

Seligman, M. E. P., Steen, T. A., Park, N., & Peterson, C. (2005). Positive psychology progress: Empirical validation of interventions. *American Psychologist, 60*, 410–421.

Seligman, M. E. P., Rashid, T., & Parks, A. C. (2006). Positive psychotherapy. *American Psychologist, 61*, 774–788.

Smith, E. (2006). The strengths-based counseling model. *The Counseling Psychologist, 34*, 13–79.

Snyder, C. R. (1994). *The psychology of hope: You can get there from here*. New York: Free Press.

Snyder, C. R., Lopez, S. J., Edwards, L. M., Pedrotti, J. T., Prosser, E. C., Walton, S. L., Spalitto, S. V., & Ulven, J. C. (2003). Measuring and labeling the positive and the negative. In S. J. Lopez & C. R. Snyder (Eds.), *Positive psychological assessment: A handbook of models and measures* (pp. 21–40). Washington, DC: American Psychological Association.

Stuart, R. B. (2004). Twelve practical suggestions for achieving multicultural competence. *Professional Psychology: Research and Practice, 35*, 3–9.

Sue, D. W. (2003). *Overcoming our racism: The journey to liberation*. San Francisco: Jossey-Bass.

Sue, D. W., Arredondo, P., & McDavis, R. J. (1992). Multicultural counseling competencies and standards: A call to the profession. *Journal of Counseling and Development, 70*, 477–486.

Sue, D. S., Sue, D. W., & Sue, S. (2006). *Understanding abnormal behavior* (8th ed.). Boston: Houghton Mifflin Company.

Wong, J. (2006). Strengths-centered therapy: A social constructionist, virtue-based psychotherapy. *Psychotherapy: Theory, Research, Practice, and Training, 43*, 133–146.

Wright, B. A., & Lopez, S. J. (2002). Widening the diagnostic focus: A case for including human strengths and environmental resources. In C. R. Snyder & S. J. Lopez (Eds.), *The handbook of positive psychology* (pp. 26–44). New York: Oxford University Press.

Part V
Conclusion

Chapter 17
Future Directions for a More Multiculturally Competent (and Humble) Positive Psychology

John Chambers Christopher and Katie Lynn Howe

With force and clarity, this book succeeds at speaking to the need for multicultural concern and commitment within the field of positive psychology. The authors of the chapters in this volume all support the idea that becoming more multiculturally inclusive is an essential task for positive psychology's future. From our perspective, becoming more multiculturally inclusive requires critically looking within the field of positive psychology in addition to extending positive psychology to groups that have been ignored or marginalized. Evaluating current positive psychological theory and its implicit assumptions (e.g., how those assumptions are Western assumptions), will reward us with deeper and more nuanced theory, research, and practice. Such a self-critique will give us the tools and framework to understand and describe positive phenomenon within different cultural, racial, and ethnic groups of origin and identity. In contrast, uncritically and prematurely applying positive psychology to different populations can potentially lead to pathologizing, stereotyping, and misunderstanding—essentially a violence to the other.

Within these chapters are varied topics and points of emphasis, all of which address particular areas and populations that need greater attention from positive psychology. Agreed among the authors collected here in this volume is the conviction that positive psychology not only has made very important contributions to psychology as a whole, but can continue to play an essential role in providing a more balanced view of human nature. There is no question among the authors in this book that positive psychology has been at the forefront in describing positive human experience and optimal functioning. Such efforts have been invaluable to the field of psychology.

J.C. Christopher, Ph.D. (✉)
Department of Psychiatry, Dartmouth Medical School,
Hanover Psychiatry, 23 S Main St, #2B, Hanover, NH 03755, USA
e-mail: johnchristopherphd@gmail.com

K.L. Howe
Lesley University, Cambridge, USA

J. Teramoto Pedrotti and L.M. Edwards (eds.), *Perspectives on the Intersection of Multiculturalism and Positive Psychology*, Cross-Cultural Advancements in Positive Psychology 7, DOI 10.1007/978-94-017-8654-6_17,

Despite these important contributions however, we and the other authors believe there is room to take this work even further. In particular, we see two main issues that have not been fully addressed by positive psychology. These issues include critically assessing the nature of the self and the nature of values, virtues, and strengths that underlie positive psychology. In this chapter we'll consider these points in more detail and explore how they might help positive psychology become more fully multiculturally sensitive.

As we see it, the primary goal for a positive psychology that is multiculturally informed is to take seriously the understandings of the positive that are inherent in other cultural traditions. However, from its inception others have noted that positive psychology appeared to distance itself in some ways from other attempts in the past to examine, as Maslow put it, "the farthest reaches of human nature," including humanistic psychology as well as philosophy, history and religion, by categorizing them as unscientific (see Downey and Chang, Chap. 1; Taylor 2001). Seemingly, there was no room in the positive psychology manifesto penned by Seligman and Csikszentmihalyi (2000) to learn from the many traditions outside of Western academic psychology that have been concerned with healing, growth, and transformation. Even within the Western perspective, provided by Seligman and others, there, at least initially, was little space for the voices and perspectives of those who represent the various sub cultures within the West. As Bacigalupe (2001) observed in his response to Seligman and Csikszentmihalyi, all the psychologists included in the special issue of the *American Psychologist* were White. Bacigalupe appeals for the inclusion of contributors to positive psychology who can rightly speak to the "manifold variety in the United States" and concludes by writing "A blind eye that continues to render large segments of society invisible cannot be compensated for by one informed eye turned only toward individuals and groups in mainstream psychology" (2001, p. 83).

Positive psychology, Seligman and Csikszentmihalyi declared, unlike philosophy, religion, or humanistic psychology, would be scientific, studied in an ostensibly culture-free or culture-neutral way. And yet, the philosophy of social science is adamant that there is no escape from culture (e.g., Bishop 2007; Christopher 1996; Richardson et al. 1999). Culture permeates and shapes all that we do in the social sciences, especially when we think we're being objective and neutral. As many authors in this book have noted, the idea of developing entirely culture-free measures, theories or interventions is seriously misguided and limited.

The result of attempting to be "culture-free" is that positive psychology, like psychology in general, has been thus far unduly influenced by Anglo-American and Northern European cultural values and assumptions. In this chapter we'd like to level the playing field. If there's no "escape" from culture, and if positive psychology has been unduly influenced by one cultural orientation, namely individualism, then it makes sense to study, learn from, and incorporate the understandings of the *positive* in other cultural traditions. In this way we will be helping to make positive psychology truly a multicultural psychology. Simultaneously, we will also help prevent positive psychology from lapsing into just another passing intellectual trend that loses its moment in the sun because it fails to speak to all of humanity.

17.1 Positive Psychology as a Moral Vision

So where do we start? To delve into these cultural roots one needs a framework to limit the range of what is considered and to provide focus. Seligman and Csikszentmihalyi (2000) contend there are "twin imperatives that a science of human beings should include: to understand what is and what could be" (p. 7). We think this is a good place to start. However, unlike Seligman and Csikszentmihalyi, we do not believe psychology has to start from scratch in answering these questions. Elsewhere we have written extensively about how these two imperatives are actually existential questions that underlie all cultural orientations and form moral visions (Christopher 1996, 2008). We've suggested in past work that philosophical hermeneutics provides a powerful way of thinking about what is at stake when we consider how human beings are products of culture. From this hermeneutic perspective we believe it is useful to think of cultures providing moral visions that rest on two pillars: one is an understanding of what the person or self is and the other normative expectations about how the person or self should be or become. Together these two pillars help to provide the folk psychologies that underlie and give coherence to all societies and all human functioning. Importantly, from the hermeneutic perspective these moral visions and their core assumptions and values need not be consciously known or articulable. Most often they are implicit. They are presupposed by the ways that we have learned to structure our lives and the social practices that we have adopted. To function successfully in life we need to have a folk psychology, even if it is implicit or tacit, and this folk psychology is a moral vision of what life is all about. Our behaviors, feelings, and thoughts always presuppose such moral visions. From this angle, all cultures provide developmental psychologies, personality psychologies, social psychologies, clinical psychologies, and positive psychologies.

In all societies much of a folk psychology will be outside of awareness. As human beings we are simply unable to articulate or consciously represent all of the rules, assumptions, and values upon which we rely. Different societies place varying degrees of emphasis upon the importance of trying to make the implicit explicit. Some societies have rich traditions in which understandings of healing and the good life are transmitted orally. And in other societies, like India and China, or more recently Europe, the United States and Canada, these kinds of understandings tend to be preserved in literate forms by trained specialists. Science, in this way, represents an extreme example. So while all cultures functionally provide positive psychologies, how they manifest can vary through different ranges of explicitness.

One of the consequences of this way of looking at the matter, is that contemporary positive psychologists trained in the Western tradition are actually operating at the conflux of cultural influences occurring at different levels. In part, as individuals, they are raised within particular societies and have taken over the folk psychologies and the indigenous positive psychology that exist tacitly within those societies. For most, this means being grounded in individualistic values and assumptions. In addition, as psychologists they have been trained explicitly in Western models of psychology which are emergent out of, but not identical with, the individualistic folk psychology of Western culture. Given the pervasive socializing that occurs within scientific training (Berger and Luckmann 1966; Kuhn 1970), and the lack of viable alternatives to mainstream psychology, we are perhaps all still influenced by the individualism that comes with the culture of psychology (cf., Fowers and Richardson 1994). It should be rightfully noted that psychologists of color, women, sexual minorities, and others often have a sense that mainstream psychological theory, research, and practice do not capture or, at times, pathologize their experience. Yet, because psychology has focused on quantitative precision at the expense of training psychologists in the interpretive and critical methods needed to discern and grapple with underlying cultural and theoretical assumptions, it is exceedingly difficult to channel intuitions about what's wrong or limited with mainstream psychology into forms capable of transforming the mainstream.

Culture then operates upon human beings at different levels of awareness or consciousness, often simultaneously, with the positive psychologist being no exception. Given this state of affairs, we believe as others have noted what makes most sense scientifically, is not to pretend that we can be objective or neutral. We can't. But instead we can begin to carefully explore and consider the widest possible understandings that have existed of the positive aspects of human nature and development across culture and across time.

Unfortunately, this was not the track taken in the beginnings of positive psychology. The movement under Seligman's guidance and with the funding of the Templeton Foundation documented their earliest endeavors. At meetings in Akumal, these senior psychologists like Seligman and Csikszentmihalyi along with promising early career psychologists developed the framework for pursuing the heart of positive psychology, the Values In Action classification system, or the un-DSM, the manual of the sanities (Peterson and Seligman 2004). What stands out to us from reading the documented history of these meetings is how little effort or time was spent in questioning the underlying assumption in the VIA framework that the six primary virtues are universally endorsed. It is one thing to see whether you can shoehorn other traditions cultural values and virtues into your own framework and quite another thing to discern the indigenous framework that has developed within local cultures and why it might differ. Surprisingly, given the resources at their disposal, the founders of positive psychology did not make a whole hearted attempt to dialogue with anthropologists, area studies experts, philosophers, historians, or scholars from non-Western traditions. Certainly, doing so would have been time consuming and it would have been messy. And given the short amount of time that lapsed between the initial funding of positive psychology and the publication of the VIA Handbook, it appears that the founders of positive psychology wanted neither. We believe this has been a huge loss to the field of positive psychology, reinforcing a kind of cultural encapsulation and discouraging the genuine dialogue with other cultures that we believe is so essential for the future of psychology.

So if we start over, we need to begin with the acknowledgment that cultures provide different moral visions. And an important preliminary task of a multiculturally committed positive psychology will be to explore these moral visions. In particular, it will be to discover the range of possible understandings about what the self is and what the self should be.

17.2 Individualism and Well-Being

We believe that at its core positive psychology is about well-being. Surprisingly, little has actually been written within psychology about the nature of well-being. There is much research though about well-being. But most of this research equates well-being with the outcome on one or two different measures of well-being. The nature of well-being is not really examined, it's assumed by what is presupposed in the measures being used. Of course, there are a variety of different interesting findings about what kinds of variables then correlate with the outcomes on well-being measures. But again, the nature of well-being, of positive psychology, has largely escaped critical scrutiny. To understand why this is problematic we turn now to briefly showing how theory and research on psychological well-being despite its pretensions to cultural neutrality presupposes one particular historically driven moral vision, individualism, and how potentially destructive that has been for those outside of the dominant majority in the United States, Canada, and Northern Europe. Current theories and research on psychological well-being, on close and critical examination, are shaped by Western individualistic moral visions of the good or ideal person (Christopher 1999; Christopher and Hickinbottom 2008; Ho et al., Chap. 4). By situating contemporary theory and research on psychological well-being in a cross-cultural and historical context, it becomes clear how they rest on particular Western cultural assumptions about the nature of the self as well as cultural values about how the self should be or what it should become.

The term individualism refers to a specific moral vision that emerged in Western history beginning with Renaissance humanism. This type of individualism essentially sees the individual as an autonomous and self-contained entity defined most essentially by personal objectives, needs, desires, and interests. The individual is the primary reality-whereas society is a derivative, second order level of reality that is simply a collection of individuals (Dumont 1986; Sullivan 1986). Individualism first emerged as a kind of political tool to wrest control of the individual away from church and king (McPherson 1962) and limit the abuses of power that could remain unchecked in the hierarchical societies of the European Middle Ages. However much these individualistic conceptions seem like common sense to the dominant cultural group in the West, they are "rather peculiar...within the context of the world cultures" according to researchers like Geertz (1983, p. 59) and Shweder and Bourne (1984).

There are clear ways in which individualism in its different guises underlies and informs the two main approaches positive psychology has taken to studying psychological well-being: subjective well-being (SWB) and Ryff's (1989) psychological well-being (PWB). Because of space limitations we will just focus here on a few examples from the predominant approach, subjective well-being (SWB). SWB consists of two general components: (a) judgments about life satisfaction and (b) affective balance or the extent to which the level of positive affect outweighs the level of negative affect in one's life. On the surface this approach to studying well-being seems void of any particular cultural bias as it allows individuals to self-evaluate and, in the case of life satisfaction measures, to (subjectively) chose what criteria or standards they use to assess their satisfaction. On keener examination it becomes clear how influenced SWB is by a disguised Western individualism. In essence, in this approach well-being is determined by the individual alone. Yet the capacity to do this kind of self-evaluation is encouraged in liberal individualistic societies, like the United States or Canada, and historically discouraged in more collectivistic societies like China. This approach to assessing well-being presupposes that the good life is freedom to choose—the freedom to pursue happiness as defined by the individual. It rests on the assumption that the self can turn inward to determine the good (either using reason or using feelings/sentiment). And it preserves the freedom from arbitrary authority in that the use of any norms or standards to assess psychological well-being run the risk of being seen as dogmatic, ethnocentric, or relative.

For instance, subjective well-being measures such as the Satisfaction with Life Scale (Diener et al. 1985) presuppose that the high scoring person is one whose life is satisfactory or fulfilling. For many in the United States and Canada, perhaps particularly in White majority culture, it is unproblematic to endorse items like "The conditions of my life are excellent" as they tap into culturally encouraged tendencies for self-promotion and stressing uniqueness. Indeed, we are in the sway of what social psychologists call the tendency to false uniqueness; in other words, the average person in the White majority assumes they are above average in intelligence, popularity, attractiveness, and so on. However, in many-nonWestern societies such as Taiwan and Japan, such self-assertions are considered immature and a potential invitation to bad luck (Bond 1986; Hu 1944; Markus and Kitayama 1991). These beliefs may also be endorsed by Asian Americans within the United States depending on level of acculturation. Generally, in collectivist cultures, one should avoid drawing attention to oneself. This cultural orientation gets captured in Japanese culture, as Markus and Kitayama (1991) point out, by the aphorism, "the nail that stands out gets pounded down." Rather than "tooting your own horn," those in collectivist societies evaluate themselves objectively while family and friends might compensate with praise. It makes a significant impact on the multicultural pursuit of positive psychology to recognize seriously how virtues such as self-expression, self-promotion, and the pursuit of self-chosen satisfactions (or even virtues) can be seen as signs of selfishness and immaturity in many collectivist cultures (King and Bond 1985; Markus and Kitayama 1991).

Individualism also influences the second component of subjective well-being: affective balance. Affective balance assumes that well-being is partially based on the predominance of positive affect over negative affect in one's life (Bradburn 1969) which bolsters the other assumption which is that happiness is the yardstick of the good life. As Taylor observed (1985) for Westerners "the good life is defined in terms of emotional satisfaction" (p. 262). In contrast, Diener and Diener (1995) found that "How a collectivist feels about him- or herself is less relevant to his or her life satisfaction than is his or her view of whether he or she behaves properly in the organized social order" (p. 662). Yet, despite such findings, leading researchers in well-being still conclude the "experience of pleasure and the achievement of a subjective sense of well-being remain at the center of the story" (Kahneman et al. 1999).

Additionally, as an approach to assessing well-being, affective balance has relied on Western emotions and has failed to include more indigenous non-Western emotions. As Hung-Bin Sheu (in press) expounded in Chap. 5, there are clear racial and ethnic differences in the affective components of well-being. Western emotions have been found to have a two-dimensional scaling solution (Russell 1980), with the first dimension consisting of pleasant/good vs. unpleasant/bad and the second dimension being of active high energy vs. inactive/low energy. Collectivist cultures such as Japan have a third dimension, one which places self-centered emotions versus other-centered emotions. Social or other-centered emotions are often not positive or negative such as *amae*, an emotion identified in Japan that is the hopeful anticipation of another's indulgence (Doi 1971/1973). The lack of identification of such social emotions in the United States or Canada does not mean that individuals living there do not experience such social emotions, rather that such social feelings are largely undifferentiated and presumably play little role in well-being, at least in White majority culture.

By seeing how individualism operates here, and by extension in other areas of positive psychology, we can start to sense why it is so essential to understand the range of ways of being human. First, our common sense,-culturally informed notions of psychological well-being are likely to be at odds with people whose cultural and ethnic backgrounds are different from ours. The authors of chapter three (Capielo et al., , Chap. 3, this volume) remind us that positive psychology's identification of strengths and virtues derive from the experiences of Euro-Americans and therefore cannot automatically be applied or extended out to the experiences of either U.S. minority populations or the 95 % of human beings who live outside the U.S. (cf., Arnett 2008). This inability to generalize is due to the multiple definitions of values that exist across cultural groups. Such differences are bound to yield different results on positive psychology measures. Second, psychological interventions necessarily presuppose some sense of what is positive. As psychological interventions, such as counseling, are increasingly applied in non-Western parts of the world, it is necessary to have some critical awareness of what is actually being exported. And even within the U.S., such an individualistic focus is likely to be problematic for clients of color, perhaps the source of their under-utilization of psychotherapy services. Third, gaining awareness of the cultural roots of our understanding of psychological well-being is a good first step in discerning our own biases and presuppositions, challenging them when we find them lacking, and learning from the wisdom in cultural traditions other than our own.

By failing to examine the cultural roots and underlying assumptions laden in its current definitions of well-being (and other constructs as the authors of this book note) means that these assumptions will operate implicitly and as kind of disguised ideology (Bernstein 1978). This is a huge problem for a more culturally-sensitive positive psychology. It means that whatever assumptions about human nature and the good life that are implicit within the reigning understanding of well-being are simply uncritically extended to cultural groups for whom they may not be relevant. At its worse such theories and measures of well-being may end up pathologizing those from other cultural traditions.

A notion of well-being that does justice to cross-cultural and historical variation requires two things: (a) a view of the self, or ontology of the self, of the "being" in well-being, that is robust enough to handle the kind of variations in selfhood that have in fact existed, and (b) the virtues that constitute the "well" part of well-being are in fact interpreted and prioritized differently across time and location, including one's socioeconomic position and other cultural variables such as gender and sexual orientation. Short of this, positive psychology will necessarily fail to respect and honor the diversity of human experience.

17.3 Variations in Selfhood and Identity

Reigning approaches in positive psychology fall short in both ways. First, within positive psychology the possibility that self and identity can vary is largely ignored. Instead it is presupposed, as with well-being, that the self is the kind of thinking subject or Cartesian self that lies at the heart of the individualism of United States majority culture. Yet in many cultural traditions this kind of "I" is seen as but one possible mode or state of identity. The distinction between individualism and the independent sense of self versus collectivism and an interdependent sense of self is by now well known within psychology (Markus and Kitayama 1991). For much of the world the emphasis upon a tightly bounded sense of self is foreign to their more relational, extended or inclusive senses of identity. Yet little consideration of this exists in the current positive psychology literature.

Moreover, in most of the world's societies and religious traditions, it is the transformation of the self and not just its satisfaction that is seen as central to well-being and the good life. In many Asian indigenous psychologies such as Buddhism, yoga, and Taoism, the more individualistic, separate sense of self is explicitly seen as both quite limited and the source of suffering. It is not just religions, however, that have envisioned a sense of self that is larger, more expansive or inclusive. Many of the seminal figures in psychology including Alfred Adler, William James, Erik Erikson, and Gordon Allport recognized the potential of radical transformation. For instance, Adler's notion of social interest equates well-being with coming to identify with ever larger wholes of which one is a part, eventually including the cosmos as a whole. And among many of the minority ethnic groups in the U.S. it is not possible to separate the well-being of individual from the well-being of the family. Given this, we find it curious that positive psychology has been almost completely silent about what is in many traditions the very essence of human flourishing and development.

As the authors in this book have elaborated, there is a pressing need for more inclusion of gender/feminist, racial, ethnic, disability, and LGBTQ theory and understanding in the field of positive psychology. In addition, paying attention to the influences of religion, social class and age on the development and manifestation are more than warranted. We believe these perspectives and orientations entail more dialogical, relational, and permeable notions of self that provide a complement to, if not a corrective, of the "bounded masterful self" (Cushman 1990, p. 599) that dominates most of psychology. For positive psychology to engage in dialogue with these important areas of psychology, in a deep and ongoing way, it will have to be more open to and explicit about these varied notions of self – further incentive to providing more critical nuance and expanding its own conceptual notion of self.

Positive psychology will need to consider that not only do the boundaries of the self or identity vary, but also the elements that are regarded as constitutive of the self differ. In other words, the way the pie of the self has been sliced varies across culture: Western psychology's tripartite division of the self into behavior, emotion, and cognition is not endorsed universally. These views of the self can have important practical consequences in that they promote particular stances towards the different aspects of the self. For instance, within some traditions, it is our emotions or sentiments that are our essential to our humanity (e.g., Mencius, European Romanticism, humanistic psychology) while in others, emotions threaten to overwhelm the rationality that is thought to separate us from lower animals (e.g., Patanjali's yoga, Plato, Freud, Cognitive Therapy). Such assumptions have massive implications in terms of how we view suffering, "the good life," and the nature of healing.

In addition, we believe positive psychology needs to be more attentive to ways that the self or agency exists at different levels of awareness. For example, while there are parts of us that are clearly consciously directed and accessible to introspection, there are other aspects of our agency that are more implicit, that are embodied and engaged in social practices. Values, virtues, and meaning can be found at both implicit and explicit levels raising issues about assessment and interventions that do not provide room for the ways that we exist at multiple levels of knowing (Christopher and Bickhard 2007; Christopher 2008; Christopher and Campbell 2008).

17.4 Variations in Moral Sources, Values and Virtues

Positive psychology must also think more deeply about the nature of virtues, strengths, and values and be able to account for the variety of virtues and values across cultures that constitute well-being. In "Character strengths and virtues: A handbook and classification" (Peterson and Seligman 2004) the strategy was to treat the presence of "our" virtues and strengths in other cultures as evidence of their "universality." Yet attempts like these in the "manual of the sanities" or in character education to shoehorn these virtues into frameworks that are purportedly universal can do a kind of violence to the local meanings these virtues have (Christopher and Hickinbottom 2008; Christopher et al. 2003). From our perspective we have not reflected enough on what it means that the virtues that constitute well-being can be interpreted differently in different socio-historical contexts before we rush to place them in our own typologies. And these critical differences in the meaning of the virtues are glossed over by the decontextualized ways the virtues are treated in mainstream theory and measures. Personal growth, for instance, is treated as a good in Ryff's (1989) approach to psychological well-being, regardless of the context in which it is applied or how it is interpreted. Moreover, we have failed to consider that frameworks, like the big 6 virtues of the VIA, are themselves culturally specific—local cultures have their own frameworks, even if implicit, for organizing virtues that we tend to ignore. These local frameworks often introduce considerations, like reference to cosmology as for instance with the Chinese meta-value of co-creativity with heaven and earth, that are outside of our realm of professional experience or comfort (e.g., Munro 1985).

As we see it there are three main dimensions to this issue. First, there are often local virtues that do not easily translate across cultures, like *fago* among the Ifaluk of Micronesia (Lutz 1988) and often these local virtues are simply ignored in positive psychology. Second, the meaning of different virtues can vary quite dramatically across cultures. In Japan, for instance, caring for a cancer patient has meant giving the patient a fake diagnosis to protect them from the truth of their condition. And third, virtues and values can be prioritized or ranked differently in different contexts. We found in our research that respect was the most important value for Turks and Belauans, while for those in the United States and Canada, who were largely White, it was ranked 37th (Smith et al. 2007). While unable to examine different U.S. ethnic groups in our study, we can imagine that they would not rank respect as low as 37th. A take home point here is that much of cultural difference comes from which values trump which in specific situations.

And finally to conclude we would like to elaborate on the point that cultures vary in what they consider the source of our values, virtues and moral sources. In the kind of that individualism that majority culture within the United States takes for granted, the individual self determines their own values and good through inward reflection in a way that would be largely unimaginable to people in ancient and premodern societies, and to many today in collectivist societies. Through his analysis of the emergence of the modern Western identity, Charles Taylor (1985, 1989) clarifies the significance of this radical change and how it occurred. Prior to the modern era, Westerners subscribed to a two-tiered vision of the world that encompassed first, a cosmological framework imbued with meaning and value and second, an understanding of ordinary life that derived meaning from these larger frameworks. For example, the ancient Greeks distinguished between *zen* (the life of necessity) which includes the domain of the home where chores take place for the purpose of physical survival and reproduction, and *euzen* (the good life) which describes the public space, the life of the polis, the realm where humans can cultivate all the truly human attributes that go beyond physical necessity (Arendt 1958). In a two-tiered system the source of values is an external source (God, the natural order, etc.). In the history of the West, socio-political movements including the Protestant Reformation, the American and French Revolutions, the Enlightenment and the scientific revolution all challenged and pushed against the inequalities in the hierarchical world views of the time in part by progressively coming to deny the existence of the larger cosmological framework and thereby eroding the legitimacy and power of the reigning structures of authority, whether they be church or king. The result is what Taylor (2007) terms the secular age, in which the two-tiered vision collapsed into one tier. Values and virtues are largely no longer seen as qualities of the cosmos that are discovered by human beings but rather as human meanings that are placed over or projected onto an objective, value- and meaning-free reality.

In response, the individual becomes increasingly invested with the autonomy, freedom, and privacy necessary to cultivate the kind of reason or inner knowing that could be a guide to what is good and what is true. In the two-tiered vision of the life, the individual discovers their identity by looking outward and determining where they are located in social and cosmic orders. In the one-tiered vision, in contrast, the individual looks within and creates their own self-defined values, interests, desires, and needs. From this new outlook, external sources of meaning began to appear as arbitrary and relativistic impositions upon the dignity of individuals to "have it their own way" and define for themselves their own view of the good, of happiness, of truth.

The ways in which this one-tiered vision shapes Western understandings of the self and our understanding of the source of meaning and values is critical for positive psychology to address. First, the two different visions lead to the priority of different kinds of virtues. When the source of identity is located inward, as it is in majority culture within Western society, then the markers for maturity, well-being, and mental health will naturally have an emphasis on values such as freedom, autonomy, and self-expression. However, in a two-tiered vision, identity is defined in a more relational or collectivist sense, and the markers of the good person will be more interpersonal. In many East Asian and Asian American groups these more interpersonal criteria for maturity and well-being are epitomized by the virtue of *filial piety*—being a dutiful son or daughter through respect and obedience to one's parents and elders. Filial piety in these groups has been historically seen as the most distinguishing marker of good character and the primary way of conveying maturing (Hoshmand and Ho 1995; King and Bond 1985; Munro 1969; Wei-ming 1985). In majority groups within Western culture, however, such an emphasis on duty and obligation to elders and parents has often come to be perceived as an impediment to optimal personal growth and fulfillment.

Second, the two different visions posit different relationships that the self has to values and meanings. The modern or postmodern self, that positive psychology takes for granted, tries to define itself and its values without reference to external sources. This is a radical and new development in the history of humanity. And because the second tier has largely disappeared for many in the majority culture within the United States, Canada, and Western Europe, meanings and values are justified by whether they lead to individual satisfaction; the satisfaction of personal desires and feelings is the highest good. One might argue that surely positive psychology has a bigger vision. Seligman (2002), for instance, distinguishes between the pleasant life, the good life, and the meaningful life with the explicit aim of limiting the role that pleasure plays in happiness. And yet probing more deeply, we find that unlike in most cultural traditions, the criteria for what constitutes the good or the meaningful are amorphous, untethered to anything outside of the individual's preferences. While Seligman suggests that the most complete life is the one that is meaningful, he is silent about what is meaningful. A dilemma arises because as a self-described scientist, he aims to provide a positive psychology that is "descriptive, not prescriptive." If psychologists and positive psychology as a field are to remain value-neutral, than they cannot suggest what kind of specific meanings are best because doing so would be prescriptive, potentially imposing criteria that might be relative and arbitrary. They are left only being able to declare that having meaning is important. As Richardson (1989) trenchantly observes, by starting with a dualistic rendering of an individualistic self set over and against a disenchanted world, psychology no longer has any resources for seeing meaning as something that is grounded in anything other than individual preference. Yet most of us find the relativism in this position troubling as it leaves little ground to reject the kind of meaning that animated the Hitlers, Stalins, and Pol Pots of the world. The dilemma that catches Seligman is part of a larger problem found in the Western cultural tradition since Enlightenment (MacIntyre 1984; Richardson et al. 1999; Taylor 1985, 2007). By presupposing the bounded atomistic self, Seligman (2002) is left having to justify how meaning and values can have authority. As he states, "I also hunger for meaning in my life that will transcend the arbitrary purposes I have chosen for myself" (p. 14).

So long as positive psychology examines happiness and character strengths from a one-tiered model alone, it will remain ill-equipped to account for cultural differences in understanding well-being and positive psychology (cf., Falb and Pargament, Chap. 10). Modernity has for the most part done away with the second tier of life, with the notion of a cosmological framework that situates us morally. Positive psychology has missed thus far how for most people in the world and for most of history, self, identity, meanings and values were configured through orientation to a cosmological framework. From their perspective, positive psychology's individually focused and defined sense of the good and meaningful is highly problematic and short-sighted. It is for this very reason that psychotherapy and counseling are criticized by many fundamentalists, both Christian and non-Christian alike, for their unquestioned humanism and contribution to the erosion of traditional cultural values. It is quite difficult for Western psychologists to realize that the emphasis upon individual choice is for many a kind of hubris that should be replaced by learning to surrender, harmonize, or adapt to God's will or the natural order. From these traditions, positive psychology's current vision of the good life will unlikely be very compelling.

17.5 Conclusion

In support of the thrust of this book to help positive psychology be congruent with the diversity that exists in the world, we have tried to encourage the reader of this chapter to engage in more reflection on the core assumptions that will necessarily underlie any endeavor within positive psychology. In particular, positive psychology needs to continue to reflect on its underlying moral vision: its notions about what the self is and should be. To not question the nature of the self in positive psychology is to continue to speak to and reinforce the Western individualistic self. If underlying notions of the self in well-being are not made explicit or critically addressed, then well-being theory, research and practice essentially leaves out all variations of the self found in the "manifold variety in the Unites States" (Bacigalupe 2001). And, moreover, it assesses and diagnoses those other traditions in terms of the Western view of the self. To not question means also to not examine and think about how configurations of the self are complicit with socio-political-economic arrangements and yield particular psychological consequences (e.g. social inequalities in health), as critical psychologists such as Prilleltensky (1989) and Cushman (1990, 1995) have noted. The stakes of creating a positive psychology in which all people have a voice are too high for us not to slow down, think, and dialogue.

References

Arendt, H. (1958). *The human condition*. Chicago: The University of Chicago Press.
Arnett, J. J. (2008). The neglected 95 %: Why American psychology needs to become less American. *American Psychologist, 63*, 602–614.
Bacigalupe, G. (2001). Is positive psychology only White psychology? *American Psychologist, 56*(1), 82–83.
Berger, P. L., & Luckmann, T. (1966). *The social construction of reality*. Garden City: Anchor Books.
Bernstein, R. J. (1978). *The reconstructing of social and political theory*. Philadelphia: University of Pennsylvania Press.
Bishop, R. C. (2007). *The philosophy of the social sciences: An introduction*. New York: Continuum.
Bond, M. H. (Ed.). (1986). *The psychology of the Chinese people*. Oxford: New York.
Bradburn, N. (1969). *The structure of psychological well-being*. Chicago: Aldine.
Christopher, J. C. (1996). Counseling's inescapable moral visions. *Journal of Counseling and Development, 75*, 17–25.
Christopher, J. C. (1999). Situating psychological well-being: Exploring the cultural roots of its theory and research. *Journal of Counseling and Development, 77*, 141–152.
Christopher, J. C. (2008). Culture, moral topographies, and interactive personhood. *Journal of Theoretical & Philosophical Psychology, 27*, 168–191.
Christopher, J. C., & Bickhard, M. H. (2007). Culture, self and identity: Interactivist contributions to a metatheory for cultural psychology. *Culture & Psychology, 13*, 259–295.
Christopher, J. C., & Campbell, R. L. (2008). An interactivist-hermeneutic metatheory for positive psychology. *Theory & Psychology, 18*, 675–697.
Christopher, J. C., & Hickinbottom, S. (2008). Positive psychology, ethnocentrism, and the disguised ideology of individualism. *Theory & Psychology, 18*, 563–589.
Christopher, J. C., Nelson, T., & Nelson, M. D. (2003). Culture and character education: Problems of interpretation in a multicultural society. *Journal of Theoretical and Philosophical Psychology, 23*, 81–101.
Cushman, P. (1990). Why the self is empty: Toward a historically situated psychology. *American Psychologist, 45*, 599–611.
Cushman, P. (1995). *Constructing the self, constructing america: A cultural history of psychotherapy*. Reading: Addison-Wesley Publishing Co, Inc.
Diener, E., & Diener, M. (1995). Cross-cultural correlates of life satisfaction and self-esteem. *Journal of Personality and Social Psychology, 68*, 653–663.
Diener, E., Emmons, R. A., Larsen, R. J., & Griffin, S. (1985). The satisfaction with life scale. *Journal of Personality Assessment, 49*, 71–75.
Doi, T. (1973). *The anatomy of dependence* (J. Bester, Trans.). New York: Kodansha.
Dumont, L. (1986). *Essays on individualism*. Chicago: University of Chicago Press.

Fowers, B. J., & Richardson, F. C. (1994). Why is multiculturalism good? *American Psychologist, 51*, 609–621.
Geertz, C. (1983). *Local knowledge*. New York: Basic Books.
Hu, H. C. (1944). The Chinese concepts of "face". *American Anthropologist, 46*, 45–64.
Hoshmand, L. T., & Ho, D. Y. F. (1995). Moral dimensions of selfhood: Chinese traditions and cultural change. *World Psychology, 1*, 47–69.
Kahneman, D., Diener, E., & Schwartz, N. (Eds.). (1999). *Well-being: The foundations of a hedonic psychology*. New York: Russell Sage.
King, A. Y. C., & Bond, M. H. (1985). The Confucian paradigm of man: A sociological view. In W.-S. Tseng & D. Y. H. Wu (Eds.), *Chinese culture and mental health* (pp. 29–45). Orlando: Academic.
Kuhn, T. S. (1970). *The structure of scientific revolutions*. Chicago: The University of Chicago Press.
Lutz, C. A. (1988). *Unnatural emotions: Everyday sentiments on a Micronesian atoll and their challenge to Western theory*. Chicago: University of Chicago Press.
MacIntyre, A. (1984). *After virtue*. Notre Dame: University of Notre Dame Press.
MacPherson, C. B. (1962). *The political theory of possessive individualism*. Oxford: Oxford University Press.
Markus, H. R., & Kitayama, S. (1991). Culture and the self: Implications for cognition, emotion, and motivation. *Psychological Review, 98*, 224–253.
Munro, D. J. (1969). *The concept of man in early China*. Stanford: Stanford University Press.
Munro, D. J. (1985). *Individualism and holism: Studies in Confucian and Taoist values*. Ann Arbor: Center for Chinese Studies University of Michigan.
Peterson, C., & Seligman, M. E. P. (2004). *Character strengths and virtues: A handbook and classification*. Washington, DC: American Psychological Association/Oxford University Press.
Prilleltensky, I. (1989). Psychology and the status quo. *American Psychologist, 44*(5), 795–802.
Richardson, F. C. (1989). Freedom and commitment in modern psychotherapy. *Journal of Integrative & Eclectic Psychotherapy, 8*(4), 303–319.
Richardson, F. C., Fowers, B. J., & Guignon, C. B. (1999). *Re-envisioning psychology: Moral dimensions of theory and practice*. San Francisco: Jossey-Bass.
Russell, J. A. (1980). A circumplex model of affect. *Journal of Personality and Social Psychology, 39*, 1161–1178.
Ryff, C. D. (1989). Happiness is everything or is it? Explorations on the meaning of psychological well-being. *Journal of Personality and Social Psychology, 57*, 1069–1081.
Seligman, M. E. P. (2002). *Authentic happiness: Using the new positive psychology to realize your potential for lasting fulfillment*. New York: Free Press.
Seligman, M. E. P., & Csikszentmihalyi, M. (2000). Positive psychology: An introduction. *American Psychologist, 55*, 5–14.
Shweder, R. A., & Bourne, E. J. (1984). Does the concept of the person vary cross-culturally? In R. A. Shweder & R. A. LeVine (Eds.), *Culture theory: Essays on mind, self, and emotion* (pp. 158–199). New York: Cambridge University Press.
Smith, K. D., Türk-Smith, S., & Christopher, J. C. (2007). What defines the good person?: Cross-cultural comparisons of experts' models with lay prototypes. *Journal of Cross-Cultural Psychology, 38*, 333–360.
Sullivan, W. M. (1986). *Reconstructing public philosophy*. Berkeley: University of California Press.
Taylor, C. (1985). *Philosophy and the human sciences: Philosophical papers* (Vol. 2). New York: Cambridge University Press.
Taylor, C. (1989). *Sources of the self: The making of the modern identity*. Cambridge, MA: Harvard University Press.
Taylor, E. (2001). Positive psychology and humanistic psychology: A reply to Seligman. *Journal of Humanistic Psychology, 41*, 13–29.
Taylor, C. (2007). *A secular age*. Cambridge, MA: Belknap Press of Harvard University Press.
Wei-ming, T. (1985). Selfhood and otherness in Confucian thought. In A. J. Marsella, G. DeVos, & F. L. K. Hsu (Eds.), *Culture and self: Asian and western perspectives*. New York: Tavistock.

Index

J. Teramoto Pedrotti and L.M. Edwards (eds.), *Perspectives on the Intersection of Multiculturalism and Positive Psychology*, Cross-Cultural Advancements in Positive Psychology 7, DOI 10.1007/978-94-017-8654-6,

Q

R

CPI Antony Rowe
Chippenham, UK
2017-04-26 22:10